MAD MATTERS

MAD MATTERS

A Critical Reader in Canadian Mad Studies

Edited by

BRENDA A. LEFRANÇOIS,
ROBERT MENZIES,

and

GEOFFREY REAUME

Canadian Scholars' Press Inc.
Toronto

Mad Matters: A Critical Reader in Canadian Mad Studies
Brenda A. LeFrançois, Robert Menzies, and Geoffrey Reaume

First published in 2013 by
Canadian Scholars' Press Inc.
425 Adelaide Street West, Suite 200
Toronto, Ontario
M5V 3C1

www.cspi.org

Canadian Scholars' Press Inc. gratefully acknowledges financial support for our publishing
activities from the Government of Canada through the Canada Book Fund (CBF).

Library and Archives Canada Cataloguing in Publication

Mad matters : a critical reader in Canadian mad studies / edited by
Brenda A. LeFrançois, Robert Menzies, and Geoffrey Reaume.

Includes bibliographical references and index. Issued also in electronic formats.
ISBN 978-1-55130-534-9

1. Psychiatry—Canada. 2. Mental illness—Canada. 3. Mentally ill—Canada.
I. LeFrançois, Brenda A., 1968– II. Menzies, Robert J., 1951– III. Reaume, Geoffrey

RC448.C32M33 2013   616.89'00971   C2012-908417-4

Text design by Susan MacGregor/Digital Zone
Cover design by Gordon Robertson
Cover image: Leef Evans, *Stanley Park Seawall Sandstone no.31*, 2010

Printed and bound in Canada by Webcom

Canadä

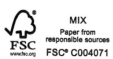

MIX
Paper from
responsible sources
FSC
www.fsc.org   FSC® C004071

Dedication

Brenda A. LeFrançois:
To my two strong and intelligent daughters, Juliette and Adèle, that you may continue to grow in your understanding of the importance of social justice, including both the activism and scholarship that are necessary to meet those ends.

To my partner in life, Dr. Jean-Marc Bélanger, whose embodied kindness and wisdom envelops me and sustains me.

To the memory of Professor David Brandon (1941–2001) whose mad academic mentoring continues to inspire me long after his passing.

Robert Menzies:
To my partner in all things, Dr. Dorothy E. Chunn, with love, gratitude, and admiration.

To the memory of my teacher, Dr. Richard V. Ericson (1948–2007), in appreciation of the remarkable legacy of critical scholarship that he handed down.

Geoffrey Reaume:
For my beloved wife, Esther Jeeyoon Lee, who lives what she studies.

In memory of Ron Wilson (1937–2005) for his friendship and "amazing grace."

Contents

Foreword

O ver recent years, there has been growing interest in mental health issues, madness, and distress in the developing international discipline of disability studies. This is encouraging, since it emphasizes the importance of an inclusive approach to such studies. This is also reflected more and more by broader recognition in disability studies of the significance of "neuro-diversity" and of the groups and people who identify with this designation.

But this book also takes us a crucial step forward through its identification of Mad Studies. While it may not be the first text to do this, it is perhaps the most significant and thoroughgoing so far. Similarly, while its focus is Mad Studies in Canada, its discussions are likely to be of international significance and assistance.

Medicalized individual models of mental illness have dominated all aspects of madness and distress in the Western world since the 18th-century Enlightenment. Over the years, they have increasingly been exported to colonize, subvert, and overshadow other cultural and societal understandings and interpretations of these fundamental human experiences. Yet we know that many mental health service users and others affected by madness and distress find such a medical model damaging and unhelpful.

This book now delineates a new subject of study, Mad Studies, which offers real hope for challenging the continuing dominance of the medical model in "mental health." It makes clear that there is a need for such enquiry and intellectual activity. Most importantly, through its approach and range of contributors, the book offers hope that Mad Studies will be a discipline that determinedly connects with activism and change. Abstracted academism is unlikely to be of much use. Studies must go with practice to make up praxis. Thus, the insights that the book can offer may provide the basis for effective opposition to psychiatrism, and a force for developing democratic and feasible alternatives to support our understandings of and responses to madness and distress at both individual and societal levels.

The psychiatric empire continues to grow, domestically and globally. Its ever-widening diagnostic categories, its increasing pretense of providing solutions to structural and social problems, and its unholy alliance with global pharmaceutical corporations have all become defining features, regardless of the good people seeking to do good things within its orbit. Intentionally or otherwise, it has become the handmaiden of contemporary neoliberalism.

Rationalist scientism of the 18th century eventually led to the two appallingly destructive and failed philosophies that marked out the 20th century: Hitler's "national socialism" and Stalin's USSR. But it is still alive and well as the justification for the present neoliberalism of the political right. This is presented as resting on the rational, objective, and scientific theories and understandings of economists, yet it actually despoils this world and stands in the way of human mutual understanding. Perhaps it is not surprising that psychiatry has become more economistic in its role, part of increasingly powerful structures forcing people into a harsh, inflexible, and pauperizing labour market and economic system. Not since the 19th century has unrestricted capitalism been unleashed on the world and its people to such an untrammelled extent. Its present global reach is unprecedented. Words such as "globalization" have had to be invented to describe it. And at its heart is a brutality and injustice that flies in the face of everything any of us have been taught is right from childhood, whether in terms of human morality, social justice, or environmental equity.

The major modern social study, *The Spirit Level*, concludes that inequality is bad for all of us. It refers to the pernicious effects that inequality has on societies: eroding trust, increasing anxiety and illness, and encouraging excessive consumption (Wilkinson and Pickett, 2009). It claims that for each of 11 different health and social issues—physical health, mental health, drug abuse, education, imprisonment, obesity, social mobility, trust and community life, violence, teenage pregnancies, and child well-being—outcomes are significantly worse in more unequal rich countries.

All this may be true. The effects of social inequality and injustice may be widely distributed. But it doesn't put the oppressors in the same relationship as the oppressed. It doesn't make it any easier for the latter to challenge the institutions and ideologies that oppress them. It still leaves the over-privileged in a much more powerful position. Historically, there seem to be few if any instances of them being prepared to stop oppressing others, or to give up their advantage in the interests of the mental health of others. More to the point, oppression and disempowerment damage all of us, and this book is a critical reminder of the increasing need to look in different places for answers to this problem. While psychiatry may be seeking to extend its empire, the destructive effects of wider political, social, and economic policies are bringing more and more people around the world to its doors.

That is why this book is both so timely and so important. It provides a counter-discourse that is desperately needed in our times. It is a counter-discourse, which, like the social model of disability of the international disabled people's movement, does not seek accommodation or understanding from dominant traditional medicalized understandings, but instead seeks to confront them head-on and provide alternatives that offer positive promise for the future.

It is no coincidence that regressive political ideologies and psychiatry are both on the rise. Equally, it is no coincidence that counter-movements have been developing related to many spheres of human identity and understanding, from environmentalism to the Occupy movement, from disability to distress. This book is a vital sign of these times. It has delineated a new subject of study and, in doing so, it offers us all much greater hope of making sense of what goes on within us and what affects us from outside, how the two interact, and how their relationship may be made a much more positive and humanistic one.

This is a *for*, not an *against* book. Not only does it offer critiques of psychiatry and associated law, public policy, media, and propaganda, and subject psychiatry's questionable "treatments," knowledge production, pedagogy, and academic activities to serious and necessary scrutiny. Not only does it examine long-standing tendencies to criminalize and pathologize madness and associate it with violence and individualized irrationality and deviance. More important, perhaps, it also explores the history, culture, and language of madness and Mad people. It highlights the diversity of Mad experience and understandings, the violence of psychiatry, the ambiguity of its reformism, and the emergence of survivor research and academic engagement. As the editors say in their introduction, the book "combines the more established understandings of Mad matters, including anti-psychiatry approaches and long-standing psychiatric survivor narratives, with an exciting and burgeoning form of activism and conceptualizations, emanating from a new generation of people ... engaging in a variety of forms of radical and Mad activist scholarship."

It does this through contributions from many perspectives. There are academic and professional experts and experts by experience—that is to say, people whose lived experiences and engagement on the basis of that underpin their standpoints and contributions. These different approaches and experiences are synthesized to offer compelling and hopeful critiques and ways forward for the future. Within these pages, we will not find a new orthodoxy, something that activist psychiatric-system survivors have long guarded against. Instead, there is food to nurture different social understandings and strategies in response both to madness and distress and to the psychiatric system.

This book delineates a new subject of study, and also signifies its coming of age. If psychiatry, for all its ambitiousness, has always seemed to narrow understanding, here is an approach that excites through the breadth of its focus and discussion. Instead of psychiatric reductionism, here all of us, whether we identify as Mad or distressed or not, get a chance to liberate our thoughts from old, unhelpful assumptions and conceptual frameworks and test out others against our own experience, knowledge, and understanding. At a time when societies are identifying more and more of their citizens as abnormal and defective, while being less and less prepared to spend money on supporting them in their difficulties, this has to be a source of hope and inspiration.

Peter Beresford

Peter Beresford, Officer of the Order of the British Empire, is Professor of Social Policy at Brunel University; Chair of Shaping Our Lives, a national network of service users and disabled people; and a long-term user of mental health services.

Acknowledgments

The following people and organizations have contributed in a wealth of amazing and vital ways to the making of this book:

- The talented and critically engaged community of contributors to the 2008 Madness, Citizenship and Social Justice Conference, Simon Fraser University, which set the stage for this project. Worthy of special mention are Anne-Marie Feenberg and Trish Graham, former Director and Program Assistant, respectively, for the SFU Institute for the Humanities; the Institute's J.S. Woodsworth Resident Scholar program and Endowment Committee (chaired by Samir Gandesha), along with its Social Justice and Citizenship working group (Adrienne Burk, Dorothy Chunn, Margaret Jackson, David Mirhady, and Bob Russell); the Social Sciences and Humanities Research Council of Canada; and the SFU offices of the President, V/P Academic, and Dean of Arts and Social Sciences.
- Our ever-inspiring colleagues and students in the School of Social Work, Memorial University of Newfoundland; the Department of Sociology and Anthropology, Simon Fraser University; and the Graduate Program in Critical Disability Studies, York University.
- Sobia Shaikh for providing detailed feedback, and the members of the Critical Race Theory and Anti-Colonial Theory Discussion Group at Memorial University who read and commented on an earlier version of some of the chapters.
- Our friends and supporters at Canadian Scholars' Press, who have embraced this project from the outset with enthusiasm and clarity of vision: Andrew Wayne (President), James MacNevin (Acquisitions Editor), Daniella Balabuk (Developmental Editor/Permissions Coordinator), Caley Baker (Production Editor), and Rhoda Dinardo (Copy Editor).
- The four external reviewers for CSPI: Nancy Hansen, Interdisciplinary Master's Program in Disability Studies, University of Manitoba; Tom Brown, History, Mount Royal College; Gregor Wolbring, Community Health Sciences, University of Calgary; and Joanne Woiak, Disability Studies, University of Washington.
- Peter Beresford, Brunel University, whose eloquent and generous words grace the Foreword to this collection.

- Leef Evans of Gallery Gachet for contributing the evocative cover image, and Lara Fitzgerald, Gallery Gachet's Programming Director, for making this happen.
- Irit Shimrat, who expertly compiled the index; and the chair and members of the SFU University Publications Funds committee, who provided the funding for it.
- The extraordinary cast of contributors to *Mad Matters*, every one of whom has advanced the causes of Mad Studies and social justice in powerful ways through words, images, and deeds.
- With the kind facilitation of CSPI, we are directing royalties earned by book sales to *Our Voice/Notre Voix* of Moncton, the Psychiatric Survivor Archives of Toronto, and Gallery Gachet of Vancouver.

Introducing Mad Studies

Robert Menzies, Brenda A. LeFrançois, and Geoffrey Reaume

"But I don't want to go among mad people," Alice remarked.
"Oh, you can't help that," said the Cat. "We're all mad here. I'm mad.
  You're mad."
"How do you know I'm mad?" said Alice.
"You must be," said the Cat, "or you wouldn't have come here."
                    —Lewis Carroll, *Alice's Adventures in Wonderland*

The madness about which I'm writing is the madness that is more or less
present in each one of us and not only the madness that gets the psychiatric
baptism by diagnosis of "schizophrenia" or some other label invented by the
specialized psycho-police agents of final phase capitalist society.
                    —David Cooper, *The Language of Madness* (1978)

As for the term, Mad Studies, it has emerged from a collective assemblage of
enunciation, from a multitude of voices. Like Nietzsche, through whom some
of those voices spoke, it is a destiny.
                    —Richard Ingram, Personal Communication (2011b)

Beginnings

Mad matters, and so does the study of madness and psychiatrization, and so too does *Mad Studies*.[1] The matter of Mad Studies—and that Mad does matter—is the express purpose of this reader; we explore here the various ways to take up the matters of "psychiatrization," "madness," the oppression and agency of Mad subjects, and the battle against psychiatry and psychiatric discourse as a way to introduce Mad Studies as an emergent field of study that matters. This is not to suggest that the matters covered in this reader are wholly new. On the contrary, many of these matters have been raised conceptually, and through actions of resistance within activist circles, within the academy and amongst radical practitioners since the very beginning of organized psychiatry in Canada and abroad. However, this reader represents the first text to consolidate Mad matters within a Canadian context, which we have done under the new umbrella of "Mad Studies." It also combines the more established understandings of Mad matters, including antipsychiatry approaches and long-standing psychiatric survivor narratives, with an exciting and burgeoning form of activism and conceptualizations, emanating from a new generation of people in Canada engaging in a variety of forms of radical and Mad activist scholarship.

In 1981, Toronto activist-survivor Mel Starkman wrote: "An important new movement is sweeping through the Western world.... The 'mad,' the oppressed, the ex-inmates of society's asylums are coming together and speaking for themselves. The map of the world is dotted with newly formed groups, struggling to identify themselves, define their struggle, and decide whether the 'system' is reformable or whether they need to create an alternative community" (Starkman, 1981; see Chapter 1). As Starkman proclaimed in 1981, so too this book proclaims over 30 years later the radical reclaiming of psychic spaces of resistance against the psychiatric domination of Mad people as a collection of chemical imbalances needing to be corrected in a capitalist system that prizes bourgeois conformity and medical model "fixes" above all. This book, in contrast, prizes the decades-long resistance of activists and allies in Canada who have sought to provide an alternative to Big Pharma and profiteers in the psychiatric system and academy who make a living labelling and medicating that which they cannot imagine or tolerate. *Mad Matters* therefore is part of a wider current that is helping to promote "Mad Studies" inside and outside post-secondary institutions. It is also intended to tap into the desire for "an alternative community" that Starkman wrote about, where people can get a sense of who they are and what madness is about without being automatically pathologized with a mental disease as happens in so many other spaces.

Mad Studies in this sense incorporates all that is critical of psychiatry from a radical socially progressive foundation in which the medical model is dispensed with as biologically reductionist whilst alternative forms of helping people experiencing mental anguish are based on humanitarian, holistic perspectives where people are not reduced to symptoms but understood within the social and economic context of the society in which they live. As such, antipsychiatry is included within Mad Studies as contributing much to our understanding of the nature of psychiatric thought and practice by helping to reveal the inner workings of a profession that has dominated interpretations of madness but which, over the past 50 years, has had critics from within and without assail its presumptions, criticisms which continue today. In this respect, we are not locating "Mad Studies" as originating solely within the community of people deemed Mad, but also as including allies, social critics, revolutionary theorists, and radical professionals who have sought to distance themselves from the essentializing biological determinism of psychiatry whilst respecting, valuing, and privileging the Mad thoughts of those whom conventional psychiatry would condemn to a jumble of diagnostic prognostications based on subjective opinions masquerading as science.

Moreover, the field of Mad Studies is relevant to a range of interconnecting social movements as well as a range of academic disciplines. These areas of thought and action circulate through this collection, precisely because of its interdisciplinary nature, its wide yet focused scope, and its importance in Canadian social policy as well as the activist community. This reader represents a collection of chapters in a growing field with interconnections across a host of disciplines and reaching out into the activist community in Canada and internationally. The importance for all forms of activism must be underscored; that is, Mad Studies is vital in informing Mad politics as well as anti-poverty organizing, queer politics, race politics, anti-colonial resistance, diaspora, and the various human rights movements, such as women's rights, children's rights, disability rights, and trans rights, among others. Furthermore, Mad Studies is reaping the benefits of its new and ongoing partnerships with other marginalized groups. In learning from our intersecting experiences of both oppression and resistance, through our identification with groups whose organized existence also threatens current forms of social dominance (LeFrançois, 2012), Mad politics can only strengthen its abilities in challenging psychiatry whilst also supporting wider resistance struggles.

The inspiration for this book comes from our encounters with the rich and innovative body of critical writing on madness, human rights, and the "psy sciences" that has been flourishing in this country over recent years. Across a range of institutional and cultural contexts, activists, psychiatric survivors, academics, journalists, and dissenting practitioners have been challenging the conventional biological paradigm of "mental illness"; exposing the systemic and symbolic violence that lie at the core of the psychiatric system; constructing radically creative ways of thinking about matters of the mind; linking the struggle against biopsychiatry with other movements organized around gender, race, disability, social class, culture, and generation; building a critical community that now spans all regions of the country; and practising mental "difference" and recovery as liberating ways of expressing our humanity and engaging in political debate and practice. In this book, we showcase an original collection of work that has emerged from these exciting trajectories of engagement, and we represent Canadian critical Mad Studies as an emerging, and increasingly vital, field of study and activism.

Historical Legacies

The contemporary Mad movement came into being during the decades of the 1960s and 1970s, an especially turbulent period in the history of the psy sciences, and in the ever-shifting relations between psychiatry, society, the individual, and the state. The post-WWII years had ushered in a powerful new wave of therapeutic discourse and practice in advanced liberal democracies worldwide. The mental health industry had undergone a quite spectacular rebirth, successfully asserting its domain over ever-widening spheres of public and private life in what Robert Castel and his colleagues would later describe as the "psychiatric society" (Castel, Castel & Lovell, 1982). Buoyed by an arsenal of new biogenetic theories and somatic technologies (among them, the first generation of so-called "antipsychotic" neuroleptics, and brain-scanning devices such as x-ray computed tomography) (Schrag, 1978), and liberated from its long-established institutional confines by a wholesale collapse of the asylum system amid the "community mental health movement" (see Shimrat, Chapter 10), psychiatry was in the process of flexing its disciplinary muscles as never before. From its first release in 1952, the American Psychiatric Association's *Diagnostic and Statistical Manual* (DSM) was already well en route to becoming North America's prime mental classification system—the go-to definer of mental pathology that it is today (Caplan, 1996; Kutchins & Kirk, 1997). If in the 1970s we had yet to become a Prozac or Ritalin Nation, Valium, Librium, and the tricyclics were flooding our marketplaces and synapses as epidemics of "depression" and "anxiety" were ominously declared (Greenberg, 2010; Lane, 2007) and prescriptions flew off physicians' pads by the millions. From our private thoughts to our love lives to the workplace to the world of entertainment and consumption, it seemed that no sphere of late 20th-century life fell beyond the mandate of mental medicine to refashion self and civilization, and to make us all happy, actualized, docile, and safe.

Yet the movement to psychiatrize contemporary culture never went unopposed. Through the 1970s and the decade that preceded it, scholars, activists, and people who would later self-identify as survivors of the mental health system began to mobilize against the advancing powers of psychiatry along a number of divergent (and often mutually colliding) fronts. As chronicled by Ingleby (1980), Pearson (1975), Sedgwick (1982), Ussher (1992), and many more, the psychopolitics of that era were volatile and complex.

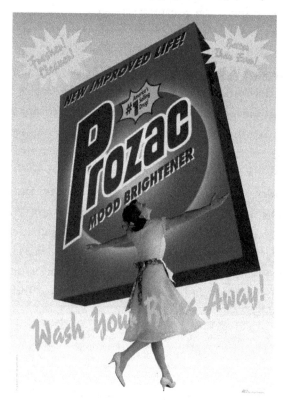

FIGURE 0.1: Prozac Laundry

In recent years Prozac's cultural currency has increased to the point of being a commonplace household staple, as spoofed in this mock advertisement.

Source: Adbusters, 2011.

To be sure, common themes galvanized the antipsychiatry movement in its championing of human rights for psychiatrized citizens, and in its opposition to the burgeoning therapeutic state and the medicalization of everyday life; from arbitrary, exclusionary, racist, homophobic, gender-biased diagnostic codes and interventions; to involuntary mental confinement and enforced "treatment"; to electroshock, Big Pharma, and the profusion of chemical straightjackets branded as therapy; and, increasingly, to systemic deinstitutionalization and the wholesale urban ghettoizing of ex-patients under the transparent deceit of "downsizing" and "reintegration."

At the same time, the sheer diversity of those people and organizations aligned against institutional psychiatry was nothing short of breathtaking. In the United States, from within the ranks of the discipline Thomas Szasz had launched his lifelong campaign against what he termed the "myth of mental illness" (1961), condemning his profession for its arrogance and coercive methods, and advancing a libertarian model of mental health care in which patients and service providers would be contractual equals and the latter would be stripped of the power to compulsorily impose social control in the name of "treatment." Scarcely less influential had been journalist Albert Deutsch's lacerating exposé of the concentration camp-like conditions of mental hospitals in *The Shame of the States* (1948), followed through the next two decades by Erving Goffman's celebrated ethnography of St. Elizabeth's Hospital as "total institution" in *Asylums* (1961); by Ken Kesey's iconic novel *One Flew Over the Cuckoo's Nest* (1962), later famously adapted to film by Milos Forman (1975); by Frederick Wiseman's devastating (and, for a quarter-century, shamefully banned) documentary *Titicut Follies* (1967) on the unqualified hell that was the Bridgewater institution in Massachusetts; and by David Rosenhan's subversive study of eight pseudo-patients who found their mental status under siege while being "sane in insane places" (1973).

On the other side of the Atlantic, radical psychiatrists like R.D. Laing (1960, 1967), David Cooper (1967), and Franco Basaglia (Scheper-Hughes & Lovell, 1987) were at the leading edge of a transnational antipsychiatry school committed to Laing's "politics of experience," the challenging premise that madness could only be understood and engaged existentially and through the eyes of those who lived it. For the European anti-psychiatrists, the objectification of so-called "mentally ill" people under the guise of science was a deeply dehumanizing pursuit that required challenging through a wholesale rethinking of human consciousness and being. Whether psychosis was, or is, an exploration of selfhood or a journey to self-actualization may remain a contested idea. But there is no doubting the impact of Laing's experiments with the therapeutic community at Kingsley Hall (Barnes & Berke, 1971), and Loren Mosher's groundbreaking Soteria Project (Mosher, 1995), and the revolutionary shift in Italian mental health policy, spearheaded by Franco Basaglia, towards patient-centred, humane, local modes of intervention (Donnelly, 1992). Then there was Michel Foucault, whose *Madness and Civilization* (1965), an iconoclastic chronicle of sanity's war on madness as the triumph of reason in the age of Enlightenment, was being read in abridged translation throughout the English-speaking world (the complete original version was only published in English in 2006 as *History of Madness*).

Simultaneously, and arguably for the first time in a systematic way, people bearing psychiatric diagnoses both within and beyond institutional settings were commencing to organize through grassroots democratic action into what was initially referred to as "mental patients' liberation," and later as the "c/s/x" (consumer/survivor/ex-patient) movement (in North America) and the "psychiatric survivor" or "service user" movement (in the United Kingdom). English-language epicentres included London, Berkeley, Boston, New York, Toronto, and Vancouver where the Mental Patients Association (MPA) evolved into a major force for human rights causes, housing and social support, and progressive democratic action of various kinds through the 1970s (Beckman & Davies, Chapter 3; Chamberlin, 1978; Shimrat, 1997). Finally, second-wave feminism embraced the aims of antipsychiatry at multiple levels. Phyllis Chesler's *Women and Madness* (1972) was perhaps the most influential book of this period, advancing the thesis that women were held to different and higher standards of reason and normalcy than were men, that the psychiatrization process was profoundly gender-biased in its premises and effects, and that the very constitution of sanity and "mental illness" in late 20th-century society was anchored in the bedrock of male normativity. Fast on the heels of Chesler's book came *Women Look at Psychiatry* (1975), edited by Dorothy Smith and Sara David, which offered an experiential, women-focused interpretation of the malestream psychiatric system through the eyes of those who had encountered, and been damaged by, it. Moreover, a wider critique of medical power and practice was flourishing, inspired in part by Ivan Illich's groundbreaking writings on "medical nemesis," the "expropriation of health," and the corrosive impact of the "disabling professions" (Illich, 1976; Illich et al., 2005).

If the 1960s and 1970s were a golden age of antipsychiatry and Mad liberation, the following two decades witnessed powerful currents of backlash and retrenchment. The sulfurous odour of counter-revolution was in the air as biogenetic psychiatry re-established its dominion in reaction to the activist breath of fresh air that was soon to be either suffocated or co-opted, depending on circumstance and usefulness to the medical model establishment of "new ideas." Thus new diagnostic systems increasingly sought to pathologize everyday behaviour in ways that reflected both the intellectual and moral corruption of participating medical professionals and academics who allied themselves with corporate drug pushers to form the most nefarious influence on the lives of millions of people categorized as "mentally ill" the world has ever seen—and all from a Western, American-centric, culturally narrow-minded perspective (Caplan, 1995; Healy, 2008; Watters, 2010). In the midst of the growth of this medical monstrosity, where pills were promoted as the ultimate panacea (Whitaker, 2002, 2010), legal rights won in the activist heydays of the 1970s and early 1980s were gradually rolled back and new laws introduced to curtail rights even further gained traction (see Costa, Chapter 14; Fabris, 2011), electroshock rose from the ashes of denunciation to become "respectable" again (see Weitz, Chapter 11), and deinstitutionalization was increasingly decried as at fault for social inequities experienced by psychiatric survivors in the community, rather than long-standing systemic prejudices that led to chronic underfunding of social supports that were supposed to go along with the release of ex-patients from institutions.

With the extension of diagnoses within revised versions of the DSM and ICD,[2] we also witnessed the widespread diagnostic labelling of children with a variety of psychiatric disorders, which are so clearly connected to controlling their thoughts and behaviour (LeFrançois, 2007), within schools, at home, and within state-run foster/residential care. For example, children who were once thought of as behaving badly have been increasingly diagnosed with conduct disorders; children—including toddlers—once seen as having vivid and creative imaginations have been increasingly diagnosed with psychotic disorders; and children who were once understood as expressing sadness or low moods have been increasingly diagnosed with depressive disorders, whilst high energy, "uncontrollable" children have been increasingly diagnosed with a range of hyperactivity-related disorders.[3] Perhaps most disturbingly, children who have survived child abuse and other forms of trauma, including state-sanctioned and politically motivated violence (Rabaia et al., 2010), have been increasingly diagnosed with a wide range of "mental illnesses," including many different permutations of those mentioned above, and have been given a cocktail of drugs to presumably match each diagnosis.[4] Paradoxically, during these decades of increased psychiatrization of children, we also witnessed the rise of the children's rights movement. This movement, and the enactment of international legislation to support the human rights of children, brought with it a proliferation of organizations run by and for children, most notably amongst politicized groups of physically disabled children and children in state care,[5] who have organized around and lobbied against the inherent adultism within society generally and within children's services specifically. However, absent from the children's rights movement, internationally, has been collective resistance in the form of politicized children's organizations formed by psychiatrized children (LeFrançois, 2010). Instead, adults, including children's rights advocates, academics, and radical practitioners, have taken up the issue of the widespread psychiatric violence committed against children (Breggin, 2001, 2002; Breggin & Breggin, 1998; Coppock, 1997, 2002; Laws et al., 1999; LeFrançois, 2007; Spandler, 1996). Dovetailing from the trend, provoked by the children's rights movement, to include children as full participants in—rather than the objects of—research studies, researchers began to document children's own narratives—with limited or no adult interpretations—regarding their experiences of distress and psychiatrization (Farnfield, 1995; LeFrançois, 2007; Spandler, 1996). Ethics review boards (not) permitting, this led to calls to engage with psychiatrized children as co-researchers within (community-based) participatory research projects (Laws et al., 1999; LeFrançois, 2006; Liegghio, forthcoming). With the acknowledgment of the agency of all children, including psychiatrized children, and fighting the tendency for adults to advocate for them and interpret their experiences from an (unavoidably) adultist perspective,[6] psychiatrized children began to demonstrate their resistance and self-advocacy in the form of writing their autobiographical stories of oppression at the hands of psychiatry (see, for example, Michener, 1998).

In other spheres as well, and at times seeming to defy all odds, the voices of dissent against the resurgent biopsychiatric industry and its confederates in Big Pharma have never been stronger. Through the latter decades of the 20th century, and into the present day, critical scholarship and activism have flourished around the world as never before. Without downplaying the very real differences in identities, political values, and forms of expression that mark (and sometimes set apart) the many strands of antipsychiatry, critical psychiatry, mental patients' liberation, psychiatric survivor activism, and Mad pride, local and global mobilizations for psychiatric citizenship and social justice in mental health have evolved into a dynamic social movement that is unquestionably here to stay. Along with these developments, a remarkable body of academic and popular writing has accumulated that forcefully refutes the dubious claims of biopsychiatry to scientific status and benevolent design—contesting, by turn, its self-referential historical narratives, its pseudo-theoretical foundations of ideas, its arbitrary nosological systems, its barren and often calamitous regimes of "treatment," and the coercive policies, structures, and practices psychiatry has devised in advancing its reach into ever-expanding fields of modern life. For their part, Canadians have figured prominently in the production of critical knowledge in opposition to psychiatric authority and human rights abuses, contributing both historical and contemporary critiques of the psy disciplines and narratives of those who encounter it as subjects and adversaries (Burstow, 2003, 2005, 2006a,b; Burstow & Weitz, 1988; Cellard & Thifault, 2007; Chan, Chunn & Menzies, 2005; Church, 1993, 2006; Cohen, 1990; Davies, 1989; Everett, 2000; Fabris, 2011; Grenier, 1999; Kendall, 2005, 2009; Kilty, 2008; LeBlanc & St-Amand, 2008; LeFrançois, 2006, 2008; McCubbin, 1998, 2003; Menzies, 1989, 2001, 2002; Morrow, 2003, 2005; Perreault, 2009; Poole, 2011; Ralph, 1983; Reaume, 2000, 2002, 2006; Shimrat, 1997; St-Amand, 1988; Teghtsoonian, 2008; Vogt, 2011; Voronka, 2008a,b; White, 2007, 2009).

Moreover, just as psychiatry has globalized its operations in this era of transnational communication, marketing and commerce, so too has the Mad movement been sharpening its tools for conviviality (Illich, 1973) and expanding its frontiers around the planet. With vibrant centres of engagement in Europe and the Americas, but ranging increasingly into the Antipodes, Africa, and Asia, psychiatric survivor activism has been gaining an ever-higher profile while organizing for systemic change and forging strategic coalitions in defence of psychiatrized people everywhere.

Grassroots advocates, community groups, and international alliances have been spreading their messages of anti-discrimination and inclusion to governments, stakeholder groups, media, and the public alike, in the process working to shift the very discourse of "mental health" from the reigning biomedical model to a paradigm of social provision, human justice, and valorization of diversity. Organizations like MindFreedom International (MFI), the World Network of Users and Survivors of Psychiatry (WNUSP), the European Network of (Ex)Users and Survivors of Psychiatry (ENUSP), Mad Pride UK, PsychRights, the Hearing Voices Network (HVN), the National Self Harm Network (NSHN), the Antipsychiatry Coalition, the Coalition Against Psychiatric Assault (CAPA), the National Association for Rights Protection and Advocacy (NARPA), and the International Network Toward Alternatives and Recovery (INTAR) maintain active lobbying, awareness, support, and mutual aid campaigns and—in the cases of NARPA and INTAR—convene regular meetings involving members of survivor-activist, educator, and research communities (Beresford, 2002; Campbell, 1996, 1999, 2005; Coleman, 2008; Crossley, 2006; Morrison, 2005; Sayce, 2000; Speed, 2005; Stastny & Lehmann, 2007). Over recent years, conferences have been hosted by institutions like the City University of New York, Simon Fraser University, Manchester Metropolitan University, Mansfield College (Oxford), and the University of Toronto.[7]

The Mad movement in Canada, which developed first in Vancouver in 1970–1971 with the Mental Patients Association (Beckman & Davies, Chapter 3) and then spread elsewhere in the years that followed (Shimrat, 1997), from the beginning included critical activism and scholarship that expressed views that were so clearly different from the medical model that formed a nascent "Mad Studies" of its own long before the term came into vogue. Alternative voices arose in print, including Vancouver's *In A Nutshell* (since 1971), Toronto's *Phoenix Rising* (1980–1990), and Moncton's *Our Voice/Notre Voix* (since 1987), all of which wrote about madness from a perspective that was, at times, radical and always devoid of the medical model dogmatism so common among mainline psychiatric publications. With the growth of the Internet and the World Wide Web, international connections, long fostered before this technological development, became much easier to engage in so that Mad movement activists and allies have connected electronically through individuals, groups, and overarching coordinating bodies such as MindFreedom International.

For Mad Studies

Since the 1960s and the first wave of the antipsychiatry and mental patient liberation movements, people in resistance against sanism and mind control have been invoking "madness" both as a means of self-identifying, and as a point of entry into the fields of power where their encounters with organized psychiatry, and their very lives, play out. Once a reviled term that signalled the worst kinds of bigotry and abuse, madness has come to represent a critical alternative to "mental illness" or "disorder" as a way of naming and responding to emotional, spiritual, and neuro-diversity. To work with and within the language of madness is by no means to deny the psychic, spiritual, and material pains and privations endured by countless people with histories of encounters with the psy disciplines. To the contrary, it is to acknowledge and validate these experiences as being authentically human, while at the same time rejecting clinical labels that pathologize and degrade; challenging the reductionistic assumptions and effects of the medical model; locating psychiatry and its human subjects within wider historical, institutional, and cultural contexts; and advancing the position that mental health research, writing, and advocacy are primarily about opposing oppression and promoting human justice.

An ancient and protean concept that English speakers have been invoking since at least the 14th century (Porter, 2002; Scull, 2011),[8] in recent years "mad" has flooded back into the language of public culture, and into the work of critical activists and scholars worldwide. For people and organizations engaged in resistance against psychiatry, to take up "madness" is an expressly political act. Following other social movements including queer, black, and fat activism, madness talk and text invert the language of oppression, reclaiming disparaged identities and restoring dignity and pride to difference. Invoking madness in the interests of resistance and critique also puts into practice Foucault's ideas regarding the "strategic reversibility of power" through the medium of discourse (Foucault, 1991; see MacLeod & Durrheim, 2002).

While no singular usage monopolizes this book, a sampling of chapter excerpts reveals several commonalities of meaning. "By Mad," write Poole and Ward (Chapter 6), "we are referring to a term reclaimed by those who have been pathologized/ psychiatrized as 'mentally ill,' and a way of taking back language that has been used to oppress.... We are referring to a movement, an identity, a stance, an act of resistance, a theoretical approach, and a burgeoning field of study." In Chapter 8 Liegghio writes: "[M]adness refers to a range of experiences—thoughts, moods, behaviours—that are different from and challenge, resist, or do not conform to dominant, psychiatric constructions of 'normal' versus 'disordered' or 'ill' mental health.... madness [is] a social category among other categories like race, class, gender, sexuality, age, or ability that define our identities and experiences." For their part, White and Pike (Chapter 17) apply the term madness "to reflect a more inclusive and culturally grounded human phenomenon that encompasses various historically and contextually specific terms such as insanity, feebleminded, mental disorder, and mental illness." Diamond (Chapter 4) describes "Mad" as "an umbrella term to represent a diversity of identities ... used in place of naming all of the different identities that describe people who have been labelled and treated as crazy (i.e., consumer, survivor, ex-patient)." In this sense, she continues, madness can be invoked "to address some of the divisions stemming from psychiatric survivor identity politics, to celebrate a *plurality of resistances* and subversive acts against sanism." Finally, in Chapter 9 Fabris chooses to differentiate between the lower-case "madness," which has no inherent critical content, and the proper noun "Mad," which he proposes "to mean the group of us considered crazy or deemed ill by sanists." In this decisive sense, for Fabris "'Mad' is an historical rather than a descriptive or essential category, proposed for political action and discussion." At the same time, the term is not uncontested amongst activists and scholars, including contributors to this book (see Burstow, Chapter 5).

However much consensus of meaning might exist among our contributors, and however widespread the term in public parlance (our Google search elicited 231 million hits for "madness" and 148 million for "mad"), we embarked on this project and decided on a title with no illusions about the controversy—and downright hostility—that the madness concept can still incite in some circles. For many practitioners of the psy professions, and for countless others who subscribe to conventional models of mental distress as biogenetic "illness," to invoke madness is to flaunt deep-seated beliefs about the nature of sanity and reason, and about the condition of being psychiatrically "sound" or "unwell." By advancing a program of Mad Studies and Mad activism, we are flagging this book politically, and we are knowingly taking up a subversive standpoint relative to the governing paradigm of psychiatric "science."

By the same token, in any project affiliated with Mad Studies, Mad movement, and antipsychiatry, participants and "stakeholders" will necessarily represent a remarkable diversity of identities and life experiences—not to mention a wide array of understandings about mental wellness and distress, and about the mental "health" system and its role in contemporary society. How to represent and promote this spectrum of Mad involvement, while maintaining a critical edge and resisting a decline into liberal relativism, remains a political and ethical challenge requiring resilience, reflexivity, the willingness to adapt, and a collective vision of the Mad movement as a living, and constantly evolving, field of political engagement and struggle for social justice.

In many respects, to propose a project of "Mad Studies" in Canada is to take an audacious step into the unknown. For one thing, the full story of Mad Studies has yet to be acted out, much less written down. As David Reville and Kathryn Church observe in their accounts of Mad Studies programming at Ryerson University (Chapters 12, 13), only in the past decade has the term begun to filter into the vocabularies of teachers, writers, psychiatric survivors, and activists in this country and beyond. Further, however we might try to capture the "essence" of Mad Studies in a book such as this, by its very nature the field is inherently in flux and thus defies any effort to pigeonhole. In this sense, the collection of essays that we have assembled here should be approached more as an interim, and decidedly partial, report than any kind of definitive survey—and, of course, its contents represent our own biases about what matters to the study of madness. For these reasons and others, we cannot even begin to capture the dizzying scope and complexity of ideas, methods, identities, points of reference, and political commitments that the project of Mad Studies embodies, or might or will embody. To claim completeness or unity of vision would be to gloss the many ongoing controversies, areas of contention, and competing understandings of past, present, and future that are represented in even a selective offering like this book.

All of this said, Mad Studies builds on a compelling tradition of critical activism and scholarship—smatterings of which we glancingly chronicle above—which has opened up a wealth of opportunity for 21st-century struggle against psychiatry in its many forms. Accordingly, the practice of Mad Studies is far more a continuation than an entirely new trajectory of inquiry and practice. In Chapter 20, Louise Tam underscores the importance of this historical legacy: "The Mad movement and Mad Studies have arrived where they are today from more than five decades of resisting against 'psy' knowledge (destabilizing diagnostic categories, naming psychiatric violence, resisting pathologization, and creating countercultures)." Additionally, Mad Studies follows in the footsteps of various other classes of "studies" that have established themselves in recent decades—among them, labour studies, women's studies/gender studies, LGBTQ studies, equity studies, sexuality studies, black studies, disability studies, deaf studies, queer studies, black queer studies, dementia studies, fat studies, religious studies, postcolonial studies, transnational studies, diaspora studies, and communication studies. In this way, it is perhaps inevitable that "Mad" would get appended to "studies" given the fertile field of specialized "studies" that has developed and the richness of work done on madness across various disciplines.

In his important 2008 paper calling for the establishment of Mad Studies as a new "in/discipline" (see also Reville, Chapter 12), Richard Ingram reminds us of the debt that Mad Studies owes to "disability studies perspectives based on a transformative revaluation of the category of 'disability'" (Ingram, 2008). For Ingram and others who highlight this key disciplinary connection, the challenge for practitioners of Mad Studies—as with disability studies, deaf studies, and their many analogs— is to pursue this project of "transformative revaluation" by carving out spaces of relative autonomy while simultaneously taking up the many "communalities" and points of intersection between parallel fields of inquiry and action. Such a pursuit must reflect the specificities of Mad experience and politics (and thus is not fully co-extensive with disability studies), just as it seeks to forge strategic coalitions with other peoples in struggle (see Diamond, Gorman, and Tam, Chapters 4, 19, and 20). In the process, studies that are madly done can "set a minimum threshold," carving out a critical topography and setting the standards by which radical theory and practice might be pursued as "alternatives to psychiatric, psychotherapeutic, and psychological perspectives" (Ingram, 2008). For those of us teaching and writing in scholarly contexts, they harbour the potential to unsettle the very way we address the subject of rationality and its alternatives, thereby "shaking the foundations of the place of reason, academia, the sum of all disciplines" (Ingram, 2012). For all of us critically engaged with the powers of psychiatry, counsels Ingram, the objects of Mad Studies are inseparable from the far-reaching aspirations of the Mad movement: "We hope that societies will recover their lost wisdom by coming to recognize once again the tremendous potential that resides in our unorthodox imaginations.... A time will come when our bodyminds are no longer declared incompetent, and are no longer regarded as accidents waiting to happen. A time will come when we can laugh and cry, love and hide, freely, and without fear. A time will come when there will be no punishment for allowing your imagination to run wild" (Ingram, 2008).

In taking up Ingram's challenge, psychiatric survivors, activists, scholars, and allies from an assortment of sites—including many of the contributors to this book—have been collectively reconnoitering the field of Mad Studies, considering its opportunities, complications, and constraints. Even at this early juncture in its life history, some common themes have emerged.

First, following Ingram (2008), Mad Studies can be defined in general terms as a project of inquiry, knowledge production, and political action devoted to the critique and transcendence of psy-centred ways of thinking, behaving, relating, and being. In this, Mad Studies is steadfastly arrayed against biomedical psychiatry, at the same time that it validates and celebrates survivor experiences and cultures. Mad Studies aims to engage and transform oppressive languages, practices, ideas, laws, and systems, along with their human practitioners, in the realms of mental "health" and the psy sciences, as in the wider culture. In Rachel Gorman's words (Chapter 19), "Mad Studies takes social, relational, identity-based, and anti-oppression approaches to questions of mental/psychological/behavioural difference, and is articulated, in part, against an analytic of mental illness."

Second, by its very nature Mad Studies is an interdisciplinary and multi-vocal praxis. From its beginnings, resistance against psychiatry has germinated in a multiplicity of sites, and it has involved people from every conceivable social position and walk of life. In the academy, as noted above, we find many mutual affinities between Mad and disability studies, and among those engaged in these pursuits. Yet in Canada, as elsewhere, critical scholarship directed at psychiatry and "mental health" is also flourishing in health studies, sciences and medical faculties, along with departments of law, sociology, psychology, history, philosophy, education, communication, English literature, cultural studies, women and gender studies, socio-legal studies, disability studies, and social work. Additionally, in keeping with its in/disciplinary status (Ingram, 2008), Mad Studies subsumes a loose assemblage of perspectives that resist compression into an irreducible dogma or singular approach to theory or practice. As Jennifer M. Poole and Jennifer Ward advise us (Chapter 6), "there are many ways to take up a Mad analysis."

Third, Mad Studies takes as its principal source, inspiration, and raison d'être the subjectivities, embodiments, words, experiences, and aspirations of those among us whose lives have collided with the powers of institutional psychiatry. By definition and design, Mad people and Mad culture occupy the analytic core, and they/we embody the very spirit, of Mad Studies. This is not to suggest that the in/discipline does not practise a coalition politics with allies who have escaped first-hand psychiatric regulation and abuse (the very line-up of this book demonstrates otherwise). Still, without the foundation of critical knowledge and action built up over many years through the grassroots advocacy of psychiatrized people, a viable field of Mad Studies would be unimaginable. In Canadian Mad Studies, the political values, canonical texts, methodologies, forms of communication, and blueprints for action—not to mention the heroes of the movement— have all emerged, in various ways, from survivor culture and history (see Burstow & Weitz, 1988; Chamberlin, 1978; Everett, 2000; Funk, 1998; Reaume, 2000; Shimrat, 1997; St-Amand & LeBlanc, Chapter 2; Starkman, 1981; Vogt, 2011).

Fourth, echoing the experiences of other social movements, relations of sameness/ difference weave their way through the language and practice of Mad Studies in complicated ways. As several chapters in this book illustrate, multiple "mental health" constituencies have emerged in Canada (as elsewhere) through the years, all of which share certain common values and perspectives, while positioning themselves variously—often spectacularly so—in their dealings with psychiatry and the "mental health" industry. In the literature of the past generation, such differences have often been presented in binary terms, usually by juxtaposing "consumer" versus "survivor" communities—with the former self-identifying as clientele of a benign but under- resourced system, and the latter aligning themselves as victims and adversaries of a fundamentally flawed and abusive industry of mind and body control (Crossley, 2006; Everett, 2000; Morrison, 2005; Speed, 2005). However, according to Diamond, Burstow, and Gorman (Chapters 4, 5, and 19), such a bifold account ignores the many layers and nuances of Canadians' engagement with psychiatry and its allied disciplines. Further, it tends to gloss the ongoing push and pull between "consumer" and "survivor" activists and organizations—a tense relationship that, as Bonnie Burstow argues (Chapter 5), cannot be reconciled by simply inserting hyphens or forward slashes, as in "c/s/x."[9] Based on her doctoral research undertaken in Ontario, for example, Shaindl Diamond (Chapter 4) finds no fewer than three distinct but overlapping communities active within the "radical" stream of the movement—respectively, the psychiatric survivor, Mad, and antipsychiatry constituencies—each with its own rich history, collective identity, ideological commitments, repertoire of discourses, and politics of resistance and change.

Fifth, Mad Studies is an exercise in critical pedagogy—in the radical co-production, circulation, and consumption of knowledge. Following Foucault, the practitioners of Mad Studies are concerned with deploying counter-knowledge and subjugated knowledge as a strategy for contesting regimes of truth (Foucault, 1980, 1991) and ruling (Smith, 1987) about "mental illness" and the psy "sciences," and about those of us who contend with psychiatric diagnoses and interventions. Further, to quote

White and Pike (Chapter 17), "In examining *how* mental health/illness is made sense of, we may also learn who is entitled to participate in the production of mental health knowledge, who has the ability, or inability, to control what becomes 'common' knowledge, and moreover, who is permitted, or not, to be seen and heard in the making of MHL [mental health literacy]." In our 21st-century age of new media we are witnessing an explosion of technologies and methods for practising critical knowledge work of this kind—among them, websites, alternative e-journals, online archives (see Beckman & Davies, Chapter 3), discussion forums, and Twitter (see generally Wipond, Chapter 18). Concurrently, public education remains a key site of radical knowledge work and conscientization (Freire, 1970), with academics pursuing Mad Studies in their role as "negative workers"—a term coined by Italian dissident psychiatrist Franco Basaglia to describe those privileged individuals who "collude with the powerless to identify their needs against the interests of the bourgeois institution: the university, the hospital, the factory" (Scheper-Hughes, 1992, p. 541). As just one illustration, in Chapters 12 and 13 Reville and Church outline a Mad history studies pedagogy that has evolved (not without resistance) at Ryerson University with a wide protocol of critical learning objectives, which bring a Mad standpoint to the teaching of history, while exploring the role of knowledge and language in both perpetuating oppression and opening up pathways to resistance (Church, Chapter 13).

Sixth, Mad Studies promotes historical memory work that can help liberate us from the particularities of the here and now, and help us connect contemporary antipsychiatry and Mad activism to the legacies of struggles past. A historical consciousness is empowering to the extent that it locates Mad people at the centre of their own narratives, while highlighting the correspondences between past and present movements, stretching our imaginative horizons of time and space, and illustrating people's capacity to change the world. Further, by breaking the frame of the present, we can come to appreciate the diversity of Mad experience, along with the many commonalities that bind seemingly disparate people together through time and space. As Shaindl Diamond argues (Chapter 4), to think and act beyond the present means "recognizing that madness is constructed differently in various historical and cultural contexts, and that there is no real basis of inherent or natural characteristics that define an eternal Mad subject." It is not surprising, then, that we find Mad people's history emerging as a cornerstone of Mad Studies in Canada (Reville and Church, Chapters 12, 13; Reaume, 2006; St-Amand & LeBlanc, Chapter 2, 2008; Starkman, Chapter 1), alongside collaborative projects like the Psychiatric Survivors Archives, Toronto (PSAT) (www.psychiatricsurvivorarchives.com) and the History of Madness in Canada website (http://historyofmadness.ca; see Beckman & Davies, Chapter 3) devoted to the recovery and preservation of "patient"- and survivor-centred history.

Seventh, along with the cultivation of historical imagination comes the need to engage the structural contexts and relations of power within which Mad subjectivities, embodiments, experiences, and engagements play out. Towards this end, White and Pike (Chapter 17) advise that we "pay attention to the socio-political and economic processes through which our common sensibilities around mental health and illness are informed, structured, and maintained." In scaffolding resistance work around systems of power—and, in particular, within formations of governance and the state—Mad Studies can learn much from the practitioners of critical, feminist, and antipsychiatry, many of whom have long been concerned with how capitalism and patriarchy frame and reproduce psychiatric subjugation (see Burstow, Chapter 5; Ingleby, 1980; Scull, 1977; Ussher, 1992). According to Tam (Chapter 20), only through a structurally informed analysis is it possible to effect a genuine paradigm shift, freeing us from the restrictive study of "discrete intersections" of identity and psychiatry to deploy a fully material analysis of "inter-institutional psy oppression" (on this point, see also Ussher's (2005, 2011) discussion of MDI theory[10]). Such an approach has become all the more compelling in the wake of the global neoliberal (counter)revolution, which began in the 1980s and continues to dominate Canadian political economy and culture into this present decade. As Morrow asserts (Chapter 23), Mad Studies must take into account the many mutual affinities between neoliberalism and biogenetic psychiatry. With its agenda of privatization, consumerism, fiscal restraint, privileging of the "free" marketplace, and wholesale retrenchment of social services, neoliberalism has paved the way for a new "shallow" relationship between the individual and the state (according to Rose (1999), the making of a neoliberal "self"). In so doing, it has fashioned a new kind of self-monitoring psychiatric consumer whose "mental illness" is purely an individual concern to be managed through self-caretaking, the administration of expert technologies and, where necessary, aggressive health interventions that proceed without any gesture towards the structural roots of human distress. In other words, observes Morrow (Chapter 23), the age of neoliberalism has ushered in the "healthification of social problems."

Eighth, and following directly from the above, Mad Studies embraces a dialectical perspective on the relations between self and society, between private and public, between subjectivities and social relations, between human agency and social structure, and perhaps most crucially for this book, between the politics of Mad identity and the imperatives of collective struggle against sanism in all its forms. In keeping with this latter commitment, contributors like Poole and Ward (Chapter 6), Diamond (Chapter 4), and Gorman (Chapter 19) invoke intersectionality theory as pioneered by feminist anti-racism scholars like Kimberlé Crenshaw (1991) and Patricia Hill Collins (2000). "Intersectionality," write Poole and Ward, "is concerned with how aspects of social identity—such as race and madness, for example—intersect with oppressions such as sexism and heterosexism." These authors note the critical need to interrogate the role of psychiatry in mediating, and amplifying, a host of crosscutting socio-economic and political forms of discrimination and oppression based on (for example) class, gender, race, (dis)ability, age, culture, nationality, and sexual identity and practice (see, also, LeFrançois, 2013). As it acts upon other institutions, and in turn is acted upon in what Hill Collins (2000) terms a "matrix of domination," the psy system cannot be studied in isolation. Just as important, people's experiences of psychiatrization vary materially, based on their ever-shifting placements along the multiple axes of the matrix. In turn, what it means to be Mad, and to face repression on its grounds, is forever contingent and hinges crucially on these same structural arrangements. For these reasons, intersectional analysis "is highly critical of dominant constructions of *madness, normality,* or *sanity,* recognizing the flawed nature of simplistic dichotomous and oppositional constructions of difference as 'dominant/subordinate, good/bad, up/down, superior/inferior'" (Diamond, Chapter 4, quoting Lorde, 2007, p. 114).

Ninth, whether it is practised on the streets, in the schools, through the Internet and print media, in the confines of courts, government offices and hospitals, or among community organizations, Mad Studies is part of a wider revolutionary project dedicated to the radical restructuring of the "mental health" industry. In the end, nothing short of wholesale transformation—to our paradigms of thought, to reigning systems of knowledge and communication, and to the institutional structures that embody and sustain psychiatric relations of power—will suffice. Granted, tactical and strategic differences inevitably abound, the voices of change are sometimes muted and suppressed, and no consensus vision of a post-psychiatric world yet exists (see Bracken & Thomas, 2005; Cohen & Timimi, 2008). Still, with its roots deeply planted in the traditions of antipsychiatry and liberation movements of the 1960s and 1970s, the struggle for social justice in and beyond "mental health" continues to be very much a project of abolition and transformation—of "nonviolent revolution," in the words of MindFreedom director David Oaks (2008). For its part, Mad Studies can help inform this project by conducting critical knowledge work, by speaking truth to psychiatric power (Brandon, 1991, 1998), by exposing the system's many contradictions, and by pointing the way forward. In so doing, Mad Studies harbours the potential to be a truly revolutionary in/discipline (Ingram, 2008), bridging the long-standing divide between scholarship and activism, theory and practice.

Tenth, if Mad Studies is to be a revolutionary project, it must also nest itself in the immediate practicalities of everyday human struggle. As we assembled this collection of essays, countless people continued to contend with the pain, anger, despair, "distress, euphoria, confusion, unusual or visionary thinking, reliving of painful memories, and alternative experiences of reality" that institutional psychiatry chooses to label as "mental illness" (LeFrançois, 2012, p. 7)—an experience that is too often compounded by that profession's ministrations (however benign the motives may often be). For those who inhabit the margins of our 21st-century civilization—the armies of lost and outcast people facing a broken system that serves up chemical cocktails and institutional constraints as a hollow substitute for care, compassion, human contact, and the basic requirements of a dignified life—Mad Studies will have little meaning if it cannot offer some sense of an alternative, some measure of hope that the present can be endured and overcome. To stay relevant and grounded—and to look at psychiatry and society, and act accordingly, from the standpoint of those who encounter power and privation in their rawest forms—is the key practical, ethical, and political challenge confronting critical scholars, writers, and activists in the realm of "mental health." Moreover, as the contributors to this book repeatedly attest through their actions as much as their words, it is likely the only one that matters in the end. To practise Mad Studies therefore means engaging our current world of suffering and injustice and seeking to change it, while simultaneously, in the words of Irit Shimrat (Chapter 10), "dream[ing] of a society brave and moral enough to eschew the whole paradigm of mental health and illness, replacing it with the creation of real community, and real help."

Organization and Contents of the Book

Informed by the issues, themes, struggles, and experiences chronicled above, this book is made up of 23 chapters contributed by Canadian activists, survivors, writers, and academics who have in various ways involved themselves in advocacy against sanism, in resistance against biogenetic psychiatry, and in the pursuit of social justice by and on behalf of psychiatrized people.

Part I, "Mad People's History, Evolving Culture, and Language," includes Mel Starkman's classic essay, reprinted from the pages of iconic survivor journal *Phoenix Rising*, on the rise of the contemporary Mad movement. Drawing from their historical work on psychiatric systems in New Brunswick (2008), Nérée St-Amand and Eugène LeBlanc explore Madwomen's encounters with the 19th-century asylum. Lanny Beckman and Megan Davies mobilize their experiences as activist and historian, in turn, to ponder the practices and possibilities of collaborative memory work. Shaindl Diamond addresses the challenge of building communities of activism in the Toronto movement as elsewhere, while Bonnie Burstow considers the politics of naming in the struggle against psychiatry.

In Part II, "Mad Engagements," Jennifer M. Poole and Jennifer Ward embrace the practice of Mad grief as a means of resisting psychiatric science's colonization of bereavement, and its pathologization of those grievers who transgress or offend; Ji-Eun Lee mines the rich legacy of writings by Canadian psychiatric survivors to chronicle the systemic, symbolic violence they have endured and overcome; Maria Liegghio draws on poignant personal experience to illustrate the power of biogenetic psychiatry to efface the identities and selves of those under its remit; and Erick Fabris reflects on the personal and professional politics of peer support in the contemporary mental health system.

Part III is entitled "Critiques of Psychiatry: Practice and Pedagogy." The four chapters compiled in this section include reflections by Irit Shimrat on the toxic sham that is the "community mental health" paradigm, and by Don Weitz on electroshock as an expression of systemic psychiatric violence. Accompanying these two critiques by long-standing members of the Canadian survivor community, David Reville and Kathryn Church tell the inspiring story of Mad education at Ryerson University.

Part IV, "Law, Public Policy, and Media Madness,"[11] includes offerings by Lucy Costa on law as a potential resource and forum for Mad activism; by Gordon Warme on the dominance of the "mental illness" paradigm and its implications for psychiatric power and human rights; by Lilith "Chava" Finkler on contesting restrictive zoning and the exclusion of psychiatric survivors from urban spaces; by Kimberley White and Ryan Pike on the contradictions of "mental health literacy" as a system initiative; and by Rob Wipond on contesting conventional wisdoms about "mental illness," and bringing critical psychiatric survivor perspectives into public view through engagement with mainstream media.

Part V, "Social Justice, Madness, and Identity Politics," concludes the book with five chapters that map the convergences and fault lines between Mad identity and political activism. Rachel Gorman offers a cautionary treatise on the praxis of Mad nationhood—on the imperative that Mad citizens pursue a critical politics in solidarity with survivors of racism, colonialism, patriarchy, ableism, and related forms of material and cultural oppression. Louise Tam proposes a paradigm shift in thinking about relations amongst racism, colonialism, and psychiatry—one that seeks to expose the raced material foundations of psychiatric power. Andrea Daley explores the charged politics of navigating queer identity within and across the psychiatrized spaces of body, intersubjective consciousness, and organizational structure. Jijian Voronka shows how Ontario's 2008 *Review of the Roots of Youth Violence* promotes a psy-centred agenda for understanding and repairing the "individual" troubles of risky, racialized, inner-city slum youth. Lastly, Marina Morrow ponders the promises and perils of "recovery" as an "alternative" paradigm of mental health practice within the shadow of contemporary neoliberalism and biogenetic psychiatry.

Continuations

Read together, the essays showcased in this book chart the many pathways through which sanism enters modern culture, along with the multiple forms of exclusion, discrimination, and human rights abuse inflicted on those of us deemed to violate reigning standards of normality and reason. Writing across a broad spectrum of topics and perspectives, the authors document the exceptional powers that biogenetic psychiatry has arrogated to itself in this 21st century—often with the open consent, if not at the very behest, of political authorities, lawmakers, opinion leaders, "stakeholder" organizations, the corporate sector, the mainstream media, and the public. As we will witness throughout the pages of this book, these powers constitute a litany of prerogatives and presumptions—among them, the right to constitute and judge mentalities; to distinguish authoritatively between "sanity" and "disorder"; to characterize the latter as an "illness" like any other; to manufacture words and systems for labelling, cataloguing, and containing Mad conduct and people; to impart discipline in the name of science; to intervene, often without consent, into the lives of others; to unleash an arsenal of chemical, electrical, and other bodily interventions under the guise of compassion and cure; and, perhaps most formidable of all, to influence the very languages, thoughtways, and social practices by which we collectively determine what it means to be "normal," worthy, and even human.

Yet at its core, this book is not just a story of biomedical psychiatry and its ever-advancing encroachment into the lives of Canadians. Navigating a remarkably wide landscape of institutional sites and human experiences, the authors are far more concerned with matters of critical engagement—with marking the cracks and boundaries of the psycho-pharmaceutical empire; with building on the legacies of mental patient liberation, Mad pride, antipsychiatry, and the c/s/x movement; with fashioning subversive vocabularies, co-operative alliances, and political strategies for the 21st century that promote individual recovery, collective resistance, and social transformation; and with finding means of speaking and writing the facts of human diversity, in all its forms, in ways that contest the biogenetic paradigm of "mental illness" and celebrate our right to be different.

In this basic sense, Mad Studies is simultaneously a continuation of the antipsychiatry project of activist organizing and dissent, a venture in the politics of Mad identity and survivor nationhood, and an exercise in Freirean conscientization directed towards all those whose lives collide with the powers of psychiatry (that is, in one way or another, well-near everyone). As several of the chapters below attest (see Diamond, Burstow, Fabris, and Gorman, Chapters 4, 5, 9, and 19), the creative tensions that exist between these different currents of the field open up exciting possibilities for mutual teaching, empowerment, partnership, and support. They also admittedly raise complications, and occasional disagreements, about how best to mobilize for change, while both searching for unity of identity and purpose, and embracing difference.

Yet while some may possibly demur, we see no irreconcilable conflicts of purpose among these intersecting objectives and pursuits. To the contrary, the Mad movement is necessarily a poly-sited venture, and the struggle for human rights in "mental health" arrays itself organically across multiple fronts, forms, and levels of involvement. As can be learned from other social movements aligned against capitalism, patriarchy, racism, colonialism, ableism, ageism, adultism, heteronormativity, and environmental desecration, there is no single script for subverting power and doing justice. Nor, as noted above, is there any unitary vision of what a post-sanist society might even look like. While the spirit of revolution is an intrinsic element of every collective struggle, so too is an embrace of immediate challenges, an engagement with the local and short term, a willingness to accept and leverage contradiction, a passion for coalition-building, and a commitment to work with and through pre-existing institutions such as law, education, and the media (see Reville, Church, Costa, and Wipond, Chapters 12, 13, 14, and 18)—and perhaps even the psy sciences themselves. To the extent that a discipline of Mad Studies can embody this kind of heterodox vision, positioning itself loosely between and around the multiple ideas, voices, and practices of Mad movement, survivor politics, and antipsychiatry activism (Diamond, Chapter 4), its place as a forum of communicative action, and a force for critical teaching and learning, is assured for many years to come.

Ultimately, as the title of this book implies, our project is grounded in the paradigm-shifting awareness that Mad Studies is about far more than the Byzantine world of psychiatry and its allied disciplines. The stakes are higher still, for to study madness is to probe the very foundations of our claims to being human. For this reason alone—and there are many more—"Mad" matters to us all.

Notes

1   This wording is adapted from the opening sentence of the introduction to Titchkosky & Michalko (2009).
2   Having originated in the 1850s as the International List of Causes of Death, the International Classification of Diseases now falls under the auspices of the World Health Organization (WHO). Its most recent iteration, ICD-10, has held sway since 1994. See www.who.int/classifications/icd/en/.
3   This is not to suggest that there are not children who experience serious forms of distress that are debilitating and painful to them. Instead, this is to stress the proliferation of diagnoses given to children who are not experiencing distress from their perspective but may be experienced as distressing to the adults that are around them. These same distressing (to adults) behaviours of children were tolerated, and seen as within the range of "normal" childhood behaviours, in earlier generations.
4   These include the same drugs given to psychiatrized adults, such as selective serotonin reuptake inhibitors (SSRIs), neuroleptics, anti-anxiety drugs, and tranquilizers.
5   An example of such a Canadian organization is the National Youth in Care Network or Youth in Care Canada. See www.youthincare.ca.
6   As such, as editors of this reader, we must acknowledge the absence of the direct involvement of psychiatrized children in this book as an unacceptable exclusion. However, the lack of involvement of children within the psychiatric survivor and Mad movements in Canada (and elsewhere)—an exclusion that the adults in our communities must take responsibility for and understand as stemming from adultism—and our own lack of access to psychiatrized children at the time of organizing and writing this text, have inevitably led to this regrettable exclusion.
7   For details on these international events, see www.sfu.ca/madcitizenship-conference/ (Madness, Citizenship and Social Justice, Simon Fraser University, 2008); http://individual.utoronto.ca/

psychout/ (PsychOUT 2010, Ontario Institute for Studies in Education, University of Toronto); www.theopalproject.org/psychout.html (PsychOUT 2011, City University of New York); www.inter-disciplinary.net/probing-the-boundaries/making-sense-of/madness/project-archives/4t/ (Madness: Probing the Boundaries, Mansfield College (Oxford), 2011); www.asylumonline.net/ (Asylum! Conference, Manchester Metropolitan University, 2011). Retrieved January 26, 2012.

8   On the English-language etymology of the terms "mad" and "madness," among other sources see www.etymonline.com/index.php?term=mad.

9   "Consumer/survivor/ex-patient." See above, in addition to (among other sources) Diamond, Chapter 4, and Burstow, Chapter 5.

10   In her book, *The Madness of Women* (2011), Jane Ussher proposes the material-discursive-intrapsychic model as a critical realist approach to the study of (women's) madness. For Ussher, MDI "moves beyond the mind-body divide or realism-constructionism divide, and avoids the unnecessary distinction between subjective and objective, or mental and physical aspects of experience" (p. 106).

11   Our reference to "media madness" is beholden to Otto Wahl's (1995) book of that title.

PART I

Mad People's History, Evolving Culture, and Language

The chapters assembled in Part I provide a point of departure for the book by chronicling both the historical and contemporary contexts of Canadian Mad Studies. These five essays address the making, telling, and celebration of Mad people's history, culture, and language through the pursuit of grassroots activism, the writing and recovery of psychiatric survivor narratives, the conduct of memory work in collaboration between historians and survivors, the practice of language politics within the struggle for social justice and survivor citizenship, and the building of critical communities in defence of human rights and against sanism.

Mel Starkman's 1981 analysis of the history of groups organized by and for "the 'mad,' the oppressed, the ex-inmates of society's asylums" (Chapter 1) was the first publication in Canada to historically analyze any aspect of this topic from the perspectives of Mad people. As such, Starkman's work is of immense importance for its originality in anticipating, long before anyone else in Canada, later histories on this theme. On this basis, we have chosen this one previously published article out of the entire collection to be republished here. This chapter forms a unique perspective from a particularly vibrant "moment" in "The Movement" when the burgeoning number of groups reflected widespread activist optimism in promoting alternatives to the psychiatric system by people like Starkman and the radical magazine *Phoenix Rising* (1980–1990) in which his article was first published. Placing Mad activism within the context of wider social movements of the time, Starkman outlines the development of what was then called the "mental patients' liberation movement" in Western Europe and North America, whilst also noting the influence of radical professionals and tensions between them and ex-inmate activists that was ongoing at the time. He then examines activist groups in several American cities and annual North American conferences concluding with reference to a forthcoming 1982 event that was about to be held in Toronto as potentially helping to build a "truly international movement."

In their essay on "Women in 19th-Century Asylums" (Chapter 2), Nérée St-Amand and Eugène LeBlanc place the life and social activism of Mary Huestis Pengilly from Saint John, New Brunswick, in the context of the social strictures and patriarchal oppression towards females deemed mad during this time period. They foreground their discussion of Pengilly's account with a discussion of the gendered experiences of Elizabeth Packard in the United States who was confined for three years in the 1860s, and Hersilie Rouy who was confined for 14 years in France beginning in the 1850s. The six months during which Pengilly was confined in 1883–1884 in Saint John are brought to life through her published diary written at this time and which she subsequently published upon release. As such, her first-person account, along with those of Packard and Rouy, reveals the abuses that women inmates endured and how this led to activism afterwards by two of the three ex-inmates. Like the more well-known Elizabeth Packard, Mary Huestis Pengilly sought to influence government officials and the wider public to improve the situation of women asylum inmates who remained confined. The chapter by St-Amand and LeBlanc thus helps to bring to a wider audience in the early 21st century the work of a woman whom they describe as a "New Brunswick hero" from the late 19th century.

Lanny Beckman and Megan J. Davies (Chapter 3) give a voice to remembrance in their collaborative project of collecting an oral history of the Mental Patients Association (MPA). Formed in Vancouver in the early 1970s and founded by the iconic Lanny Beckman, the MPA was a radical political network that provided alternative services in the form of peer support. This was the first such group of psychiatric survivors in Canada, and the first formal group of its kind in the world, that provided "work, homes and a sense of belonging and empowerment to ex-patients" and insisted "on the merits of peer support," the "use of participatory democracy for organizational decision-making," and "paid jobs ... decided in open elections." Through a narrative dialogue, Beckman and Davies walk the reader through the process of creating a documentary about the history of the MPA. This includes a discussion of the MPA's radical political understanding of psychiatry including the "ways in which mental health is connected to discrimination, marginalization, and proximity to poverty" and an analysis of "issues of gender, sex, professionalism, health, poverty, class, and powerlessness," all having been derived from the lived experiences of those members who had been hospitalized and had experienced discrimination and stigma first-hand. This documentary, and the chapter that discusses its making, provide us with an important foundational history of the psychiatric survivor movement in Canada.

Shaindl Diamond's Chapter 4, on what constitutes a community among activists who work from a perspective that is critical of psychiatry and practices anti-sanist politics, is based on her ethnographic doctoral study in Toronto. Through first-person interviews, she identifies this community as belonging to the "psychiatric survivor constituency"—"the heart of the political community" or "the Mad constituency" with a focus on "positive understandings of Mad identity and experience" and "the antipsychiatry constituency"—that seeks the abolition of psychiatry. Diamond writes that there are people who choose not to be a part of any of these groups but who are also interested in critiquing psychiatric power in their lives. Her chapter brings particularly important attention to the reasons why most racialized people are not involved in the above constituencies and choose instead to resist psychiatric interventions from within other communities, such as amongst racialized women, who are more understanding of racist and patriarchal experiences. In her interviews, a number of Diamond's participants critique the tendency to reduce a particular constituency to a specific identity, such as "Mad," and thus isolate this experience from wider interrelated forms of oppression with which it needs to be connected. Her chapter concludes with ideas about ways in which different communities might work together to address barriers between personal and political engagement so as to transform society collectively.

Bonnie Burstow's "A Rose by Any Other Name: Naming and the Battle against Psychiatry" (Chapter 5) is a contemplation of the power of words to both perpetuate psychiatric power and contest it. Inspired by the intersecting currents of feminism, antipsychiatry, popular education, and community activism, Burstow advances an analysis that both invokes Dorothy Smith's work on "regimes of ruling" (1987, 2005) and is reminiscent of Gramscian theories of language, power, ideology, and praxis. For Burstow, language about psychiatry and madness is a central terrain of struggle. Psychiatry is a hegemonic practice whose talk and texts have colonized not only "scientific" discourse, but also the commonplace language of everyday life—and even, alarmingly, the ways that resistance movements and critical communities conceive and speak about mental and spiritual diversity. Within the shadow of neoliberalism— and the seductively libertarian ethic of individualism and consumerism that it has unleashed—the so-called "mentally ill" have been turned into "users" and "consumers" in the public imagination, while "[p]sychiatry emerges as a benign merchant, doing nothing more than extending choices to a population once denied choice." By the same token, as the contents of this book collectively bear out, this "language of the ruling regime" has scarcely gone uncontested. Through the past generation, what Burstow refers to as "semantic resistance" has also flourished. The words and texts of resistance are to be found both in the oppositional politics and "refusal" language of the antipsychiatry movement, and in the celebratory identity politics and "reclaimed" discourses/vocabularies of the Mad (pride) movement. While acknowledging the critical role and many accomplishments of both these movements in speaking truth to psychiatry and advancing human rights, Burstow also admonishes activists and scholars to beware the dangers of effacing one language of resistance with another—and to be ever-vigilant against the infiltration of psy language into critical discourse, against the bowdlerizing of resistance language through hybrid terms like "consumer/survivor," and against, conversely, the false partitioning of people in struggle by conjunctively naming them "consumers *and* survivors." In the final analysis, for Burstow, the stakes of these struggles in the politics of naming could not be higher. "Progressively," she asserts, "psychiatry is pathologizing normative everyday life, and as such, *everyone* is in jeopardy."

CHAPTER 1

The Movement[1]

Mel Starkman

Editor's Note: Mel Starkman was the first person in Canada to advocate for the creation of an archive on Mad movement history in the early 1980s. Not long after this article was published, he was confined in Queen Street Mental Health Centre, Toronto, where he was an in-patient and outpatient for 13 years from 1982 to 1995. During this time, the Public Guardian and Trustee discarded Mel's personal archive of primary source material, which he had collected on the history of the early Mad movement in Toronto. In 2001, Mel Starkman co-founded the Psychiatric Survivor Archives, Toronto, an organization with which he continues to work a decade later.

An important new movement is sweeping through the Western world. The "mad," the oppressed, the ex-inmates of society's asylums are coming together and speaking for themselves. The map of the world is dotted with newly formed groups, struggling to identify themselves, define their struggle, and decide whether the "system" is reformable or whether they need to create an alternative community.

The great majority of groups in the mental patients' liberation movement (or psychiatric inmates' liberation movement) use self-help tactics, educating themselves and a fearful public in the tactics of confrontation and co-operation, and learning what is possible and what is not. So far, there has been only minimal coordination among groups, but in spite of this, different groups in different cultures have arrived at a virtual identity of purpose.

The roots of the problem faced by psychiatric inmates can be traced back to the 15th century, and the death of the Age of Faith, replaced by the Age of Reason. Until that time, "madness" was seen as an inexplicable, divine visitation, to be tolerated, pitied, and sometimes even honoured. But with the growth of reason, it needed to be *explained*—and could not be. Madness and the madman stubbornly refused to yield to reason and to science; 500 years later, they still have not yielded, and the efforts of our society to label, categorize, and "treat" fruitlessly continue. Psychiatric inmates are victims, not of their "madness," but of these (no doubt well-intentioned) efforts to pigeonhole them and solve their problems in a "scientific" way.

The mental patients' liberation movement can trace its beginnings to several sources. Much of its emphasis on consciousness-raising derives from the feminist movement, particularly from that movement's realization of the folly of medical treatment for so-called "neurotic" symptoms. For example, in Canada in the 1890s, a Dr. R.M. Bucke, Medical Superintendent of London Psychiatric Hospital, performed gynaecological operations to relieve "hysterical" symptoms in women. He saw a close connection between gynaecological deformities and psychiatric conditions, and he was far from alone in this belief. (Consider the meaning of "hysterical"—it derives from *hysteron,* the Greek word for "uterus.") In the 1960s, women began to reject such treatment, seeing it as harmful, oppressive, and sexist.

A second source was the movement among radical professionals in the early seventies, inspired by R.D. Laing among others. These professionals tried to interpret schizophrenia as an altered mode of consciousness rather than as a pathological condition. They developed critiques of society—Marxist, existentialist, and so on—that de-medicalized "mental illness." However, they still tended to invalidate the inmate experience, and approach the problem in ideological terms.

The gay liberation movement also had its impact. For a long time, homosexuality had been considered to be a psychiatric illness, and the rebellion of gays against that definition did much to force people with other psychiatric labels to question the validity of the terms applied to them.

The idea of self-help, as practised in other settings, was a further stimulus. Until the middle of the 19th century, self-help was a common way of life. Individuals, small groups, and entire communities looked to their own resources, and constructed lifestyles to match those resources. (Even today, communities such as the Mennonites practise self-help in the old way.) But around 1850, a culture of professionalism developed. Teachers, lawyers, and doctors began to be seen as experts; they developed mystifying languages that the average person could not understand. They became leaders of society, deferred to by everyone, and answerable only to each other. Their claims to "science" were not questioned by a population who did not know what they were talking about.

Since the clients could not understand what the professionals were doing, they were thrown back on faith; they still are. For example, a 1979 position paper of the Canadian Psychiatric Association states:

> The essence and very existence of the healing professions depends on the element of trust in the relationship between the person (hereinafter referred to as "patient") requiring treatment and the professional consulted. (Canadian Psychiatric Association, 1979, p. 78)

The faith, however, works only in one direction; professionals routinely ignore the perceptions of their clients. For example, consider the studies of psychologist Larry Squire on ECT. *Virtually every subject* reported memory loss; Dr. Squire states, nonetheless, that memory loss does not occur. Or consider psychiatrist Vivian Rakoff's review of *Blue Jolts* (a compelling collection of inmate experiences, also reviewed in *Phoenix Rising*, vol. 2, no. 1):

> We require more sobering examination of our errors and at this stage some-
> thing more helpful is needed in our approach to the sick than the notion that
> "sanity is a trick of agreement." The book's only effect may be to alarm some
> people who could benefit from our imperfect services. (Rakoff, 1979, p. 494)[2]

Attitudes such as Dr. Rakoff's explain why the Ninth Annual International Conference on Human Rights and Psychiatric Oppression expressed itself as it did in its press release:

> We demand ... an end to a way of thinking which calls our anger "psychosis,"
> our joy "mania," our fear "paranoia," and our grief "depression." (1981, p. 3A)

In other fields, people began to take power back from the professionals. Credit unions, run by members, took control of money away from bankers. Tenants' associations sprang up, as did organizations of people on public assistance, and of other groups persuaded that the "professionals" did not always know what was best. Vietnam protesters took war out of the hands of professional soldiers. Anti-nuclear protesters stated loudly that the scientists were not always right. And this philosophy affected the infant psychiatric inmates' liberation movement; in fact, many of its founders came from these other groups.

The last source was the mental hygiene movement, started in North America in the 1930s by Clifford Beers. The movement took upon itself the task of speaking for "patients," but eventually became an institutionalized structure, trying to educate people to adjust to our society. Beers, himself considered to be "manic depressive," refused to work with self-help pioneers, possibly, according to his biographer, because he wanted to maintain his own position as the "advocate of the insane" (Dain, 1980, p. 304).

Beginnings

The radical therapists made their move at the beginning of the seventies. Their perspective is illustrated by a quotation from a 1973 issue of *Rough Times* (originally titled *Radical Therapist*):

> Psychological oppression is a pervasive aspect of modern capitalism. The
> choices of bourgeois existence are madness, total apathy and conformity.
> (*Rough Times*, 1973, p. vii)

At about this time, interaction began between the radical therapists and ex-inmates. Active collaboration lasted until the mid-seventies, when the ex-inmates came to feel that their own experience was being invalidated by these therapists as much as by the more conservative professionals. The uneasy marriage fell apart. Its demise was hastened by the new fad of middle-class people seeing psychiatrists for "life enhancement" and "personal growth," and by the springing up of trendy therapies such as Erhard Seminars Training—a "new age" psychotherapeutic practice used during the 1970s and 1980s—and primal therapy. At the same time, cult groups such as Scientology, that criticized psychiatry in the hope of supplanting it with their own quasi-religion, were causing ex-inmates to wonder if perhaps their so-called enemies—the psychiatrists—were less harmful than their so-called friends.

One of the earliest spokespersons for the mental patients' liberation movement, and still an activist in that movement, was Judi Chamberlin. Her book, *On Our Own: Patient-Controlled Alternatives to the Mental Health System* (1978), is based on her own experience. In her introduction she sums up the concerns of the movement:

> For too long, mental patients have been faceless, voiceless people. We have been thought of, at worst, as subhuman monsters, or, at best, as pathetic cripples,[3] who might be able to hold down menial jobs and eke out meager existences, given constant professional support. Not only have others thought of us in this stereotyped way, we have believed it of ourselves. It is only in this decade, with the emergence and growth of the mental patients' liberation movement, that we ex-patients have begun to shake off this distorted image and to see ourselves for what we are—a diverse group of people, with strengths and weaknesses, abilities and needs, and ideas of our own. Our ideas about our "care," and "treatment" at the hands of psychiatry, about the nature of "mental illness," and about new and better ways to deal with (and truly to help) people undergoing emotional crises differ drastically from those of mental health professionals. (Chamberlin, 1978, p. xi)

Europe

The mental patients' liberation movement sprang up at roughly the same time in Europe and North America. One of the earlier European groups was a Dutch group, Clientenbond in de Weizijnzorg. Clientenbond is now providing alternative options of care (not "treatment") and adjustment to society, and advocating strongly on behalf of inmates and ex-inmates. Their areas of effort are wide, and have created something close to an alternative community within a society they see as unredeemable. As well as providing direct services of a support and educational nature, Clientenbond is applying grassroots pressure to the whole society, trying to change policies and attitudes. In particular, they are trying to change traditional attitudes and opinions held by psychiatrists, psychologists and social workers—attitudes which Clientenbond members believe impede the course of treatment for many members. (Hepburn & Deman, 1980, p. 17)

Clientenbond is only one example of a thriving European movement, which includes groups in England, France, Italy, Belgium, West Germany, Great Britain, and other countries. The British groups are loosely organized in the Federation of Mental Patients Unions, which is organized mainly around the issue of inmates' rights. The entire continent is involved in the European Network for Alternatives to Psychiatry, founded in Brussels in 1974. The network functions primarily as an information exchange, and involves ex-inmates, radical professionals, and lawyers working in the field.

North America
Clientenbond and other European organizations tend to be national in nature. In Canada and the United States, probably because of the much greater size of the countries, regional activity is more common; groups tend to exist on a local, state, or provincial basis. As well, North America has developed, along with organized groups, individual charismatic personalities operating on their own with a small group of devoted followers. The effectiveness of these individuals (such as Toronto's Pat Capponi) is mixed; they are very effective at commanding media attention, but often represent a highly individualized perspective rather than a democratically arrived at collective viewpoint.

In Canada, and to some extent in the United States, the mental patients' liberation movement has developed ties with other self-help groups (such as Toronto's BOOST—Blind Organization of Ontario with Self-Help Tactics—or Boston's Disabled People's Liberation Front). These organizations share a common goal: to demonstrate that existing power structures must adjust to the realities of "consumers'" rights to make decisions about programs and structures that directly affect their lives. The strength of such coalitions has been dramatically demonstrated; for example, the Ontario Coalition on Human Rights for the Handicapped has profoundly affected the scope of human rights legislation in Ontario through the co-operation of the mentally, physically, and emotionally handicapped.

The mental patients' liberation movement in North America has passed through a number of phases. The first was that of working with radical therapists, who were virtually the only people providing a perspective different than that advanced by the main body of psychiatrists.

However, as already mentioned, this was an uneasy alliance, and many inmates and former inmates moved on to the second phase—withdrawal into self-directed groups. They practised self-education and total democracy in an effort to avoid the kind of hierarchy of power that they had experienced as inmates. There was an almost total lack of structure, and an emphasis on collective decision-making and action. Priorities at this stage were consciousness-raising and politicization. At the same time, many groups were attempting to provide the kind of support to people that was lacking within the psychiatric system. Experiments were launched in alternative housing, alternative crisis assistance, and alternative social support. Houses were rented, storefronts were opened, and rights issues were addressed.

Much of the North American movement is still—through necessity or choice—in this second stage. The third phase began when some groups began to attract substantial funding. The groups getting grants went, in some respects, in different directions from the grantless. Total democracy and lack of structure came up against the hard reality of managing sizeable amounts of money. Funded groups were, on the one hand, in a better position to address such concerns as housing and employment and, on the other hand, less inclined to be purely political in nature, and to make a priority of radical protest against the psychiatric establishment.

Consequently, certain issues arose within the movement. Was it possible to collaborate in some efforts with professionals and established voluntary agencies, or would the movement of necessity continue to be isolated and totally anti-professional? These questions have not yet received a decisive answer.

As an illustration of the development of the mental patients' liberation movement, it may be helpful to look at the development of movement groups in several North American cities.

New York

In 1948, a group of people in New York started WANA (We Are Not Alone). It was formed by inmates of Rockland State Hospital. Volunteers in the community found the group a place to meet, but in the process "transformed the group from a self-help project to a new kind of psychiatric facility" (Jordan Hess, in Chamberlin, 1978, p. 87). Professionals were hired, and by the early 1950s "most of the original founding group of ex-patients quit in disgust" (ibid.). WANA became Fountain House. One of WANA's members commented on the change:

> There was a feeling of solidarity and companionship in WANA that deterio-
> rated when the professionals got involved. For a while, the ex-patients con-
> tinued to run the club. We raised our own money (by holding bazaars, for
> example), and we voted in new members. But eventually the administrators
> decided to take that power away from us. Instead of the members deciding
> who could join, when new people came in they were interviewed by the staff,
> who decided if they were "suitable cases." WANA was unique because patients
> ran it—that was abolished when it became Fountain House. (ibid., p. 78)

Soon afterwards, a group of New York ex-inmates formed the Mental Patients' Liberation Project (MPLP). A storefront was opened on West 4th Street, "a really funky neighbourhood" (Markman, 1981). By the mid-seventies the storefront had disappeared. However, before MPLP died it issued a Manifesto of Mental Patients' Rights, one of the first in existence. Another, more radical, group also formed, calling itself the Mental Patients' Political Action Committee. This group attended a conference on lobotomy, and also disrupted an orthopsychiatric conference.

When Project Release appeared on the scene, it was an example of what Judi Chamberlin calls the separatist model—a real rather than a false alternative to the discredited "mental health" system—run totally by ex-psychiatric inmates. Project Release sees itself not as providing services, but rather as a supportive community.

> It is an important distinction, because the concept of a service implies the existence of two roles, the server and the served. No matter how much a group may attempt to break down such roles, some residue of them always remains when a group is delivering "services." The concept of community, on the other hand, implies interaction.... The separatist model is by far the most radical of alternative services, but it is also the model that promotes the greatest degree of ex-patient confidence and competence. (Chamberlin, 1978, p. 95)

Project Release was formed around the issue of single-room occupancy hotels in Manhattan's Upper West Side. Many ex-inmates and others on welfare were housed "in totally inadequate and unsafe conditions" (ibid.). At first, Project Release got office space from a tenants' organizing committee; later it got a room in a neighbourhood Universalist church. Its activities spread to publishing *A Consumer's Guide to Psychiatric Medication* and working on a patients' rights manual.

In late 1976, Project Release obtained a $10,000 foundation grant, with which they rented an apartment and opened a community centre. The centre is busy from late in the morning until late in the evening, seven days a week, with a communal meal in the evening. No one is designated as "staff." Passive participation is discouraged, and each member is required to serve on one or more of the committees responsible for activity areas. As Project Release's statement of purpose says:

> Professional supervision creates a dependency pattern which is a cause of recidivism. In the informal programs of Project Release, members seek to extend acceptance and cooperation, letting each individual set his/her own pace in tasks and responsibilities. Project Release feels that this form of self-help is a strong antidote to the anxiety of isolation and helplessness induced by society and psychiatry. (Chamberlin, 1978, p. 96)

Project Release avoids structuring as much as possible, "preferring occasional confusion to impersonal efficiency" (ibid., p. 97). Staff/client relationships are nonexistent. No one receives a salary. Rather, the concept is one of community, of people caring about people and helping each other.

Today Project Release has a mailing list of over 2,000, and all the social service agencies in New York call on the group for representation on "mental health" questions.

Kansas

The Kansas City story really begins in New Haven, Connecticut. In 1968, Sue Budd had helped start a social club on a psychiatric ward. The club was very antipsychiatry in tone. There was some help from professionals at first, but basically Sue ran the club. Sue's husband, Dennis, tells it this way:

> [The social club] was loosely supervised by a social worker, who saw Sue and me every week. And Sue ran the club. It was most successful. It had a membership of ten to twelve. We shunned the help from the mental health association that was offered to us. A lot of people who were sent to our club were dismissed as hopeless by the staff. A lot of them improved while they were with us.
>
> Then Sue's boss moved to Kansas City and we decided to move with her. After she left, the Connecticut Mental Health Association laid down some rules and regulations for structuring such social clubs. Among these rules and regulations was a stipulation that no current or former mental patient should be a director of the club, because it was a hindrance to their returning to normal society. Sue attempted from long distance to fight this, but there was no way, and the club was too weak and it died. Sue was in a rage, a total rage, over this, and that was what provoked her to get politically involved. (Budd, 1981)

Meanwhile, in 1972, a group of students and faculty at Kansas University's School of Social Work formed the Kansas Council for Institutional Reform, in response to the commitment of a white student by her mother because she had been dating a black man. She was released after an organized legal effort. The council started a monitoring process, and produced a model commitment law that was introduced into the legislature in the spring of 1973.

Sue and Dennis started a Kansas chapter of a group that had been active in Connecticut—the Medical Committee for Human Rights. It produced a Mental Health Task Force, which lasted two years. The task force became involved with a group of ex-inmate nursing and boarding home residents, and undertook what was called a Resocialization Project. Although the project was formed to resocialize the residents, it ended up empowering them by raising their consciousness of their oppression.

One of the residents was informed that the operator of one of the homes had been confiscating residents' support cheques. Protesters and reporters from the local TV station sneaked into the home and exposed the conditions; the house was shut down as a consequence. But shortly afterwards funding for the Resocialization Project was cut off. Ironically, Dennis says, this happened one day after the project had been nominated for an award by the director of the local community mental health centre.

These events caused a fight between the radical professionals and the ex-inmates in the Medical Committee for Human Rights. The radical professionals won, and a number of the ex-inmates split away from the committee. These ex-inmates were approached by the university group, the Kansas Council for Institutional Reform, and joined forces with them; the name was later changed to Advocates for Freedom in Mental Health.

California

Events in California began with the founding of *Madness Network News*, which began as a newsletter and developed into the main publication of the movement in the United States. Some of the staff founded NAPA (Network Against Psychiatric Assault) as a political arm of the paper, and gradually the two groups became separate.

The first meeting of NAPA in 1974 was attended by more than 250 people, in spite of a city-wide bus strike. It got underway with a vengeance. Several committees were struck and went into action, including a Drug Action Committee, which in less than a month was confronting the American Orthopsychiatric Association. Immediately afterwards, NAPA held a public forum to present an antipsychiatry play. The Legal Action Committee began working with a senator and an assemblyman to introduce legal amendments providing for the right to refuse surgery. An anti-shock campaign got underway, along with a wide-ranging variety of seminars. NAPA, through Howie the Harp, organized a Coalition of Social Support Income Recipients.

By 1976, NAPA had also moved into attacking "slave labor" ("Slave labor," 1976, p. 7) in hospitals, and was helping organize courses in alternative perspectives on psychiatry. By 1979, NAPA was part of the Coalition Against Forced Treatment.

At the same time, California filmmaker Richard Cohen produced *Hurry Tomorrow*, a powerful documentary about conditions on a so-called "progressive" psychiatric ward at Norfolk State Hospital.

More recently on the California scene is BACAP (Bay Area Coalition for Alternatives to Psychiatry), bringing together NAPA and other California groups.

Annual Conferences

As groups sprang up around the United States and began to find one another, they looked for ways to get together, share information, and support one another. The result was the First National Conference on Human Rights and Psychiatric Oppression, held in Detroit in 1973. (The name has since been changed twice—first to "North American Conference" and then to "International Conference"—to reflect a widening geographic participation.)

At that first conference, some important things happened. Resistance developed among the ex-inmate participants to the idea of a structure being advanced by professional attendees, and the resulting dynamics produced a very unstructured, free-floating conference; the pattern has largely held ever since. There were no plans made to hold a second conference, but during the intervening year a Kansas group (Advocates for Freedom in Mental Health) and a New York group (Mental Patients' Liberation Project) decided to organize one in Topeka, which advertised itself as "Psychiatric Capital of the World."

The Topeka Conference began the tradition of organizing a demonstration as part of each conference, as well as continuing the idea of lack of preplanned structure. Movement veterans tend to remember Topeka as a high point in the organization of the movement, as a "beautiful" (Budd, 1981) conference.

In 1975, the conference moved to San Francisco and a much more structured format. Reactions were so strong that the conference formulated an exclusionary rule to keep out professionals, who had been largely responsible for the structuring.

The 1976 Boston Conference was therefore totally unattended by professionals. This was the conference that produced the movement's first and only position paper— the first unified statement by the American movement as a whole, which emphatically condemned commitment and forced treatment. The conference also decided to relax the exclusionary rule, allowing professionals to attend the second half of the next conference.

Consequently the 1977 conference, in Los Angeles, was split into two with ex-inmates only for the first half and professionals included in the second half. Again the experience was considered unsatisfactory, and the rule was altered to once again exclude professionals, unless they were sponsored by a legitimate antipsychiatry group. The rule has been basically unchanged since then.

The 1978 conference in Philadelphia, 1979 in Florida, 1980 in San Francisco (see *Phoenix Rising*, vol. 1, no. 2), and 1981 in Cleveland have continued to serve as a unifying force, not only to the North American movement, but to groups around the world. The participation of groups outside this continent is still limited, unfortunately, by the cost of crossing the ocean, but at least a little European representation happens, and there are hopes for the future.

Next year [1982], the conference will be held in Toronto, Canada—physically not far from the United States, but symbolically a large step. It heralds even more progress towards a truly international movement.

Notes

1 This chapter was originally published (December 1981) in *Phoenix Rising: The Voice of the Psychiatrized*, 2(3), 2A-9A, and is adapted here with the author's permission. This chapter does not follow the capitalization of "Mad" used throughout the rest of the book, and instead retains the style used in its original 1978 printing.

2 At the time of writing, Dr. Rakoff was chairman of the Department of Psychiatry, director and psychiatrist-in-chief of the Clarke Institute in Toronto.

3 Editor's note: The term "cripple," as used here is considered offensive by people with disabilities and allies, and thus is generally not used in this way any longer among Mad activists. For a discussion of terminology, see Simi Linton, *Claiming Disability: Knowledge and Identity* (New York University Press, 1998), Chapter 2.

Women in 19th-Century Asylums:
Three Exemplary Women; A New Brunswick Hero

Nérée St-Amand and Eugène LeBlanc

The 19th century constitutes an important period in the history of psychiatric institutions, particularly in the Western world. The notion that an individual suffering from a mental disorder should be removed from his or her home and community to be placed in confinement was commonplace, in Canada and elsewhere. The population was led to believe that recovery could only happen once this individual was placed in a controlled environment, meaning, of course, a psychiatric institution (Warsh, 1989, p. 10). "No insane man recovers at home," wrote Dr. Waddell, Superintendent of the New Brunswick asylum from 1849 to 1875 (LeBlanc & St-Amand, 2008, p. 16). In such a context of institutional "care," women were especially likely to be committed, as insanity and hysteria were thought to be characteristic of feminine lives (Mitchinson, 1991, p. 280).

The purpose of this text is to focus on three women's written experiences with 19th-century psychiatry. This chapter will begin with an overview of the state of psychiatry, with a special focus on the realities of women within the asylums. We will then describe the experiences of two women who challenged these harsh realities in the United States and in France. Then we will focus on the journal that Mary Huestis Pengilly wrote during her six-month commitment to Canada's first asylum, in Saint John, New Brunswick. The analysis of her writings and of her subsequent activist role in Eastern Canada will illustrate her persistent attempts to change the system, both from within the institution and throughout the rest of her life. Based on these three women's personal experiences and the way they challenged male-dominated psychiatry, we will be able to appreciate the politics of madness in a context of industrialization (St-Amand, 1988). We conclude that they were true activists espousing humanitarian values and that they were precursors of the feminist movement, defending voiceless psychiatrized people and, in particular, of the more widely diffuse Mad movement of today. Their historical examples serve as an important reminder that today's Mad activism did not start in the late 20th century but has harbingers long before contemporary time with, among others, the three women discussed in this chapter.

Psychiatry in the 19th Century

Foucault reminds us that asylums "enabled the growth of a microcosm where all the great massive structures of bourgeois society and its values had their own symbol: the relationship between family and children structured around the theme of paternal authority; the relationship between fault and punishment around the theme of immediate justice; and the links between madness and disorder around the theme of social and moral order. It was here that the origins of the doctor's power to cure were to be found" (Foucault, 2006, pp. 507–508).

In the industrial era, asylums were used as instruments of social control for people who violated norms of conduct. Refusal to participate in the workforce was considered a serious enough offence for people to be committed. Promiscuity, disruptive behaviour, or financial irresponsibility were also reasons invoked to lock up people, put them in cages, and other coercive ways of controlling their behaviour (St-Amand, 1988, p. 60). For example, the New York State Lunatic Asylum was the site of the invention of the "Utica crib," generally referred to as the "crazy crib." It was heavily used in the 19th century to confine patients. Based on a French design, it was then modified to incorporate slats that gave it an appearance similar to a child's crib (Camp, 1976).

In such a context, women's deviation from accepted norms was severely repressed and punished. Feminist historians argue that "hysteria was a psychological response to the limitations placed on

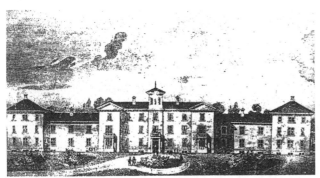

FIGURE 2.1: New Brunswick's Lunatic Asylum

Opened in 1848, the New Brunswick Lunatic Asylum was home to more than 20,000 patients, including Mary Pengilly, before institutional care was decentralized in the province in 1985.

Source: *Dare to Imagine: From Lunatics to Citizens*, 2008.

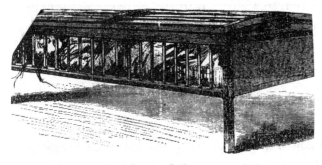

FIGURE 2.2: The Crazy Crib

The "crazy crib" was just one among many forms of physical restraint inflicted upon the inmates of psychiatric institutions like the New Brunswick Lunatic Asylum at the time of Mary Pengilly's confinement.

Source: *Dare to Imagine: From Lunatics to Citizens*, 2008.

women's lives. The family was changing and so was women's place in it. Added to this pressure was the lack of alternative roles for women outside the home. Hysteria in such a context became an option or tactic offering particular women … a chance to redefine or restructure their place within the family" (Mitchinson, 1991, pp. 280–281). Elaine Showalter reports that in 19th-century asylums, women were secluded in locked cells five times as frequently as male patients (1985, p. 81). The conditions in which women found themselves during the 19th century can be illustrated through the recorded experiences of three women—Elizabeth Packard, Hersilie Rouy, and Mary Huestis Pengilly—who were hospitalized against their will, abused, and eventually released. They left us with testimonies of their ordeals.

The Case of Elizabeth Packard (1816–1897)

> *I should not hesitate one moment which to choose, between a confinement in an insane asylum, as I was, or being burnt at the stake. Death, under the most aggravated forms of torture, would now be instantly chosen by me, rather than life in an insane asylum.*
>
> —Elizabeth Packard (1866, p. 48)

Married to a Presbyterian Calvinist preacher, Elizabeth led a quiet life for many years even though she did not agree with her husband's conservative ideology and beliefs. Eventually, she began to question his opinions on child rearing, family finances, and slavery. In 1851, the state of Illinois, where they lived, opened its first psychiatric hospital. A law was passed that required a public hearing prior to any involuntary commitment, but with one exception: in a husband-wife situation the public hearing was not required. In 1860, Elizabeth's husband judged her to be "slightly insane" and made arrangements for her commitment. She spent three years in the state's asylum, but always refused to consider herself insane (Packard, 1882, p. 74). She wrote numerous notes during her years of confinement and upon her release.

> Yes, I am getting friends, from high and low, rich and poor. I am loved and respected here by all that know me. I am their confident, their counselor, their bosom friend. O, how I love this new circle of friends! There are several patients here, who are no more insane than I am; but are put here, like me, to get rid of them. (Packard, 1866, p. 96)

After some months in the asylum, Elizabeth was transferred from the best ward to the worst, where she had to live with the most distressed women. She stayed there for more than two years, until her discharge. In that unit, her life was very difficult, so much so that she would have preferred death to this kind of confinement:

> Prison life is terrible under any circumstances. To be confined amongst raving maniacs, for years in succession, is horrible in the extreme. For myself, I should not hesitate one moment which to choose, between a confinement in an insane asylum, as I was, or being burnt at the stake.... My life was exposed, both night as well as day. I have been dragged around this ward by the hair of my head; I have received blows that almost killed me. My seat at the table was by the side of Mrs. Y, the most dangerous and violent patient in the whole ward, who almost invariably threatened to kill me every time I went to the table. I have had to dodge the knives and forks and tumblers and chairs which have been hurled in promiscuous profusion about my head, to avoid some fatal blow.... From this 8th ward I was not removed until I was discharged, two years and eight months from the day I was consigned to it. (Packard, 1866, pp. 48, 111)

When considering Packard's comments, above, about being confined among "raving maniacs," the issue of stereotypes and distancing oneself from one's peers within the asylum arises. Concepts of pride for Mad people did not exist in any organized form during the 19th century. Instead, to be labelled "mad" was a form of social death. Packard sought to advocate for Mad people with whom she had feelings of solidarity given her own experiences, even while she did not view herself as Mad. It was clearly crucial to her own sense of legitimacy in the wider world, and undoubtedly with herself, to be seen as different from "raving maniacs." Thus for people like Elizabeth Packard and Mary Pengilly to embrace their mad labels as positive is outside the historical context of the world in which they lived. Furthermore, the coercive environment in which these women found themselves, the *atmosphere of terror* that existed inside these institutions (Cellard & Thifault, 2007, p. 25) lent itself to violence that was not of their making. The great majority of people were not dangerous when admitted into totalitarian institutions (St-Amand, 1988, p. 122). Many became violent, and this institutional violence was recognized, if not encouraged, by the employees. New Brunswick's asylum superintendent clearly acknowledged these abuses in his 1900 *Annual Report*: "The old-time abuses which surround the name asylum with so many associations odious to the public mind arose from barbarously crude conceptions of treatment" (Dr. Georges Hetherington, Superintendent, *Provincial Lunatic Asylum—Annual Report 1900*, p. 15, in LeBlanc & St-Amand, 2008, p. 38).

Packard's children exercised pressure for her release and because of their persistence, she was discharged in 1863. Upon hearing this news, her husband left the house where the couple had resided and took their children and all their possessions, including her personal ones, to another city. Elizabeth had to go through a long court battle in order to gain custody of her children. She also had to prove her sanity; the jury took six minutes to decide in her favour. Here again can be seen the distancing effect of an ex-inmate not wanting to be viewed as mad at a time when such a label had incalculable personal and political consequences for an individual so labelled. There was no Mad pride movement in the 1860s for Packard to turn to for support and the concept itself would have been completely alien to her as she lived at a time when mad equalled bad, including amongst asylum inmates. It is expecting too much of her, and other mad people from this period, to think of themselves as being, what is in the early 21st century called "Mad positive." To be declared sane for Packard was not just a strategy to ensure credibility for her legitimacy as an activist, though this was likely a factor too; it was undoubtedly how she felt about herself. Throughout the rest of her life, she published several books and was responsible for 34 bills protecting women from undue hospitalization and treatment. She was the founder of the Anti-Insane Asylum Society, a precursor to the mental patients' liberation movements. She passed away at age 81 (Wikipedia, 2012).

The Case of Hersilie Rouy (1814–1881)

> How can you destroy the future of a woman and allow her liberty to be assaulted simply because she carries her head high?
>
> —Hersilie Rouy (Appignanesi, 2008, p. 91)

Born in Milan in 1814, Hersilie Rouy was the "illegitimate daughter" of astronomer Henri Rouy with whom she lived in Paris until his death. A gifted pianist, she was committed to the asylum at age 40 because of her half-brother's manipulation: he wanted to become sole inheritor of their father's fortune. She describes her admission process and the way she was diagnosed:

> He (the doctor) saw me only for a minute or two and sentenced me on the strength of doctor Calmeil, who sentenced me on the strength of a doctor who had never seen me at all, who took me away as a favor to somebody else, on the strength of what they had told him. (Appignanesi, 2008, p. 90)

Once inside the asylum, when asked by her doctor to play the piano, she refused. Hersilie was consequently given the diagnosis of "incurable pride." When she protested against her incarceration, her doctor responded: "Your delusion is total, and all the more dangerous and incurable in that you speak just like a person who is fully in possession of her reason" (Appignanesi, 2008, p. 91).

Hersilie's many letters to the Ministry of the Interior convinced the government to launch an inquiry into her commitment. She eventually met the Inspector General of Asylums: "They came to test my thinking, my beliefs, to see if there were grounds for keeping me in perpetuity.... How can you destroy the future of a woman and allow her liberty to be assaulted simply because she carries her head high and has the audacity to want to live from her own talent and her own writing? I have been buried alive" (Appignanesi, 2008, p. 91).

She left first-hand accounts of her experiences, a legacy of a unique insight into the experience of treatment from the patient's perspective (Wilson, 2010). Hersilie Rouy was released after 14 years of undue confinement and then received a lifetime pension to compensate for her unjustified internment. She died in 1881 (Appignanesi, 2008, p. 93).

The Case of Mary Huestis Pengilly (1821–1893)

> *This journal may emphatically be called the book of the poor, as I who write it am poor. Poor in purse, but rich in sympathy for my fellow being, rich in the possession of courage sufficient to tell the truth, when by it a public good is accomplished, even though by it I have endangered my life, and may get the reputation of interfering with a business not my own. Wherever I may meet a sufferer, whether man or woman, rich or poor, I cannot hold my sympathy.*
>
> —Mary Pengilly (1885, pp. 34–35)

When the Great Fire of 1877 destroyed Saint John, New Brunswick, Mary Pengilly went to live in Lowell, Massachusetts (Pengilly, 1885, p. 26). There, she put pen to paper and wrote about the "laws of health." Passionately dedicated to this undertaking, she went through some sort of psycho-spiritual experience. She became so enthused by this manuscript that she ceased to eat for a few days. Her five sons, who still resided in Saint John, became apprehensive. One of them, a pharmacist, arranged for her to be committed to the Provincial Lunatic Asylum in Saint John, New Brunswick (Cusack, 2006, p. 4). Mary was 62 years of age. The year was 1883.

During her six-month incarceration, Mary kept a secret diary that described the abuses and disrespect she witnessed (LeBlanc, 2006, p. 1). "They will not allow me to go home, and I must write these things down for fear I forget. It will help pass the time away. It is very hard to endure this prison life, and know that my sons think me insane when I am not." She noted that, "If I were committed to the penitentiary for a crime I would not be used any worse than this" (Pengilly, 1885, p. 28). Mary and the other patients/inmates were locked in their rooms at night. She wrote: "I remember telling the Doctor, on his first visit to my room, that I only needed biscuit and milk and beef tea to make me well. He rose to his feet and said: 'I know better than any man.' That is all I heard him say, and he walked out, leaving me without a word of sympathy, or a promise that I should have anything" (Pengilly, 1885, preface).

Mary wrote about the terrible food: "And here we have such horrid stuff. Dark colored, sour bakers' bread, with miserable butter constitutes our meal; there is an oatmeal porridge and cheap molasses for breakfast, but I could not eat that.... When I first began to realize that I must stay here all winter, I begged the Doctor to take me to his table, or change his baker. 'I cannot live on such fare as you give us here.' His reply was: 'I don't keep a boarding house'" (Pengilly, 1885, p. 6). During her seven months of forced stay, she documented many abuses and contradictions of the daily life within the walls of the asylum:

> There is a Miss Short here—a fair-haired nice-looking girl.... I did not think her much out of order when she came, but she is now. She has grown steadily worse ... she tears her dress off, so they have to put leather hand-cuffs on her wrists so tight they make her hands swell. I say: "Oh, Mrs. Mills, don't you see they are too tight. Her hands look ready to burst—purple with blood." She paid no heed: "It doesn't hurt her any." Yesterday she tied a canvas belt round her waist so tight that it made my heart ache to look at it. I am sure it would have stopped my breath in a short time; they tied her to the back of the seat with the ends of it. (Pengilly, 1885, p. 23)

> This day, I remember, was worse than common days of trouble. I had been excited by seeing one of the most inoffensive inmates pushed and spoken to very roughly, without having done any wrong. They attempted to comb that poor girl's hair; she will not submit, begs and cries to go down there. I go to the bathroom door and beg them to be gentle with her. Mrs. Mills slammed the door in my face. She is vexed at any expression of sympathy. Again I hear that pitiful cry ... they had taken her in a room to hold her on the floor, by those heavy, strong nurses sitting on her arms and feet, while they force her to eat. I can't endure the sight. (Pengilly, 1885, p. 22)

As time went by, Mary learned how to manipulate the system; she understood the asylum's unspoken code of survival: conform outwardly but manipulate when possible or necessary: "I love to cheat Mrs. Mills, to get the heat put up in the ward, since it is very cold in February, and the institution hardly seems to be heated at all. I am regulating the comfort of this ward but they don't know it" (Pengilly, 1885, p. 5).

Mary's plight was quite intense. She went about caring for 40 other women who resided in the same ward with her. She witnessed abuses and disrespect from staff and tried her best to console the abused, the disillusioned.

I often sit beside her and she tells me of her mother, and wants me to go home with her.... She does not seem a lunatic and she is neglected.... I soothed her as I would a child in trouble, until she ceased her raving, and then questioned her to discover the cause of her disease. She is a well-educated, intelligent lady. She seems to have a temper of her own, which has been made more than violent by her stay in this ward. If the ladies (in her village) would only come here and study the needs of these poor victims of insanity and make better arrangements for their welfare, they would find a higher calling than exhausting their energies working for bazaars and leaving us to the care of those who care nothing for us and will not learn. Too much temper and too much indolence rule here.... I have taken her in my heart as my own; she is so good a girl, wasting her precious life here for amusement of others—I don't see anything else in it. (LeBlanc & St-Amand, 2008, p. 52)

A reading of her journal reveals her to be quite compassionate and generous, dedicating her days to the well-being of her colleagues and friends. She was very alert, had a good grasp of the situation and suggested other ways of caring for her fellow human beings: "If the doctor would question the patients and their friends as to the cause of their insanity, they might, as in other cases of illness, know what remedy to apply" (Pengilly, 1885, p. 9).

Until every individual shall have learned of the wretchedness that is endured in lunatic asylums, hospitals, until petitions are sent to the Legislature and Governors to make new laws and rules for public institutions, that the poor be made comfortable through the public treasury, the pen of a woman shall write and her books shall go as messengers over land and sea, to vindicate the rights and redress the wrongs of the poor." (Pengilly, 1885, p. 25)

Mary foresaw that there was a central role for the psychiatrized in leading the staff and mental health officials on how to conduct their business, and in this she was exemplary and visionary:

I will teach them to think theirs is no common servitude—merely working for pay. But a higher responsibility is attached to this work of making comfortable those poor unfortunates entrusted to their care, and they will learn to know they are working for a purpose worth living for.... My graduating lessons have cost me dear; but they have proved rich blessings. I will not fear! (Pengilly, 1885, p. 23)

After being released from the asylum, Mary met with the province's Lieutenant Governor to make her case, and gave him a copy of her journal. "I would like to

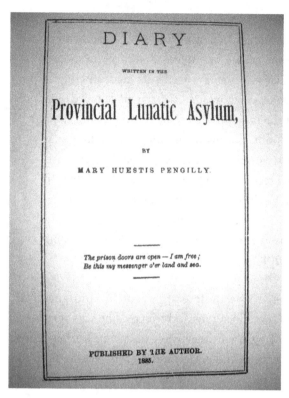

FIGURE 2.3: Mary Pengilly's Diary

Mary Pengilly's diary is an iconic depiction of a woman's existence in a Canadian "lunatic asylum" in the late 19th century. To read the diary first-hand, visit the Canadiana Collection at http://historyofmadness.ca (CIHM 11978).

Source: *Dare to Imagine: From Lunatics to Citizens, 2008.*

devote my remaining years, as far as I am able, to better the condition of those poor sufferers in the asylum." Governor Wilmot answered: "I hope you will, for I think it will be well for them to have your care, and I will do all I can to assist you" (Pengilly, 1885, p. 9). The Lieutenant Governor did nothing! Mary's desire to reform practices at the asylum never took place and in the end she continued selling her diary—which, after her death, was left unpublished for over 120 years (LeBlanc, 2006, p. 3). For the introduction she had stated: "This little book is humbly dedicated to the Province of New Brunswick, and the State of Massachusetts ... that it may be read in every state of the Union, as well as throughout the Dominion of Canada, that it may help to show the inner workings of their hospitals and asylums, and prompt them to search out better methods of conducting them, as well for the benefit of the superintendent as the patient" (Pengilly, 1885, preface). For the next nine years after her discharge, Mary travelled throughout North America, selling her diary and poems to advocate for changes within mental institutions regarding the invisible "unfortunates" who were forgotten inside. Mary Pengilly died in Dubuque, Iowa, in 1893 (Cusack, 2006, p. 4).

Concluding Remarks

These three women, contemporaries living in different countries, started their lives as normally as any women could in those days. Two of them had children and it seems that both played their mother role in a way that fit within the gendered expectations women lived with during the 19th century; the third was an artist living off her talents. The three had different life circumstances but with similar experiences in terms of their relation to the male-dominated societies they lived in, the doctors who impacted their lives, and the psychiatric system that treated them. All of them were brought to the asylum because men wanted them committed. Mary's sons wanted her treated. Hersilie's half-brother did not want her around, nor did Elizabeth's husband. All three, like the majority of people admitted in the 19th century, were declared insane by male medical experts who labelled them crazy, reflecting society's attitude towards women. Whether or not they were "mad" by their own definition or anyone else's, their experiences as individuals who were treated as such within the asylum system also reflect the overwhelming prejudice at this time towards genuinely distressed people for whom no tolerance was shown for their mental differences within conventional society.

In Mary's case, she neglected to eat for a few days during a psycho-spiritual experience while working on an important project. Her pharmacist son had her committed. As for Elizabeth, her rigid-thinking Calvinist preacher husband had her committed after a heated argument; Hersilie's half-brother knew that "crazy people" lose their legal right to inheritance. The initial frameworks are different but the struggles they all had to go through are similar: to fight against an unfair system that seems to agree that women are hysterical, irrational, and without legal rights.

Through their testimonies, these three women have certainly advanced the cause of the oppressed. The antipsychiatry movement that came into existence more than half a century later certainly inherited some of the dynamism, the values, and the strategies that these women had invented for their own defence and for the cause of oppressed people, particularly women.

Elizabeth was a victim of her husband's religious bigotry and supreme sense of male entitlement: he refused to accept the fact that his wife could think for herself and could develop her own ideas and values. Once inside the institution, all three had to struggle fiercely in order to be released, and upon their release, the ordeal continued. They used their personal experience in order to change the system, maintaining their dignity and convictions amidst a world of challenges and injustices. Even if they lost practically everything, they continued to fight. The injustices they endured for months or years gave them extra motivation to change an unfair system. Mary's "rich in spirit" attitude shone through her actions, both when she met the Lieutenant Governor and when she travelled throughout Eastern Canada to defend the rights of the underprivileged. Their legacy can be summarized in the words of Susannah Wilson:

> Psychiatric medicine functioned as an integral part of an essentially misogynistic and oppressive society. Delusional utterances can be read as meaningful when read as metaphorical expressions of real suffering and as strategies to ensure the survival of a self under threat. These narratives therefore constituted an act of resistance on the part of the women who wrote them, and they

prefigure the feminist revisionist histories of psychiatry that appeared later in the twentieth century. (Wilson, 2010, preface)

To what extent has the psychiatric system changed? Is Mary's message still relevant? We suggest that these women's exemplary courage and determination continue to inspire those who believe that psychiatry, and not only asylums, need radical transformation. And *Our Voice/Notre Voix* (LeBlanc, 2006) is keeping Mary Pengilly alive by recognizing contributions to the advancement of a transformed psychiatry. In recognition of her example, the Mary Pengilly Award is offered regularly in New Brunswick by *Our Voice/Notre Voix* to a psychiatrized person who has written his/her life story, in order to facilitate publication of their document.

CHAPTER 3

Democracy Is a Very Radical Idea

Lanny Beckman and Megan J. Davies

R adical historian Max Page (2001) tells us that "memory-work," and giving a voice to remembrance, is an essential democratic act (p. 116).[1] Oral histories are perhaps the most fundamental of primary documents, less constrained in form and less controlled by the researcher who sets out to collect them, for spoken memories resonate with life (Thompson, 1978). This chapter is the story of a collaborative project that has tried to share ownership of history, and in the process to address questions of voice, interpretation, responsibility, and audience (Borland, 1991; Kearns, 1997; Sangster, 1994). Scholars might present these as methodological concerns, but they are really issues of power, and they become particularly pertinent in projects that engage with narratives of suffering, discrimination, and social and economic marginalization (Kerr, 2003).

The Project

Megan: I am a social historian of British Columbia health practices. Over the past decade I have collected oral histories about counterculture homebirth and midwifery in the 1970s and 1980s and about home health in the pioneer Peace River country (Davies, 2011 and forthcoming). My recent research on mental health has been as a member of a pan-Canadian History of Madness in Canada/Histoire de la folie au Canada website (historyofmadness.ca) project on the history of deinstitutionalization. In June 2010, along with Geertje Borshma (University of British Columbia) and Marina Morrow (Simon Fraser University), two of my *After the Asylum/Après l'asile* colleagues, I was looking for stories of the Mental Patients Association (MPA), a radical self-help group that formed in Vancouver during the turbulent years of the early 1970s, when Greenpeace took a boat to Amchitka and Prime Minister Pierre Trudeau invoked the War Measures Act. But most particularly, I was searching for Lanny Beckman, the reputedly reclusive and certainly elusive individual who appeared to have been at the heart of the organization over the first years of its existence.

Lanny: I was leading a quiet life as a semi-recluse when this Megan J. Davies person banged down my front door. She said she wanted to interview me about an organization called the Mental Patients Association, which she claimed I founded in 1970. She said I had boxes of early MPA documents in my basement—how she knew this I have no idea, but she was right. The boxes touched off a sense memory and then the whole history of MPA flooded back in sensuous detail.

After a stint in Vancouver General Hospital's psychiatric ward in 1970, I founded the MPA rather than continue my PhD studies in psychology at UBC (I left with an MA). The tragic reason I started the organization was that three people in the day program I was attending after I was discharged from hospital committed suicide, all on the weekend when we didn't meet. These grim events were the kernel from which the organization grew. And it grew very quickly. The origins of the group were extremely exciting, but let's skip ahead to 1974 when I left. At that point MPA was a thriving community with hundreds of members, a paid staff of 25 ex-patients and allies, 50 beds in MPA accommodation, and an annual budget of $150,000. We garnered a lot of media attention in the early years, which we used to radically defend the rights of people called mental patients, something that really had not been done before.[2]

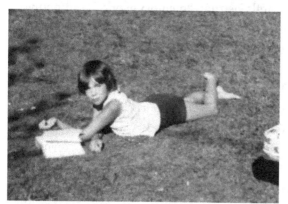

FIGURE 3.1: Megan, 1970

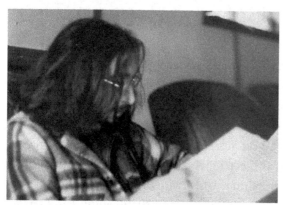

FIGURE 3.2: Lanny, 1970

Both the MPA documentary project and this chapter are illustrations of knowledge exchange, bringing together academic research and experiential understandings from the "lifeworld." In 1970, Lanny Beckman was founding the MPA and living in one of Vancouver's well-known alternative households—the left-wing York Street Commune in Kitsilano. Meanwhile, Megan Davies was an eleven-year-old bookworm already in love with the study of history. Forty years later, a shared regard for the craft of writing and a radical public history project resulted in this chapter.

Source: Megan Davies and Lanny Beckman

From 1975 to 1990, I was the publisher of New Star Books, a Vancouver socialist-feminist press. It seemed that every time we published a book, Ronald Reagan got more popular. Currently I am polishing the final draft of a manuscript, "What's Wrong with Psychology," that I have been writing for the past 40 years.[3]

Megan: I spent a lot of time over the summer months of 2010 thinking about the MPA, the 1970s, and the June interviews. The MPA consumer/survivor advocates and allies that we had interviewed were the first in Canada—and among the first in the world—to form a politically active support network, providing work, homes, and a sense of belonging and empowerment to ex-patients (Chamberlin, 1978; Shimrat, 1997).[4] It felt important to convey to the MPA founders that they had created something brave and magnificent. And I wanted to tell other people about the early radicalism of MPA—its insistence on the merits of peer support, its use of participatory democracy for organizational decision-making, and the manner in which paid jobs were decided in open elections.

The MPA founders had expressed profound, experiential-based interpretations of the history of the mental health system. We couldn't ignore these insights and, in fact, the notion of "shared authority" rests at the heart of current thinking in the field of oral history (Frisch, 1990; High, 2009).[5] Marina and Geertje were of the same mind, agreeing that a collaborative project would mirror aspects of what MPA did for members and might result in a mutual or negotiated understanding of why and how the organization evolved, and a fresh appreciation for personal and collective achievements.[6]

Oral historians stress the shape-shifting pathways of their projects and this one was no exception. Arthur Rossignol, a 17-year-old summer visitor, enchanted by Lanny's radicalism, suggested that we work with his friend Nick Nausbaum to transform Lanny's interview audio into a short educational video.[7] I agreed, and found myself in new methodological realms. One Friday night Nick and Arthur polished off a dozen of my chocolate chip cookies, then left for a party, gently but firmly abandoning me to edit our iMovie solo. Telling Lanny's tale of the early MPA through images and sound brought his story into close personal relief and helped us become friends and allies. Lanny sent me his top-10 movie list and a literary doodle on the threat posed to the American Empire by gay marriage and the construction of a mosque two blocks from Ground Zero. I knit him a pair of socks while working my way through Bergman, Altman, and Allen. When the finished piece was uploaded to YouTube in December, I was inordinately proud of what we had produced and newly appreciative of the possibilities of making public history through a shared conversation that involved storytellers, scholars, and teenagers.[8] In other words, I saw participatory democracy as a model for working with the MPA founders on a historical project (Polletta, 2002).[9]

The MPA project group includes seven survivors, and two allies who worked for MPA in the 1970s.[10] In February 2011 we had our first meeting in Vancouver. Responding positively to the "Lanny & the MPA" video, the MPA founders decided to create a collaborative documentary about the organization's first decade of existence. We determined that participants would select the segments of their interviews, which in turn would comprise the basic building blocks for the documentary. When the project group gathered again in April I showed the participants a rough iMovie version of the selected interview clips grouped into topical baskets. During our May meeting the group placed interview "topics" on a documentary storyline that traced the birth of the group in 1970, the flowering of the MPA community, and the changes of the late 1970s and early 1980s. At the end of June, Marina led a discussion to refine a core project values statement that the two of us had roughed out.

Arthur Giovinazzo, a keen member of the documentary group, helped search out archival footage and photographs.[11] I commissioned Nick and the younger Arthur to create original music and hired Lily Ross-Millard, a high school film studies graduate, to begin editing interview footage over the summer. As the project developed, we retained Catherine Annau, a documentary filmmaker, to help shepherd what she referred to as "the violently underfunded documentary" to completion, and Craig Webster, a professional film editor, to mentor the project. In October 2011 Catalin Patrichi, a talented young film graduate from York University, joined the project and began editing in earnest to give the film its first shape. Illustrators Willie Willis and Jeffrey Ho added their talents to animate Lanny's audio sections of the production, and Catalin and I sifted through a B-roll of historical footage and stills for images strong enough to give punch to the powerful interview segments. In a fanciful yet commonsensical fashion, I found that Lanny's contributions to the documentary echoed what he had done for MPA 40 years ago. Strategist Lanny pushed Marina and me to set up a project meeting with the present MPA executive director, sensibly suggesting that we take Patty Gazzola (née Servant), an MPA founder, along for ballast. Organizer Lanny mapped out our first plans for launching the documentary. And in June 2011, Musician Lanny let me record him on the guitar for the documentary soundtrack, realizing a dream that Nick and I had been holding on to for months.

Lanny: The day before the "recording session," Megan and I and another friend went to a Vancouver Canadians baseball game. They are a lowly Class A team. Vancouver is a lousy sports city. The only major league sport it supports is hockey, and Canadian football, if that's a sport.

En route I stopped to pick up Megan at the current headquarters of MPA. I'd had no contact with the group for decades. Inside, I met David McIntyre, the executive director, who seemed happy to meet me and was eager to tell me about MPA's growth over those many years. The organization now has over 200 people on staff, an annual budget of $15 million, and is doing good on an impressive scale (Motivation, Power and Achievement Society, 2011).

Megan: What was nice about that moment was that it wasn't scripted. It just happened. Lanny's unexpected arrival at MPA caused a stir through the office, and the executive director was swiftly produced to meet this mythical figure. Lanny was plainly discomforted by the attention,[12] but in my remembrance the moment is equal parts tender and amusing: two earnest men, a decade on either side of me in age, one dressed for the office and the other for the baseball game, discuss MPA and its practical role in reducing the obscene fact of homelessness.

The project evolved through a series of meetings held at Vancouver's Gallery Gachet, a Downtown Eastside social justice arts space just a few blocks from the MPA offices. Looking critically at the progress of the project, I believe that we did our best to let creative decisions rest with the group while we put into place the necessary logistical and professional scaffolding. But this was not a perfect process. Lanny and I have a standard joke about the need for redistribution of our unequal energy levels, but in fact this has a real impact on what each of us can contribute to the documentary. Similarly, there are great gaps in power, income, confidence, and in access to technology and funding between the academics on the project and the MPA founders whose lives have intersected with the mental health system. And if history were nonlinear, I would press rewind and have the group interview each other with Geertje, Marina, and myself there to share our questions. Perhaps it would be useful for us to be interviewed as well, but I don't think so. This is their story (Gondry, 2008).[13]

Systems of Knowledge and Historical Understandings

Megan: From the beginning of the *After the Asylum/Après l'asile* project there was an understanding that our work—and particularly the aspects that connected to the website—would transgress the academic/community divide. We wanted to encourage community participation and give equal value to experiential knowledge and knowledge traditionally defined as "expert." Like the pages created by members of the Parkdale Activity and Recreation Centre (PARC), which will depict the history of the first drop-in centre in Toronto's psychiatric ghetto, the documentary project met our goal of creating inclusive research.

Within academia, embodied knowledge of the "lifeworld" is no longer the poor second cousin to textual knowledge that it was a decade ago. Current health literature demonstrates the effectiveness of involving community stakeholders, creating a research exchange rather than a one-way consultation process (Beal et al., 2007; Beresford et al., 2006; Dennis Jr. et al., 2009). This approach is always going to be more challenging when dealing with the past, but Keith Carlson's work with the Stó:lo Nation and Daniel Kerr's collaborative analysis of homelessness in Cleveland point to the richness of such endeavours (Carlson, 2009; Kerr, 2003).

Lanny: I usually don't like the concept of esoteric knowledge, but when it comes to "mental illness" it is all but impossible to understand the experiences if you haven't known them personally. The result is a brew that usually contains four bitter ingredients: the pain of the disorder, the loss of work, the threat of poverty, and the stigma of shame.

Alarming statistics on the current "epidemic of mental illness" abound, but let's use BC's Mood Disorders Association (MDA) as a lens to suggest the scope of the problem. Founded 25 years ago as a non-profit, non-professional self-help society, this struggling, underfunded organization now has groups in 52 cities and towns outside the Greater Vancouver and Victoria areas (Mood Disorders Association of British Columbia, n.d.). Imagine living in Vanderhoof, BC, population 4,064, and leaving your home only once a week to attend the MDA meeting.

Almost everyone with a mood disorder label has a spotty work record, often leading to long-term or permanent unemployment. What comes first is the attempt to hide the fact from one's boss and fellow workers. In almost all cases the person is ultimately forced to quit, take a leave of absence, or is fired. Next to homelessness, unemployment and the spectre of poverty are the biggest practical problems facing people with psychiatric labels.

"Mental illness is an illness like any other." This brave little slogan has been fighting the stigma of mental illness for eons. Sadly, it hasn't worked and is unlikely ever to because it's not true and everybody knows it. Aside from the fact that mental illness is the only illness for which you can be involuntarily incarcerated, it is obvious to all that something that goes very wrong with your mind falls into a naturally different category from something that goes very wrong with your pancreas. No one would say that pancreatic cancer is an excuse for bad behaviour, though 40 percent of respondents in a recent poll said mental illness often is (Canadian Medical Association, 2008, p. 4). And the synonym "sick," when spoken in anger ("You're *sick!*"—never used to refer to physical illness), is one of the strongest epithets of hate in the language. Also, unlike almost all other illnesses, there is not a single physical test for any psychiatric disorder.

Megan: Storytellers have an everyday knowledge of social places and situations and an ability to convey events as tactile and multi-faceted. They are content experts.[14] As Stacy Zembrzycki (2009) notes, their factual knowledge allows them to pick up on subtleties that the interviewer has not registered (p. 231). But there is something much stronger than simple factual knowledge happening with the MPA interviewees. They bring to the project a lived understanding of how the organization met the desperate need for shelter against stigma and prejudice, and thus hold content within an appreciation of systemic inequity. I relate this to the alarm I experience when I am cycling home at night and a man yells at me from a passing car that is suddenly 10 inches too close. What I am feeling is a woman's fear of rape, an awareness that is always present and is a measure of the bounded lives of women. But the incident is so much an aspect of my daily life that I don't even mention it when I arrive home.

Lanny: Moreover, because MPA was an explicitly political organization, most former members have an analysis of ways in which mental health is connected to discrimination, marginalization, and proximity to poverty. People came to MPA—particularly those who had been hospitalized—as isolated individuals, but they brought with them their own knowledge of discrimination and stigma. And the little world of our organization opened up their, and my, understandings of issues of gender, sex, professionalism, health, poverty, class, and powerlessness. So the MPA founders bring this political analysis to the documentary project.

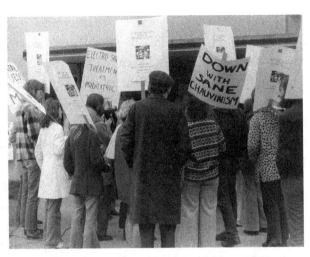

FIGURE 3.3: MPA at Work and Play, 1973

Although direct political action was a small part of the MPA's activities, the organization is noteworthy for having held North America's first antipsychiatry protest on March 30, 1973, at Riverview Hospital. In this image one documentary project team member holds a placard reading "Down With Sane Chauvinism."

Source: Eve Hamilton

When MPA started in the early 1970s, radical politics were in the air, so it was widely acknowledged, in the lingo of that time—people really did talk this way—that oppression existed and therefore so did oppressors and the oppressed. This feels very dated today, but at that moment MPA's politics seemed natural. The media were fascinated with us, and we took that opportunity to fight publicly against the oppression faced by mental health patients. Indeed, the name of the organization—the Mental Patients Association—was chosen as a conscious radical act—an inversion of language, think of "queer studies" today, that would be described now as *in your face*. Thus the name itself was an attack on stigma.

Megan: At the beginning of August, our teenage film editor confided that she had fallen in love with the people whose lives were moving across her computer screen. The interviewees had become her heroes. Lily, I surmised, understood much better than I that a documentary is powered by emotion. Because this was the story of their lives, the MPA founders shared Lily's affective response to the tale we were telling, but I came to appreciate that they also regard the history of their former organization in a functional fashion. They are interested in creating a public document that both preserves and presents the history of the MPA. From their perspective there is the possibility of telling the whole story as well as laying out the particulars of the past. On a personal level, my response to the MPA founders was not that far removed from Lily's, but as a scholar, I am located in a very different place from both other parties in the project.

Historians are empiricists who gather primary materials from the past to create a foundation and then build upwards and outwards by considering context and theoretical possibilities. In the end, we regard the historical edifice we have constructed as a careful arrangement of interwoven arguments and imaginative interpretations, rather than a set of emotions or definitive facts. As project historian, I was willing to revisit the way in which I use theory, analysis, and synthesis, but not to abandon these elements of my craft. That would be like not setting the table for supper. I think the historian will be present in our documentary, inserting relevant detail and situating the organization within the broader context of the period. Although concepts drawn from disability research and theories of therapeutic landscapes, third spaces, and radical social capital will not be used explicitly, they will be evoked to underscore the way in which the early MPA inverted the traditional power structure of the mental health system and created a Mad-positive space in the deinstitutionalization era (Oldenburg, 1989; Oliver, 1992; Putnam, 1995; Williams, 2007).[15]

And shared authority means learning about what intellectual tools are useful to non-academics. Over the winter I sent Lanny a short article from the *Radical History Review* about the democratic potential of radical public history. Framed in a discussion of the urban streetscape of Atlanta, Georgia, and written in plain language free of theoretical jargon, Max Page's piece (2001) is a succinct and powerful plea for a public history that speaks beyond the lecture halls of academia and aims, "to impact the present political situation through investigations into the past" (p. 115). Page's writing is as relevant to the history of MPA as two subsequent articles that I posted to Lanny, likely culled from the journal *Health & Place*, which employ the concept of therapeutic landscapes to interrogate the spatial aspects of madness. He was too kind to say so to me, but I heard through the Mad grapevine that Lanny hated these publications.[16]

Lanny: "Hated" might be too strong a word. I recall one article that dwelt on the "spatiality of therapeutic landscapes." Maybe it's not too strong a word. It is a common practice and failing in academia, which I experienced when I studied psychology, to use jargon to render intelligible ideas difficult to follow. Physicists talk about striving for "elegance" in their theories (Greene, 2000), meaning the briefest description of the broadest band of phenomena, e.g., $E=mc^2$.[17] I think of elegant language as being poetic. Both the language of psychology and of the two articles that Megan sent me are at poetry's opposite pole. I liked the Max Page article (2001) from the *Radical History Review* and found it interesting to read about how his ideas apply to Atlanta, a real place and one you do not associate with radicalism. Page reminded me again that there are good guys in every corner of society, and though we might not have much power now, the progressive ideas stay in circulation, incubating.

History, you might say, is the final draft of journalism, but actually historians do important work because they come along and make small stories part of the historical record. Our documentary is an opportunity to make the past public and is revealing not just to an imagined viewer but to the participants themselves. There on the screen is Patty Gazzola, who came to MPA as a young single mother four decades ago, now explaining her role in negotiating mortgages with the Canadian Mortgage and Housing Corporation for MPA-owned houses. This is MPA at its best—a place where members developed their intelligence to deal with the real and complicated world to promote the welfare of the community as a whole. Because of Patty, people who needed homes got them (not as halfway houses—halfway to what?) for as long as they wanted to stay.

Megan: As Lanny's response to Patty's videotape demonstrates, the kind of historical understanding I witnessed with the MPA documentary participants was sometimes political, but always intensely personal, linked to key individuals and events and underscored with strong feelings.[18] Asked why they agreed to help create a history of MPA, the founders stressed the profound importance of MPA, its ongoing relevance, and their distress with the way in which the organization had changed. Avi Dolgin, a former MPA housing coordinator, told the group that, "I want to tell the MPA story because it was one of the most exciting things I had done.... Lanny Beckman was a man with a vision, and I grabbed hold of his coat and said, 'Let me come along. I want to build with you'" (Notes, MPA Documentary Meeting, April 6, 2011).[19] Alex Verkade said, "Because the old MPA saved my life," and Ian Anderson continued by stressing the acceptance and the healing that characterized the organization and the treasured friendships he made there (Notes, MPA Documentary Meeting, April 6, 2011). John Hatfull added, "I have the vain hope that if we talk about it enough maybe we will find a way to recreate MPA the way it was. I always thought it was a great idea, I loved it, and I thought it helped more people than any other group" (Notes, MPA Documentary Meeting, April 6, 2011). When I visited Jackie Hooper in October 2011 and posed the same question, she replied, "I wanted to be part of the project. MPA meant so much to me at the time. I was very suicidal, and of course it helped" (Personal communication, October 29, 2011).

Encounters with this kind of "living history" are sometimes destabilizing for me, because, as British historian Raphael Samuel points out (1994), "It plays snakes and ladders with the evidence, assembling its artifacts as though they were counters in a board game. It treats the past as though it were an immediately accessible present, a series of exhibits which can be seen and felt and touched" (p. 197). But historians working with storytellers need to be open to non-academic ways of interpreting the past. This is particularly important when we work with stories of people who have been psychiatrized. Without due sensitivity to questions of ownership, we risk simply adding a new chapter to the categorization and disempowerment that characterize the life history of a person with mental health difficulties.

Lanny: I understand the distress the old timers feel about the conservative changes that MPA has undergone since the 1970s. But change was inevitable.

MPA was radical in two ways: it publicly criticized the policies and institutions that harmed psychiatric patients; and internally it was democratic to a fault (one wag suggested MPA's history could be titled *Met to Death*). At the same time, the organization provided services, which cost money, which came from government. For a while the grants came with few strings attached, but with the advent of neo-conservative governments, both types of radicalism were whittled away. At some point the name was changed to Motivation, Power and Achievement Society.

From a distance, I have no criticism of what MPA has become. The opposite, in fact. It provides very needed services to people who very much need them.

Mental patients' liberation, an idea that MPA pioneered in Canada, has been excluded from the broader history of 1970s social justice groups because it did not fit the same mould as feminist and gay rights organizations and therefore did not share the same (partly) successful emancipatory future. Unlike feminists and gay activists, and not to deny the existence of a small Mad movement (Shimrat, 1997), the great majority of people with mental health labels don't want to celebrate the experience that so defines them. With radical mental health groups like the early MPA left out of the historical record, it is easier for mainstream groups like the Canadian Mental Health Association and the Mental Health Commission to define the current mental health agenda.[20] In collecting, recording, and disseminating the story of MPA's early days, Megan's various projects might inspire radical action in an unforeseeable future; they will increase the likelihood of progressive changes in attitudes and policy. At worst, they'll have expanded the portrait of a hopeful and interesting moment in Canadian mental health history.

Megan: Lanny, who perhaps should entertain the notion of a third career as a Canadian historian, is pointing out an important gap in the historiography of 1970s social protest movements (Anastakis and Martel, 2008; Adamson et al., 1988; Aronsen, 2011; McKay, 2005; Owram, 1996; Palmer, 2009).[21] My daughter Mab agreed. Why did her English 12 teacher not talk about Mad liberation when he told his class about second-wave feminism? Surely people like Lanny, who hold a lifetime of experience negotiating a difficult world, Mab argued, should be regarded as Elders in the same way that they are in First Nations communities (Personal communication, August 25, 2011).

Other members of the documentary group shared the notion that our film should inspire and educate. Alex Verkade told the group that he wanted our film to be shown to mental health patients "so they can do things other ways," but cautioned that the film should be accessible to everyone (Notes, MPA Documentary Meeting, May 4, 2011). We all loved Arthur Giovinazzo's idea that, "Somewhere out there is today's Lanny Beckman ... a sixteen-, seventeen-, eighteen-year-old who is going to get inspired and start their own version of MPA" (Notes, MPA Documentary Meeting,

May 4, 2011).[22] A documentary that sends youth an envelope with the story of a once-upon-a time peer support group that inverted the power structures and created a Mad-positive space appeared delightfully revolutionary to the group.

Another set of people that the group thought could benefit from the teachable moments provided by the documentary are mental health workers. Ian Anderson asked if the film would be made available to non-profit organizations (Notes, MPA Documentary Meeting, May 4, 2011). John Hatfull regarded the service provision constituency as critical, arguing that, "Primarily I think we should aim it at professionals to show them what they are not doing that takes the soul out of mental health" (Notes, MPA Documentary Meeting, May 4, 2011).

The documentary project connects to several areas of scholarship that illuminate oppression and social injustice. Oral history is a field with its own progressive tradition of challenging centrally held beliefs and authoritative knowledge systems (Shopes, 2003). Similarly, ownership is a core value of path-breaking research being done by British psychiatric survivors, which builds on emancipatory disability methodology (Oliver, 1992). And there is also a link between this project and a new Canadian field being nurtured by a group of young historians. Like survivor researchers, ActiveHistory.ca present their field as one with public responsibilities to listen, to respond, and to foster change.[23] The MPA founders have made it clear that they are operating within a framework that links radical, activist history with a survivor sensibility. The experiential knowledge of group members, and the political understandings they gained from their tenure at MPA, means that if we can produce a documentary that the group considers authentic, it will inevitably challenge exclusion on individual and societal levels (Sweeney, 2009).

This kind of knowledge translation is common academic currency today, and programs that support this work have been a good source of funding for *After the Asylum/Après l'asile* projects. We have already used project research on two secondary education sites (Davies & Marshall, 2010; Davies & Purvey, 2010) and are currently creating a set of learning objects for post-secondary educators.[24] Along with the MPA documentary, these will be freely shared with educators and students via our website. Animated group discussions about how to market our film demonstrate that this is not just academic parlance and, indeed, the first time I met Lanny, he said that he agreed to speak with me because he liked the progressive teaching materials I had created for high school students.

Conclusion

Megan: I presented the workshop address on which this chapter is based in a celebratory manner, as if to suggest that these kinds of collaborations are easy. An observer at our February 2012 group screening of Catalin's first rough cut would have been right in reading pride and satisfaction on the faces of the MPA founders. But I would have been wise to pay closer attention to Michael Frisch's assertion (2003) that shared authority is a "necessarily complex, demanding process of social and self discovery" (p. 112). A 2011 summertime snapshot brings this point into sharp focus. Geertje and I were visiting Dave Beamish, one of the MPA founders,[25] when his building manager, clearly concerned, asked me to persuade Dave to take his medication. To my mind the manager's request narrowed Dave's identity down to that of a "mental health patient." Of course I know about Dave's mental health history, but I regard Dave as a research partner, and in fact he was someone I had come to care about and fiercely admire over the course of the project, for Dave loved MPA and fought harder than anyone to try and stop it from changing. The manager's worry was undoubtedly genuine, but I was so frustrated at the seeming intractability of the stigma conveyed in that conversation, that writing about it months later still makes me cry.

Few historians who are passionate about connecting scholarship, community, and social justice have the opportunity to work alongside people who hold history, and I have been extraordinarily privileged in this regard. And I have learned to accept our chaotic project meetings with their limited organizational structure, persistent technical problems, and erratic attendance as characteristic of the organic nature of an oral history endeavour and charmingly reminiscent of the shape-shifting, crisis-ridden style of the early MPA. But it is the testing moment that I sketch out above that I believe is the most instructive. When historians engage directly with narratives of suffering and systematic inhumanity, every step they take needs be traced with an awareness of power and appreciation for the democratic potential of *memory-work*. The real responsibility is not just to get the story *right* in academic terms, but to facilitate both a process and a product that the MPA founders believe to be authentic.

Lanny: I was initially skeptical about the idea of collaboration between Historian Megan and early MPA people—and if the collaboration proved not to work that would have been okay with me. But my skepticism really proved to be wrong. I don't think Megan, Marina, and Geertje could have done this project without us, because they needed access to our *theories* (and the consultants' honorariums we received were not merely tokens), and of course it would not have happened without them. Beyond all of that, the project of revisiting our distant memories has been an unexpected pleasure.

MPA was an attempt to create a utopian community in an era when people had radical utopian dreams, but it is too easy to interpret calls for a return to the early MPA model as nostalgia. Rather, the radicalism of MPA should be seen as an idea that is still worth fighting for, even though we live in conservative times. We were self-consciously trying to change the world and saw ourselves as agents of history writ small. Equality, democracy, and social justice were bywords of the period, and at MPA we tried to give life to both the words and the ideas they represented, scripting them into the everyday life and activities of the group.

This is October 31, 2011. Since the economic crash of 2008 I've been asking the logical question: Why are there no demonstrations on Wall Street? I'd come to think the idea was futile and that the spirit of collective rebellion lay in a seemingly permanent coma (see above). Then, just like the Arab Spring, Wall Streets sprung up everywhere.

Depression has taught me that hopes, like bones, grow brittle with age. I'm habitually careful not to raise either of them too high. But here's a giddy exception. It's just possible that the spreading protests are early steps on a long road towards something the world has never known—democracy, which is a very radical idea.

Acknowledgments

We would like to thank organizers of and participants in the May 2011 Storytelling and History: Encounters in Health graduate workshop at the University of Ottawa's AMS Nursing History Research Unit for the opportunity to present an earlier version of this paper, and the following groups and individuals for support and input: Colin Coates, Mab Coates-Davies, the York Gender History Group, and our colleagues on the Translating History/Shaping Practice Project. CIHR funding for *Open Doors/Closed Ranks: Mental Health after the Asylum* made the documentary project possible. Most of all, we would like to express our appreciation to the rest of the MPA documentary project team: Ian Anderson, Magdelanye Azrael, Dave Beamish, Geertje Borshma, Avi Dolgin, Patty Gazzola, Arthur Giovinazzo, John Hatfull, Jackie Hooper, Marina Morrow, Irit Shimrat, and Alex Verkade.

Notes

1 Radley's (1999) work on patient narratives also connects with this understanding of the power of owning stories, arguing that patient narratives can also be read as efforts to "de-colonialize" the body claimed by biomedicine, recover personal identity, or at least stand as testimony to the sense of personal alienation that the sick role creates.

2 Throughout this paper we variously refer to such people as psychiatric survivors/consumers/mental health patients/mental patients/ex-patients/the psychiatrized/the Mad/and people with mental health difficulties. This is because we don't have the right language; as someone said, everyone is searching for idiom of distress. So when we use one of these terms think of it as being in imaginary quotation marks.

3 Epistemic and related problems that call into question the findings of psychological research include: conscripted undergraduate subject bias; the many-membered cult of statistical significance; lying to subjects unpersuasively and not lying to subjects unpersuasively; experimenter bias and many other instances of broken microscopes; null-hypothesis publication bias; the "decline effect." These compounding problems, added to the elusive complexity of psychology's subject matter, have so far blocked the formulation of anything that could credibly be called a scientific theory—unless the bar is set extremely low.

4   Historical analysis of MPA is limited and there has not yet been scholarly work on the organization. For personal recollections of the MPA see Lanny Beckman's interview section in Shimrat (1997) and Judi Chamberlin's recollections of her time in Vancouver (1978). The organization's tabloid newspaper, *In a Nutshell*, is a good source of institutional history, but researchers should also note early MPA publications: *Madness Unmasked* (1974), *Antipsychiatry Bibliography and Resource Guide* (1974), *Head On: A Self-Help Model* (1978), *Head On Into the Eighties* (1983). Among the many media sources on the early MPA are a 1973 CBC documentary and the 1977 National Film Board documentary, *Mental Patients' Association*. In 2001 the current MPA produced a documentary, *In a Nutshell: Stories of the MPA Society.*

5   Presented first in 1990 by American historian Michael Frisch (1990) in his seminal work, *A Shared Authority: Essays on the Meaning and Craft of Oral and Public History*, as operating within the confines of the interview process, the concept has evolved and expanded in meaning to include the entire oral history process (High, 2009).

6   Fletcher and Cambre (2009) make this last point about creating digital stories (p. 115).

7   "Lanny & the MPA," is part of *More for the Mind: Histories of Mental Health for the Classroom* (Davies & Purvey, 2010).

8   Sharing authority involves opening up possibilities for a collective conversation and a project that allows all parties to expand their skill set and knowledge base. Oral historians now involve storytellers in determining project design, protocols, and products (Kerr, 2003).

9   Francesca Polletta (2002) took this approach in her oral history work with veteran community activists in the United States, modelling her research methods on the organizational methods that had been employed by her subjects in the 1960s. It was probably at this moment that Megan's fantasy of being elected documentary coordinator by the MPA founders—but just for six months!—was born.

10 The MPA founders are as follows: Ian Anderson, Dave Beamish, Lanny Beckman, Avi Dolgin, Patty Gazzola, Arthur Giovinazzo, John Hatfull, Jackie Hooper, and Alex Verkade. Magdelanye Azrael and Irit Shimrat have also participated in the documentary project.

11 Unfortunately, due to the high cost of obtaining archival footage from CBC Toronto and the National Film Board, the vast amount of media material about MPA is not available for community projects such as this. This is particularly unjust given the fact that many members of the documentary group freely gave their time for interviews in the 1970s.

12 Lanny, now 68, leads a quiet private life and is noticeably ill-at-ease with the publicity given to a chapter of his distant past. He insisted on being the junior author, so the published chapter will come as a surprise.

13 Michel Gondry's (2008) slim volume on community filmmaking is inspirational regarding shared authority in community filmmaking. Gondry's "utopian idea" includes a focus on the everyday, accessible ideas, community ownership, and emotional connection to the material. Gratification comes not from an external voice of assessment, but from the participants collectively admiring and appreciating what they have created (pp. 7–8).

14 We are not suggesting that the MPA founders hold "the truth" about the organization. Oral history, in particular, underscores the elusive attribute of truth itself, for the story is not just what happened, it is also what the respondent believed took place, and what the long line of memory has constructed as occurring.

15 We are making fleeting references to wide and important areas of scholarship here. Oldenburg, Oliver, Putnam, and Williams are major voices in their respective areas of research and theory,

but there are many rich secondary resources that will be useful in the interpretation of the history of MPA.

16   Megan found that her fourth-year students had much the same reaction to a set of academic articles about Vancouver's Downtown Eastside. They were able to fully engage with Dara Culhane's (2009) chapter recounting the life stories of three women of the Downtown Eastside, but they found two other assigned articles entirely inaccessible (Masuda & Crabtree, 2010; Robertson, 2007). In Megan's view, all of the readings were equally analytical, but Culhane had simply submerged theory and argument into a compelling set of personal histories.

17   Brian Greene uses this phrase in his book *The Elegant Universe* (2000).

18   Megan saw this highly personal and emotive perspective on the past on the fascinating BBC Capture Wales digital history website. Retrieved from www.bbc.co.uk/wales/arts/yourvideo/queries/capturewales.shtml.

19   Lanny says he is flattered by what Avi says but he still wants his coat back.

20   From a survivor research perspective our documentary should use history to challenge the current focus of mainstream Canadian mental health on stigma, treatment, and recovery (Sweeney, 2009).

21   Aronsen's (2011) book on alternative Vancouver in the period (ironically put out by the press that Lanny helped create) looks at Greenpeace, the anti-war movement, the Vancouver Free University, and the Four Seasons Park occupation. But Aronsen shows little interest in radical Vancouver community efforts that connected health and social justice and makes no mention of MPA. Similarly, McKay (2005) does not include Mad liberation in his analysis of the history of the Canadian left in the period when MPA was created, giving space to neo-Marxism in Quebec, the Waffle movement and the NDP, and variable elements of feminism.

22   Lanny particularly liked this notion since he was actually 27 when he started MPA.

23   ActiveHistory.ca. Retrieved from http://activehistory.ca/about/. There is an obvious link here as well to the work of activist ethnographers like Gary Kinsman (2006).

24   Post-secondary education webpages from the *Translating History/Shaping Practice: Community-Informed Teaching Resources on Mental Health* project are currently in development.

25   As I tried to explain to the building manager, Dave Beamish has had an illustrious career in the mental health world. He was a coordinator at MPA, then was involved with innovative MPA programming that brought MPA ideas and people into Riverview Mental Hospital, the provincial psychiatric facility. In the early 1980s he worked with Fran Phillips, his MPA friend and colleague, to found Pioneer House in New Westminster—a residential establishment run on MPA principles. In the same decade Dave also served on the Westcoast Mental Health Society and the national board of the Canadian Mental Health Association. Dave died in December 2011.

CHAPTER 4

What Makes Us a Community?
Reflections on Building Solidarity in Anti-sanist Praxis

Shaindl Diamond

While biological psychiatry continues to gain social and economic power at a rapid rate, there is a worldwide movement that is questioning its theories and interventions, turning them around, and examining approaches to understanding and responding to human experience in alternative ways that empower people who are conceived of as Mad (MindFreedom Ghana, 2005; MindFreedom International Global Campaign Committee, 2011; Salie, 2010; Tanasan, 2011). This movement is made of up smaller political communities in different locations around the globe that come together on the basis of political orientation, priorities, experiences, identity, culture, and history (MindFreedom Ghana, 2005; MindFreedom International Global Campaign Committee, 2011; Tanasan, 2011). Each of these communities consists of people representing different backgrounds and experiences, but who share a common concern about how people who are defined as Mad within dominant culture are being treated, particularly under the current psy regime[1] known as the "mental health system." This worldwide movement has many different goals emerging from particular communities based on specific local contexts, but each recognizes itself as part of a larger global group of people committed to questioning how human experience is understood and treated under the surveillance of the psy disciplines (MindFreedom International, 2011).

This chapter focuses on one such community located in Toronto, Canada. It draws from a critical ethnography I conducted focusing on the ideological underpinnings, empowerment, and social change goals in the community, as well as the actions and strategies used by members to meet these goals (see Appendix 4.1 for information about participants).[2] From the outset, I was interested in developing an in-depth understanding of some of the barriers blocking community members from meeting shared visions of empowerment and social change. During the data collection process, I learned that one aspiration that most community members share is to build stronger alliances with others and to develop more effective strategies for solidarity work. In order to achieve this hope, I realized the importance of understanding the differences in how community members theorize problems stemming from psychiatry and other sanist institutions,[3] how they go about creating change in the world, and how they respond to these ideological and strategic differences. The purpose of this chapter is to provide a small glimpse into some of the patterns of tension that exist among differently situated people in this Toronto-based community and offer some ideas as to how we can move towards a paradigm that draws on the strengths of the community in ways that nurture solidarity work.

Describing Community Constituencies

I have come to conceptualize the Toronto community as being made up of three main constituencies, which overlap a great deal in their goals and ideologies, but also have distinct ideological and strategic trends in their approaches to community activism. I refer to these three constituencies by the names most frequently used by people who associate with each: the psychiatric survivor constituency, the Mad constituency, and the antipsychiatry constituency.[4]

The psychiatric survivor constituency is at the heart of the political community, representing those who are most deeply affected by the practice of biological psychiatry and sanism[5] in dominant culture. It cannot easily be defined by a common politic, because it is not organized around a shared political ideology. Rather, psychiatric survivor initiatives tend to prioritize connecting people who have experienced the psychiatric system and improving the conditions in their lives, alleviating pain and suffering, and finding ways to meet their needs. Peer support and consciousness-raising initiatives are seen as foundations of the community, where people can come together to provide mutual support and question the disempowering rhetoric they had been forced into accepting. There is also a major focus on curtailing forced psychiatric interventions, ending stigma and discrimination, and creating accessible survivor-positive employment opportunities, affordable housing options, and other non-psychiatric alternatives. Psychiatric survivors have been actively involved in the development of organizations that work towards the realization of these goals, such as the Ontario Council of Alternative Businesses (1993–present), which over the years has worked at sustaining consumer/survivor-run businesses and providing support to new ones (Church, 1997); the Gerstein Crisis Centre (1990–present), a non-medical service established to provide a place for people in crisis to spend time and to sleep instead of going to hospital; and Sound Times (1992–present), a drop-in centre that was originally established by professionals but has for many years been run by people who have first-hand experience of psychiatrization.

The Mad constituency is a newer phenomenon within the community that reflects contemporary complexities, divisions, and theoretical trends. It evolved out of the psychiatric survivor constituency, and in many ways can be viewed as an extension of it, although given the unique ideas put forth by many of those who identify as Mad,

I feel that a distinction between the two is merited. Most notable is the shift from focusing on psychiatric oppression to the development of positive understandings of Mad identity and experience. Mad is frequently used as an umbrella term to represent a diversity of identities, and it is used in place of naming all of the different identities that describe people who have been labelled and treated as crazy (i.e., consumer, survivor, ex-patient). There are many different interpretations of what Mad means and what the Mad constituency is about, but there is a common emphasis on the oppression faced by people who have been oppressed as crazy. It is a term that covers a wide spectrum of discourses about madness and liberation. Many of the concerns central to the psychiatric survivor constituency are also central within the Mad constituency, such as fighting for accessible employment and affordable housing; but in the Mad constituency, there is a greater emphasis on exploring and celebrating individual experiences of madness and developing Mad culture. Mad Pride in Toronto is a key example of an initiative that strives to bring together a multiplicity of different experiences and perspectives in celebration of a developing Mad culture (see http://madpridetoronto.blogspot.com for more information).

The antipsychiatry constituency is based on a rich history of resistance efforts led by ex-patients, ex-inmates, psychiatric survivors, academics, and professionals (Burstow & Weitz, 1988; Shimrat, 1997; Starkman, 1981; Weitz, 1986). The primary goal of this constituency is to abolish institutional psychiatry, or at least undermine the power and authority it is granted in large part by the state. To support this goal, antipsychiatry activists often draw on the theoretical and empirical work of professionals and academics who are critical of psychiatry, as well as the personal experiences of psychiatrized people who have had negative encounters with the psychiatric system. It differs from the psychiatric survivor and Mad constituencies in its main organizing principle, which is focused on political ideology rather than identity politics discourses about shared experience. While the perspectives of psychiatrized people are often placed

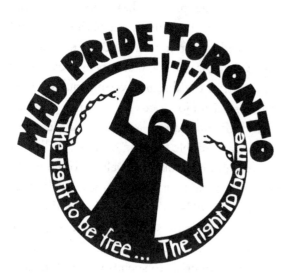

FIGURE 4.1: Mad Pride Toronto Logo

In this chapter, Shaindl Diamond chronicles the history, politics, and culture of Mad Pride in the city of Toronto. As with other social movements involving historically marginalized people (black pride, gay pride, fat pride), psychiatric survivors worldwide have embraced the idea that celebrating one's identity and heritage can help to erase stigma and overcome oppression.

Source: Mad Pride Toronto

front and centre, the constituency is open to all people who are interested in undermining psychiatric dominance and includes both those who have been psychiatrized and those who have not. Examples of antipsychiatry groups based in Toronto include the Ontario Coalition Against Electroshock (1982–1987), Resistance Against Psychiatry (1989–present), and the Coalition Against Psychiatric Assault (2003–present).

The above-mentioned constituencies include many ideological and strategic trends emerging from the political community in Toronto, but there are also many people who do not identify with any of these constituencies who nonetheless have a stake in resisting psychiatric oppression and sanism. While speaking to people actively involved in the community, it became clear that many activists are concerned about the under-representation of certain groups of people at events organized for psychiatric survivors, Mad people, and antipsychiatry activists. While psychiatric ideology is widespread within many communities in Toronto, it cannot simply be assumed that people outside this political community do not have a critique of psychiatry and other sanist institutions. To the contrary, people in various communities across Toronto are organizing in different ways against psychiatric oppression, albeit not always in collaboration with established psychiatric survivor, Mad, or antipsychiatry groups, and not always using the same language as psychiatric survivor, Mad, or antipsychiatry activists.

Areas of Contestation

In my ethnographic encounters, community members often pondered questions about why stronger coalitions do not exist among the various communities that are particularly vulnerable to psychiatrization. Many different topics came up in my encounters related to differences in priorities, needs, identities, experiences, and strategies. Questions about identity and experience were front and centre in explorations of divisions among differently situated people. This is not surprising, given that identity politics have been a hotly contested area since this community came into being (Reaume, 2002). In the early days of the Toronto community, identity debates were often centred on terminology such as *patient, ex-patient, psychiatric prisoner, psychiatric inmate,* and *ex-inmate* (Reaume, 2002; Shimrat, 1997; Weitz, 2002). While these terms are still in use, new terms, such as *psychiatric survivor, Mad,* and *consumer,* have become much more common, although many of the same underlying tensions persist, rooted in different ideas about institutional psychiatry and one's position in relation to the institution.

The development of the consumer constituency in the last 30 years has had an enormous impact on the community and has been met with mixed reactions. With the development of government-funded consumer initiatives and consumer positions within mental health organizations, the term has become widespread and is now used by many who are associated with psychiatric survivor initiatives. Some psychiatric survivors are protective with respect to the use of language and are upset about how commonplace the term *consumer* has become within the community. They believe that the term fails to communicate the reality of psychiatric violence or coercion, but rather evokes notions of choice and freedom (Giannakali, 2007; Weitz, 2002). On the flip side, some psychiatrized people to whom I spoke resent the stance of some psychiatric survivors, which is perceived to be harsh and critical of those who identify as consumers in the community and who do not relate to the more radical terminology.

In debates over language, survivors have correctly understood that they are fighting partly over understandings of themselves and the context in which they live. Yet, as Reaume (2002) explains in his article about community terminology, while some psychiatrized people involved in the community continue to grapple with the question of which term best represents collective and individual experiences of psychiatric survivors, in practice, the meanings of terms are fluid and change in different contexts. For example, Reaume (2002) points out that while the term *psychiatric survivor* originated with a radical critique of the psychiatric system, now many people who are not as radical in their vision embrace the term, sometimes even attributing different meanings to it, such as the implication that one has survived mental illness rather than the psychiatric system. Likewise, in an interview, Jeremiah Bach pointed out that many people use the term *consumer*, not because it necessarily fits with their ideological perspective, but because it is the term they are most familiar with because of where they are situated vis-à-vis the community. Clearly, while there are specific intentions and meanings behind terminology, language is used in multiple ways by psychiatrized people, reflecting different perspectives and experiences of psychiatry.

While often identity politics debates centre around language, people are in actuality debating much more than meanings of identity labels. The consumer movement is linked to particular strategies and connections to government and the psychiatric system. Some survivors, such as David Reville, described the consumer development as an opportunity for survivors to influence change from within the system, while getting paid for their labour, by participating in forums where real policy, program, and funding decisions are made. In this way, the consumer development is considered a step towards gaining power and influence in government and the psy complex where people can implement real change. At the same time, Reville and some others viewed it as a threat that has in some ways diluted the collective vision and energies of psychiatric survivors—a strategic action taken by governmental institutions to make them appear accountable to psychiatric survivors without really addressing underlying problems. Major concerns emerging from the community are co-optation, further division among psychiatrized people, and the weakening of grassroots initiatives. These tensions are not easily resolvable, and any approach has its trade-offs. The benefits that have come from the consumer constituency are very real, such as the development of employment and housing options and alternatives to traditional psychiatry. Yet, the effect the consumer constituency has had on radical political action remains a sore point for many.

Beyond the survivor/consumer divides, in the wider population of psychiatrized people, other tensions exist around how to conceptualize psychiatric oppression. My encounters with racialized psychiatrized women taught me that psychiatric survivor identity politics do not fit with all people's experiences of the world. This was clear in a conversation I had with Rora, a racialized woman who understood that she was oppressed by psychiatry, but viewed this oppression as deeply intertwined with the racist and sexist violence she had endured throughout her life. She knew about the psychiatric survivor constituency, but felt more connected to a community of racialized women who she believed understood her experience in the context of racist-patriarchy. Additionally, through my experiences in the feminist community, I have encountered feminist and anti-racist initiatives that deal with issues of psychiatric oppression within the larger context of combating racism and patriarchy, without necessarily having strong ties to the psychiatric survivor constituency. For example, the Toronto Women of Colour Collective has included issues of psychiatric violence in events about violence against women, without forging more formal connections with other psychiatric survivor groups. Another event I was part of in December 2010 was organized by THRIVE, the Multicultural Women's Coalition Against Violence and Oppression, to address violence against racialized women, where I facilitated a group about psychiatric violence against women. Most of the women who attended were psychiatrized and understood their experiences of psychiatric oppression as inseparable from issues such as immigration, motherhood, domestic violence, and racism, yet most did not identify with the psychiatric survivor constituency.

Many of those who identify primarily with the term *Mad* hope to address some of the divisions stemming from psychiatric survivor identity politics, to celebrate a *plurality of resistances* and subversive acts against sanism. The Mad constituency offers people places to connect in their resistance against sanism while decentring psychiatry and making space for divergent perspectives on the role of institutional psychiatry. According to some, the potential for people to understand the construct of normal as an oppressive ideal can open up more realms to Mad activism. As Erick Fabris explained to me in an interview:

> No longer will people just simply assume that [Mad] people ... need to eventually be corrected somehow or they will simply go unmanaged and unruly. They won't be able to assume that anymore, because there's going to be a rhetoric that says ... they don't need to be fixed at all.... This is going to be coming from consumers. This is going to be coming from ordinary folk who don't have anything against government or business.

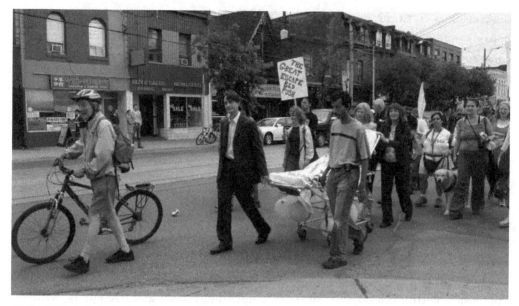

FIGURE 4.2: Mad Pride Toronto March

In this Mad Pride Day "bed push," which took place on July 14, 2007, participants wheeled a gurney along Queen Street West in Toronto to raise public awareness about the use of force and lack of choice for people ensnared in the Ontario mental health system.

Source: Sound Times

Fabris, Ruth Ruth, and Charlie expressed the belief that opening up the Mad constituency could ultimately help Mad people gain greater credibility in society, as more people from various social locations and political affiliations come to view madness as acceptable and understand it as simply part of being human. However, what some people view as a radical embracing of diverse localized resistance efforts, others view as relativism, where a multitude of perspectives are considered equal, regardless of what dominant values are left unchallenged. For example, Hope feared that this dynamic sets the community up to privilege those perspectives, identities, and actions least disruptive to the hegemonic order, thereby further marginalizing critiques of psychiatry and other sanist institutions. Her concern is that when community initiatives take a relativist approach to radical inclusion, this often leads to weakening critiques of the psy complex and other sanist institutions and leaves dominant power relations based on other forms of oppression unquestioned.

Community members who critique Mad identity politics frequently point to examples of essentializing notions of madness and experience as an issue of concern within the Mad constituency. Indeed, there are some Mad people who favour notions of Mad identity based on cultural or biological etiologies of madness. For example, Ricky explained that particular dimensions of Mad experience, such as hearing voices or living highly variable emotional states, which may or may not have genetic and/or biological causes, can serve as a foundation for Mad culture. This appears to be a comfortable and even empowering narrative for some Mad-identified people, who focus on how Mad people are oppressed under structures that do not accommodate them. On the other hand, Louise Tam fears that this type of approach can essentialize difference in ways that compromise more complex ways of understanding people's experiences based on historical, social, and material contexts. Like Tam, others argued that this orientation of Mad identity places *Mad* at the centre, surpassing all other individual or group identities in decontextualizing and homogenizing ways. For example, Jackie explained to me in an interview:

> If we just celebrate madness, whatever that is, we are forgetting about the ways many women have been persecuted for being crazy because of their reactions to violence. That won't do for those of us who are being diagnosed and drugged because of trauma.... It is important to put our experiences back into context instead ... recognizing and naming the specific dimensions of oppression.

Essentializing both Mad discourse and psychiatric discourse has the potential to obscure how processes of racialization, gender, class, disability, sexuality, and other processes shape and define madness. The experiences and narratives of many marginalized Mad people demonstrate how madness is shaped by a complex system of power relations, and narratives that fail to address this reality can alienate individuals whose identities are shaped by this very understanding.

I do not wish to overstate the presence of racist, sexist, ableist, adultist, and otherwise oppressive attitudes and dynamics within psychiatric survivor and Mad organizing, for in comparison to other realms in society, many psychiatric survivors and Mad people strive to be inclusive, aim to embrace difference and diversity, and at the very least, are well-intentioned in their work. Nevertheless, it is evident that awareness about marginality within community spaces varies a great deal among people and that sometimes a general lack of awareness allows for the reproduction of hegemonic power dynamics, even within spaces that are constructed to challenge the dominant social order. As such, it is important to recognize, acknowledge, and change the ways in which dominant cultural values are left unquestioned or unchallenged within spaces that strive to be anti-oppressive and inclusive to all psychiatrized and Mad people, even when this means examining our own ways of thinking, behaving, and relating to others in demanding and difficult ways.

The ideology-based approach of antipsychiatry activists poses its own challenges, as community members who do not have first-hand experience of psychiatrization attempt to work with those who do have this experience in pursuance of their ultimate goal of psychiatry abolition. Their approach offers a counter-hegemonic perspective on how psychiatric dominance works in the world without relying on an identity politics or standpoint approach. The inclusion of those who have not been psychiatrized, along with those who have this first-hand experience, is viewed as a benefit by those who want the community to branch out and garner more support to build stronger political networks among radical political communities. Furthermore, as Florence pointed out in an interview, some antipsychiatry activists believe that an emphasis on psychiatric hegemony can lead people to consider the effects of psychiatric dominance on differently situated people, including those who have not been psychiatrized. On the other hand, some psychiatric survivors and Mad people assert that those who have not been psychiatrized often lack the insight needed to respond with the respect and sensitivity that is appropriate when addressing the experiences, needs, and desires of those who have been psychiatrized. This brings into question the legitimacy of some initiatives stemming from the antipsychiatry constituency, particularly among those who do not agree with the long-term objective of the abolition of psychiatry or specific approaches taken by activists in pursuance of this goal.

The principal concern among these critics is that the work emerging from groups that include those who have not been psychiatrized will marginalize the perspectives of psychiatrized people and fail to respond appropriately to their everyday lived experiences. Some psychiatrized people feel that antipsychiatry is, and perhaps always was, too far removed from the lived experiences of psychiatrized people, given that the constituency's roots are in part embedded in the academic and professional realm.[6] For example, some psychiatric survivors and Mad people I spoke to believed that the antipsychiatry stance ignores their positive experiences of support in favour of a total rejection of the system. Others argued that antipsychiatry activists are striving for an unrealistic goal, which if achieved would leave many people in desperate need of help without state-sponsored supports they are currently able to secure. For example, Rudy and Bach were concerned about psychiatrized people losing support from social assistance programs for people with disabilities, employment programs available for those who are labelled as mentally ill, and disability accommodations in education and employment settings. All of these programs require psychiatrized people to have psychiatric diagnoses as proof that they are disabled and in need of assistance. Some community members felt that activists who are not dependent on these programs do not take seriously the implications of getting rid of the psychiatric system when it is so deeply intertwined with other state institutions. Others critiqued antipsychiatry for its centring of psychiatry as the main source of oppression shaping the lives of psychiatrized people, rather than equally considering how other forms of oppression influence people's experiences of psychiatric oppression and sanism.

Many antipsychiatry activists, including those who are not survivors, are aware of these critiques, are concerned about negative perceptions of their work, and care about being accountable to psychiatrized people. For example, Florence and Don Weitz recognize the immense power of psychiatry, the dependence of state programs on the psychiatric paradigm, and the lack of viable alternatives for people without financial resources; but they conceptualize these problems as part of the larger problem of psychiatric hegemony that needs to be remedied. The antipsychiatry constituency has a long and hard road ahead in its journey towards the abolition of psychiatry. This is a complex venture in consciousness-raising. People do not and will not easily understand antipsychiatry, given that the psy complex is an empire backed by enormous money-making industries, and that it has the public relations advantage of serving the vested interests of many who inhabit positions of privilege and command massive resources to finance subtle and pervasive propaganda in its support (MindFreedom Media Campaign Committee, n.d.).

Tensions will always exist between those who would reform current institutions to ease immediate pain and suffering and those who would transform society to meet human needs in alternative ways that intrinsically respect the dignity and welfare of all. Important questions to consider are: How do we react to these differences? And how do we come to the realization that these political visions can work together to serve the interests of human justice? There are no easy answers to the complex process of bringing people together; but we must grapple with these difficult questions, as everybody is needed if we are going to make changes in the direction of eliminating sanism and psychiatric oppression.

Towards a Paradigm for Anti-sanist Community Praxis

The diverse narratives of community members make it abundantly clear that not all people experience psychiatry in the same way, and in part, the diversity of experiences that people have with the psy complex accounts for the different solutions people view as appropriate in their healing, empowerment, and social change work. Still, many are determined to figure out ways to address tensions and build stronger solidarity networks. Without minimizing the significance of different experiences, understandings, roles, and access to privilege among differently situated community members, I propose that there are ways of fostering empathy and understanding across difference that are useful in attempts to develop analysis and strategy that account for the many different (partial) truths emerging from a multiplicity of standpoints.

A starting point is to emphasize a clear understanding that being psychiatrized, or being perceived as mentally ill, has consequences in the world we inhabit that are often unjust and vary depending on one's economic and social marginality and privilege. However, it is equally important to emphasize that sexism, racism, ableism, audism, classism, ageism, adultism, misogyny, transphobia, and heterosexism are entrenched in social and political institutions that rule, including psychiatry, which inevitably shape the everyday experiences of differently situated people, putting some people at greater risk of violence and marginality. These oppressive processes are each infused with one another, are inseparable, and are completely integrated into the social and material world. Hegemonic ideologies shape and define all of our lives, albeit in different ways depending on how we are situated vis-à-vis dominant culture.

The political community in Toronto has a rich array of ideological and strategic approaches to draw upon in our work, and I believe that many important principles that can ultimately help us build stronger solidarity networks are found in the fabric of existing ideological and practical approaches. For example, we can draw on elements of identity politics, recognizing that an analysis of the everyday lived experiences of marginalized people leads to knowledge about systems of domination that shape all of our lives, while rejecting the premise that we can rely on the perspective of any single marginalized group to develop a more holistic understanding of how systems of domination are at work. We also need to go beyond bringing together many different perspectives, to subject each experience or perspective to a process of critical interpretation and theorization, taking into consideration its historical and material basis, before it can become part of the foundation for solidarity and struggle (Mohanty, 2003).

The paradigm I am suggesting views institutional psychiatry as a tool within the larger "matrix of domination" (Hill Collins, 2000) that helps monitor and regulate those who disrupt hegemonic social relations and institutional processes, while always considering how it responds to people differently based on various dimensions of power. In other words, the threat of being labelled as mentally ill and treated against one's will foregrounds the analysis and strategy developed within the community, but pays attention to how the presence of this threat differs in people's lives, depending on their social locations and individual histories. As such, it also foregrounds how the psychiatric system is shaped by and interacts with other ruling institutions that are likewise complicit in processes such as colonization, capitalism, heterosexism, ableism, ageism, and patriarchy. It insists that resistance efforts are based in the recognition that all people are implicated in, and affected by, psychiatric dominance, drawing on an analysis of how various systems interact with one another to shape the lives and experiences of individuals in diverse ways. It is highly critical of dominant constructions of *madness, normality,* or *sanity,* recognizing the flawed nature of simplistic dichotomous and oppositional constructions of difference as "dominant/subordinate, good/bad, up/down, superior/inferior" (Lorde, 2007, p. 114). While every attempt is made to understand and contextualize why some people find essential notions of Mad identity to be empowering, this approach rejects any universal claims made about Mad people or madness, recognizing that madness is constructed differently in various historical and cultural contexts, and that there is no real basis of inherent or natural characteristics that define an eternal Mad subject.[7] It recognizes and values the many different forms of resistance against psychiatric dominance, but avoids liberal tendencies that exalt all perspectives and actions as equal, as it analyzes their particular social, historical, and material foundations, recognizing where various beliefs and actions come from. It encourages reflection on how diverse perspectives and experiences fit within the larger comprehensive whole.

I also want to acknowledge here other practical logistical concerns, mentioned to me by community members, that need to be front and centre in building community initiatives. For one, creating community materials in clear and easily understandable language, ideally in multiple languages, is a very important goal (Geoffrey Reaume). We need to reach out to parents, grandparents, teachers, and neighbours who may be completely uninterested in radical social transformation, but who have the potential to understand anti-sanist goals because of what they have witnessed or experienced in their own lives, and because they can relate to experiences of human suffering (Florence). Accessibility, however, goes beyond expressing political analysis in ways most people can comprehend and relate to. It also means finding ways to dismantle other barriers to participation, including making event fees optional or sliding scale, providing free child care and transportation, using wheelchair accessible spaces, providing ASL interpretation, creating spaces for specific marginalized groups to strategize at larger events, and, if possible given the resources available, creating multilingual environments (Jenny Blaser and Shoshana Erlich). These are all small but important pieces in the larger project of creating accessibility within the community, and while there are financial barriers to building inclusive spaces, finding the resources to do so helps to demonstrate a real commitment to the liberation of all differently situated psychiatrized and Mad people (Erlich, 2011).

All of these principles lay important groundwork for creating conditions that can foster solidarity within and among political communities that are interested in fighting back against psychiatric oppression and sanism in their many insidious forms. However, even if community members are inspired to regroup based on emerging critical insights from many different sources, much hard work remains. The hierarchies that shape our social world and the desire by some in marginalized groups to achieve respectability within the dominant social order make powerful teammates to hold us back. We need to hold on to radical transformative visions in the midst of all these hegemonic dynamics. Even when people find it necessary to collaborate within the psychiatric system to meet the immediate needs of psychiatrized people, a lot is lost if it means they give up on the larger vision of what the world could potentially become.

As bell hooks (2000, p. 110) writes, "To be truly visionary, we have to root our imagination in our concrete reality while simultaneously imagining possibilities beyond that reality." In line with these words, I am proposing that we keep working towards a vision that is based on our commitment to anti-sanist, anti-racist, feminist, anti-imperialist, disability, trans, anti-adultist, deaf, and queer liberation. I am optimistic that the community can progress towards the commonly held goal of engaging with others to end the pain and suffering inflicted on psychiatrized and Mad people. My optimism is based on my first-hand knowledge of the strengths, courage, and commitment of all three constituencies in the Toronto-based community to end the oppression imposed by a sanist society that uses psychiatry as a tool. But in addition to psychiatry, there are many tools in the master's house (Lorde, 2007). The paradigm that I am offering urges us to bring together the whole arsenal of tools, to examine them to better understand how they are wielded against us, keeping the master's power in place—tools, administered against us, often together in combination. We can blunt these tools and even dispose of them by reaching out and embracing all who are injured. By working together we can dispose of these tools forever and in their place create implements to nurture growth where we now have destruction. It is the knowledge we gain by truly listening to each other and linking arms to save each other that will inspire in us the vision and perseverance to work together to abolish suffering inflicted by sanism and psychiatric oppression within the context of a racist, ableist, patriarchal, heterosexist, transphobic, adultist, ageist, and classist society. I am confident that we can use our exemplary strengths, experiences, talents, and caring to help us move towards the realization of transformative visions of peace and well-being for all.

Notes

1 Throughout this chapter, I use terms such as *psy disciplines*, *psy professionals*, and *psy regime* in reference to the various disciplines and professionals that accept and implement the theories and practices of biological psychiatry. It is not sufficient to simply refer to psychiatry, given that in contemporary times, many related professions including psychology, social work, and nursing are greatly influenced by the psychiatric paradigm and are in many ways complicit in maintaining psychiatric hegemony. Nikolas Rose was the first to use this term (Rose, 1999).

2 As a researcher, I believe that it is important to be transparent about my social location in relation to my work. This chapter is based on parts of my PhD dissertation, which was inspired by my involvement in community activism. I was first drawn to this community because of the experiences some of my close friends and family members had with the psychiatric system and my understanding that we all suffer in the context of a society that medicalizes oppression. I am also a psychotherapist, trained in counselling psychology, who is committed to resisting the medicalization of humanity. Today, my interest in the community is to participate in transformative projects that work towards eradicating systems that further marginalize people, and to participate in building communities that are founded on values of equality, nurturing, and support.

3 While the psychiatric paradigm currently dominates contemporary thinking about human experiences, other institutions play a role in reinforcing the marginalized position of those who are deemed as mad. For example, people often experience discrimination in education, employment, or health care due to their "mentally ill" status, and these institutions often serve as entry points into the psychiatric system. Furthermore, it has not always been the case that psychiatry has been the dominant institution theorizing and controlling madness. For example, up until the end of the Middle Ages, madness was largely understood as a spiritual phenomenon, often viewed as demonical possession, and was controlled and suppressed using such methods as torture, exorcisms, and judicial murders (Porter, 2002).

4   The way I am conceptualizing this community emerged from my ethnographic work, and its organization makes sense from my vantage point, but I would like to acknowledge that it does not represent the only way this community can be conceptualized. While it serves as a useful organizing tool in my understanding of the community, I am aware that differently situated community members might come up with a different community model based on priorities and understandings that vary from those inherent to my understanding. What I am offering here is one perspective on this community, a glimpse at areas of contention within, and some ideas that can hopefully help us nurture stronger solidarity networks, with the ultimate goal of building a stronger political community addressing the needs of psychiatrized people and other marginalized people.

5   Sanism is a term widely used within the community that refers to the inequality, prejudice, and discrimination faced by people who are constructed as "crazy" within dominant culture. Perlin (2003, p. 683) defines sanism as "an irrational prejudice of the same quality and character as other irrational prejudices that cause and are reflected in prevailing social attitudes of racism, sexism, homophobia and ethnic bigotry."

6   In the 1960s, when biological psychiatry was first becoming a major force in the theorizing and treatment of madness, dissenting psychiatrists began to speak out against the medicalization of human emotion and perceptual experience, bringing forth important questions about how historical and social context shape the psyche and about the social control function psychiatry plays in the organization of society (Foucault, 1962; Goffman, 1961; Laing, 1960; Scheff, 1966; Szasz, 1960). In many cases, these theorists opposed physical interventions used in biological psychiatry and instead advocated for talk therapies or other types of alternatives. Many of these theorists were labelled as antipsychiatry and are recorded in the history books as antipsychiatry professionals, despite the fact that many did not meet the criteria of today's antipsychiatry activists to merit this label (that is, holding a political position for the total abolition of psychiatry), and despite the fact that many outright rejected the antipsychiatry labelling of themselves. Nevertheless, they developed theories that have had a major impact on what is known today as the antipsychiatry constituency, as well as particular strains of thought popular within both the psychiatric survivor and Mad constituencies, and their work is often considered foundational to the contemporary antipsychiatry movement.

7   This perspective does not altogether dismiss critical Mad approaches to science, described by participants, that are interested in developing better understandings of biological processes associated with different states of consciousness and diverse emotional and perceptual experience, but rather rejects the overly simplistic biologizing of human experience and the erasure of social, material, and historical context that is endemic in psychiatric theory and practice. See Chapter 3 of my doctoral dissertation for further discussion (Diamond, 2012).

Appendix 4.1: Participant Information

A total of 40 people participated in this research by taking part in one or a combination of the following research activities: a Freirian codification group with psychiatric survivors and Mad people (n=9), a focus group with community activists (n=14), a focus group with members of my research support team (n=3), semi-structured one-on-one interviews (n=17), and unstructured interviews or conversations (n=7). All research activities took place between May 2008 and August 2010. In this chapter, the following 16 participants are cited:

Charlie*
David Reville
Don Weitz
Erick Fabris
Florence*
Geoffrey Reaume
Hope*
Jackie*
Jenny Blaser
Jeremiah Bach
Louise Tam
Ricky*
Rora*
Rudy*
Ruth Ruth
Shoshana Erlich

A combination of pseudonyms (marked with * in the above list) and real names is used throughout this chapter, reflecting how participants wished to be represented in the research.

CHAPTER 5

A Rose by Any Other Name:
Naming and the Battle against Psychiatry

Bonnie Burstow

Gazing into my computer screen, I am looking right now at a poster for Toronto's Mad Pride 2011, where it is my honour to be speaking shortly. I see words that are well within my comfort zone, many that even delight me—terms like "Mad pride," "survivor," and "rights." I see others that create an unmistakable disjuncture—phrases like "mental health awareness discussion." I am aware that such phrases belong to an entirely different discourse—indeed, one which is in critical ways incompatible with the discourse bodied forth by the words quoted earlier; and I wince at a mixture with which I am familiar but that inevitably concerns me. I also think back to first receiving an invitation to write a chapter for this important book. The opening lines read, "Would you like to contribute a chapter to a book on madness? We are presently developing an edited collection of essays tentatively entitled *Mad Matters*" (R. Menzies, personal communication, November 21, 2010). As someone who uses very different words and conceptualizations, this too created a disjuncture, albeit a minor and resolvable one. Again I am reminded that as a species, we live in and through words, that words matter. It is precisely because words matter—matter more than it is convenient to take in—that I chose to write a chapter about the significance of words in the battle against psychiatry.

A biographical note—an academic in my late sixties, I come from a family intruded on in devastating ways by psychiatry. I have been an active member of the antipsychiatry movement for over 30 years. Correspondingly, like Diamond (see Chapter 4), I see myself as part of a complex community with quite different constituencies, though one held together by a common cause—we all of us take serious issue with psychiatry.

The backdrop of this chapter is psychiatric discourse and psychiatry as what Dorothy Smith (1987, 2005) calls "a regime of ruling." The purpose of the chapter is to explore the various ways in which different parts of our community challenge and offset psychiatry discourse and the discourse that reinforces it. What is every bit as significant is to see ways that we fall into that discourse. It is not to trace a history, albeit inevitably history will enter in, for our choices stem from and create history. It is rather to get a general picture of the strengths and weaknesses of our semantic choices and to help us make more judicious choices. In this, I am guided by the lessons of feminism as well as by popular education. Insofar as our "ontological vocation" (Freire, 1970) is to name the world in order to change the world, it is critical to keep reflecting on our discourse, for we need discourse that serves us. Minimally, we need to remember that, as Audre Lorde (1984) puts it, "the master's tools will never dismantle the master's house."

The Backdrop: Psychiatry as a Regime that Names the World

Every day throughout the world, individuals have spiritual crises, have hard times. Maybe they have lost their way. Maybe, as happened with my father (an ECT survivor), they were a breadwinner who fell into financial distress, found themselves unable to part with their last dollar. Maybe they are a mother who casts an uneasy glance at the pile of dirty dishes and cannot bring herself to budge. At this point, the people in question are in distress. Should psychiatry enter in, by invitation or otherwise, in the blink of an eye the story alters—alters dramatically. The person is now "mentally ill" and in need of "treatment." Herein lies her entry into a regime of ruling.

That psychiatry is a regime of ruling is clear. It is a mammoth industry ensconced in law. It is the only profession allowed to incarcerate people who have committed no crime. Its words, indeed, are backed up by law, have the force of law. A person is "schizophrenic" or is "of danger to self or others" because someone in this industry has uttered what Austin (1961) calls a "performative utterance"—something essentially true by virtue of the right person uttering it. Its central concept is "mental illness," and that concept is hegemonic; it is seen far and wide, from the ditch-digger to the bank president, as referring to an actual illness. Psychiatry and its discourse are hegemonic because we believe in doctors, because "mental disorder" is embedded in law, because there are bureaucracies in every major city devoted to it, because the work of researchers throughout the globe is predicated on it, because a massive

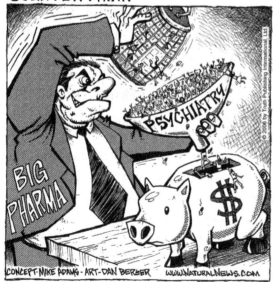

FIGURE 5.1: Big Pharma

In this cartoon, Mike Adams and Dan Berger have collaborated to depict the collusion between psychiatry and the pharmaceutical industry.

Source: Mike Adams, The Health Ranger of www. NaturalNews.com, 2006.

amount of the public purse is spent on it, because a veritable army of state officials—
"nurses," "doctors," "police," "social workers"—are paid to deal with it, because it
is actively propped up by the ever-growing multinational pharmaceuticals, indeed
even the World Bank. Colbert (2001) is undeniably correct that there is no marker for
"mental illness." In the face of an industry this formidable, however, such facts have
little traction. Nor do decisive critiques such as those of Mirowski (1990) and Brown
(1990), which expose the diagnoses as fundamentally flawed conceptualizations. The
credibility and the "work" of the institution continue.

Now as Szasz (1997) and others have pointed out, medicine is hardly the first
profession to exercise control over the madness turf. And so to historians the attention
that we pay medicine may sometimes seem overblown, for a new regime will eventually
replace it. Informed though this vantage point is, however, psychiatry is what is before us.
What faces us at this moment in history, moreover, is unprecedented—an ever-growing
industry, which is worldwide and which manufactures progressively more labels and
captures more and more people in its net. What we have—and this is rendered invisible
when we look at nothing but the perhaps kindly doctor or nurse facing the patient—
is a government-entrenched regime of ruling, with billions of people performing the
"work" of the institution, with all of that ruling mediated by texts. There are simple
texts such as the "patient's chart." There are higher-level governmental texts such as
mental health laws (which, among other things, enable people convicted of no crime
to be incarcerated). There are professional texts such as the *Diagnostic and Statistical
Manual of Mental Disorders*, which establishes "diseases" and "diagnostic criteria"
and whose words govern lower-level texts. With all these texts and the ruling so clearly
mediated by words, words cannot be seen as innocent; words could not matter more.

Real problems in the real world may be traced back to this regime of ruling.
Correspondingly, there are many battles to be waged as we contend with the damage
caused; and the community of which I am a part has been waging them—whether
it be the battle for independent advocacy or making a case for non-medical support
services. Even if it does not materially chip away at psychiatry, all of this is important,
as it leads to what I have called "attrition" (see Burstow, 2010). This notwithstanding,
it would be a mistake to underestimate psychiatry's demonstrated ability to fold other
discourse and other services into itself. Bottom line—as long as the medical model
remains hegemonic, as long as the average person believes in "mental illness," we
cannot appreciably stem the tide of psychiatry; and as long as we cannot stem the
tide, irrespective of whether we achieve independent advocacy or not, irrespective of
whether or not there are sensitive psychiatrists, legions of people will continue to be
harmed. Hence the importance of waging this battle conceptually as well as in the
manifold other ways that we do.

Unquestionably, part of the conceptualization work facing us involves creating
critiques that problematize the discourse underpinning this regime. Our community has

produced many such critiques—often stunning critiques—and they should continue. There is another level of semantic resistance, however, that also matters, arguably that matters far more. The point is, despite excellent critiques, psychiatric discourse remains hegemonic. The average person in the street speaks of "schizophrenia," of "mental illness" or "symptoms" of this or that "mental disorder." When we talk this way, irrespective of our intentions, we are performing our designated role in the work of psychiatry. Just like the nurse who picks up a chart, we are activating it; we are helping it to exist. On the other hand, when our talk is psychiatry-resistant or even psychiatry-free, we do something very different, potentially even revolutionary. Simply by how we speak, in other words, we are either tacitly upholding or undermining psychiatric rule. To varying degrees and in varying ways, we as a community (the resisting community already referred to) have been doing both.

Their Language, Our Language

We are all of us familiar with psychiatric language. It includes words like "mental health," "diagnosis," "mental illness," specific diagnoses like "schizophrenia," words like "patient" and "doctor." The government bureaucracy under which "mental hospitals" fall uses similar words, albeit these days it also uses ones like "consumer." While the government and medical terms are not always identical, for the most part they are interchangeable, with both constituencies drawing on the other's words, albeit with the government veering more to the bureaucratic and consumer-oriented. People in the "resisting" community in turn have generated and continue to generate their own sets of words, all to varying degrees commenting on or displacing the terms of the regime. Some are meant to normalize what psychiatry is seeing as aberrant. Others constitute a more obvious refusal of the psychiatric term. I call both of these types "refusal terms." Additionally, we employ terms that haunt the popular imagination, while technically belonging to a regime of ruling that predates psychiatry. I am calling this last set "reclaimed terms."

What follows is a table of terms, in no way intended as exhaustive. The first two columns contain expressions employed by psychiatric professionals and their government counterparts, respectively. The third and fourth contain words that replace the medical and government terms. Some are markers of identity and should not be seen as responsive only. Nonetheless, they are also words that our community uses in their stead—same denotation, as it were, different connotation and conceptualization. While I gleaned the "refusal" and the "reclaimed" terms from documents that have appeared at different times in history, I would add, all are still in use.

The words contained in column four (the refusal terms) largely originated in the antipsychiatry movement. Some, such as "survivor," have been widely adopted throughout the community, as have terms like "patients" when enclosed in quotation

TABLE 5.1: Terminology

Medical Term	Government Term	Reclaimed Term	Refusal Term
committal	committal		incarceration
depressed	depressed		sad/low energy
diagnosis	diagnosis		label
electroconvulsive therapy	electroconvulsive therapy		shock
hallucination			hearing or seeing what others do not see or hear
hospital, psychiatric facility	hospital, psychiatric facility	loony bin	psychoprison
medication, psychiatric medication	medication, psychiatric medication		psychiatric drugs
mental disorder, mental illness, mental disability	mental disorder, mental illness, mental disability	disability	a way of being or processing that psychiatrists do not see as "normal"
mental health	mental health		sense of well-being
mentally ill, mentally disordered	mentally ill, mentally disordered	Mad, lunatic, psycho, crazy, nutter	troubled, having emotional problems, having problems in living, having a spiritual crisis
mental patient, psychiatric patient	consumer, consumer/survivor, user	Madman, Madwoman	psychiatric survivor, psychiatric inmate, "patient"
recovery, remission	recovery, remission		feeling better; alternatively, recently acting in a way psychiatrists prefer
suicidal ideation	suicidal		thinking of killing self
symptoms	symptoms		ways of being or coping that others find problematic, sometimes also the person themself
treatment	treatment		intervention/assault

marks. I include this particular one to draw attention to a common strategy in the community—placing the regime's words in quotation marks, thereby at once using it and marking it as problematic. Others such as "psychoprisons" and "incarceration" have more or less remained the exclusive domain of antipsychiatry. To varying degrees, all of the words contained in column four are "fighting" words, many of them pointedly exposing the pernicious underbelly of what is passing as innocent. Significantly, "incarceration" and "inmate" stand in sharp contrast to "committal" and "patient." What is thereby exposed is that medicalized words are covering up something not inherently medical—control and imprisonment. This exposure, it should be pointed out, is highly reflective. As a movement enormously sensitive to the meaning of words, the antipsychiatry movement has long protested the use of medical words to camouflage incarceration and control. "Euphemisms such as 'mental patients,' 'mental hospitals,'" writes the Phoenix Rising Collective (1980, p. 2), "obscure the facts: that 'mental hospitals' are in fact psychiatric prisons ... that 'psychiatric treatment' is a form of *social control.*"

The terms in column three (the reclaimed terms) have been employed historically by the antipsychiatry movement (who can forget the Mad Market?), although for political reasons antipsychiatry activists who do not identify as part of the Mad movement tend not to use these words today. Overwhelmingly, these words are now associated with the Mad movement, with the word "Mad" particularly focal. I call them "reclaimed words" because, in the popular imagination, most have been traditionally associated with something dangerous—the madwoman, say, in the attic who will kill you any chance that she gets. What the community is doing is essentially turning these words around, using them to connote, alternately, cultural difference, alternate ways of thinking and processing, wisdom that speaks a truth not recognized (as in Cassandra, the mythological figure), the creative subterranean that figures in all of our minds. In reclaiming them, the community is affirming psychic diversity and repositioning "madness" as a quality to embrace; hence the frequency with which the word "Mad" and "pride" are associated. While not strictly speaking belonging in it, also in the third column is a term that is in a large measure responsible for bringing academic credibility to our various perspectives—"disability." While on the face of it this is a ruling regime term—hence its inclusion in columns one and two—in employing the term the community intends it in the "critical disability" sense, with disability, that is, seen as a social construct, and as such is reclaiming it.

Despite ongoing conceptual, semantic, and tactical disagreements between the antipsychiatry movement (mostly associated with the words in column four) and the Mad movement (more associated with column three), I would suggest that all of the terms in columns three and four are useful. That is, they have advantages and disadvantages, but the advantages are compelling. The downside of the antipsychiatry discourse, note, arises precisely from its most sterling strength—it is oppositional, it speaks truth to power, and for that reason alienates officials and even some potential allies. Correspondingly, it can be upsetting to survivors who do not see themselves as harmed, who view psychiatry as a benign or rapidly improving resource. These, I would add, are reasons for sensitivity, but they are not reason to dispense with these words, nor reason to tone them down, nor even reason to bypass the ones not yet adopted by the community as a whole. Ultimately, what is most distressing about these words is that they do indeed speak truth; they show what no one exactly wishes to look at, and given that the regime of ruling dispenses something less than truth, they are direly needed. In short, they keep us honest. They keep us on track. And they are the surest safeguard against co-optation. Moreover—and herein lies their greatest strength—they intrinsically stem from and foster critical analysis.

For different reasons the "Mad" language is also a "win." It facilitates celebration and pride. It gives permission to explore the forbidden regions of our mind. It promotes acceptance of difference. It acts as a link to history (see Dellar et al., 2001). It at once reframes and pokes fun at the images of "crazies" that lurk in the popular imagination, including the minds of doctors and nurses, and legislators—and make no mistake about it, ominous gendered, classed, and racialized images underpin the legal concept of dangerousness. The downside—and there is a sizeable downside— precisely because it dwells in the cultural and the existential (both highly important in themselves), is that this discourse can easily slide into liberalism, displacing the structural. What is related, when the words and concepts of a community fail to explicitly target the regime with power over it—and mostly, such is the case here—the regime in question can accommodate, provide space for celebration and consultation, offer minor concessions, and yet not appreciably change anything. Correspondingly, in the absence of a more targeted discourse, such discourse acts as a slippery slope where words and analysis become progressively less political.

This being the case, while the words in both columns three and four are being theorized as valuable, I do not see them as equal. Insofar as stemming the power of psychiatry—including "the shrink within"—is the aim, for the most part, the words in column four are more reliable. Correspondingly, even while supporting a culture of difference and freedom, words in column three can either assist or jeopardize that fight, depending on the analysis behind them and the care with which they are deployed.

And Their Language Is Our Language

Whatever vigilance may sometimes be needed in employing them, and whatever disagreements we may have with respect to them, the terms in both columns three and four serve us in significant ways. Not so for all the language used within our community. What is not surprising given the hegemony involved and the personal history of survivors, the terminology in columns one and two—the language of the ruling regime—is also alive and well, one might even say thriving in the community. I just attended Mad Pride 2011, and exciting though it was, what hit me like a thunderbolt is that terms such as "patient," "consumers," "users," "schizophrenic," and "multiple personality disorder" were repeatedly used (I stopped counting after 40 occurrences), with these terms blending in easily with Mad discourse. More generally, groups not only incorporate these words into their literature and announcements, as seen in the advertisement referred to at the beginning of this chapter, they are found in the very names of movement groups, indeed in the names given to entire constituent movements. Consider in this regard, "Patients Council," "Lothian Mental Health Service Users Movement," and "National Mental Health Consumers Association." Names such as this stand in sharp contrast to resisting names such as "MindFreedom International" (an international Mad movement organization), "Lunatics' Liberation Front" (a Canadian organization that identified as both "Mad" and "antipsychiatry"), and "Coalition Against Psychiatric Assault" (a Canadian antipsychiatry organization), or even names that are not overtly oppositional but keep the establishment at arm's length (e.g., "Support Coalition International"). For whatever reasons they are chosen—and we all of us make choices under circumstances not of our choosing—words such as "users" and names such as "Patients Council" signal that there is no real problem, indeed that psychiatry, the government, and our community are partners; moreover, they are equal "stakeholders" (another commonly used term) creating services together. In the process, analysis and resistance are compromised.

The issue is particularly serious when it comes to names designating people who are or have been "in the system." Throughout our community, the antipsychiatry part excepted, names such as "users," "consumers," and "patients" are commonplace. You hear these words at Mad Pride festivities. You find them in great abundance on websites (see the website of the Consumers Health Awareness Network, Newfoundland and Labrador, http://channal.ca). Now to be clear, individuals have a perfect right to identify how they wish; and when anyone, including an antipsychiatry activist, tells a person what they should call themselves, they are being presumptuous. That said, it is serious—not minor—when an organization within our community openly designates survivors in this way. It is still more serious when a plethora of our organizations do. Such practice activates the language of the regime of ruling and in so doing, however innocently, becomes complicit in it.

Nowhere is this more obvious than the popular word "consumer," embedded in the website cited above. When governments around the world introduced the language of the marketplace—and such this is—they were doing something shrewd, to say the least. By displacing overtly medical model terms with this seemingly innocuous and arguably uplifting discourse, they created the erroneous impression that critiques of the medical model were now less relevant. Correspondingly, they placed on the table a term that is not inherently demeaning, which creates the impression that the designee is free and in control. It announces to the world that oppression is not happening, that "psychiatric treatment" is simply one among a smorgasbord of approaches to psychological well-being that the "consumer" may consider. Ironically, the comparatively innocuous nature of this governmental nomenclature makes the name all the more dangerous. Psychiatry emerges as a benign merchant, doing nothing more than extending choices to a population once denied choice. And quite understandably, many of the people targeted become excited by the terminology and take it up. Who cannot understand Hook's (in Hook, Goodwin & Fabris, 2005) attraction to it when she states, "If I am 'consumer/survivor' of the mental health system, it means that I have choices, that I am an active participant in my treatment." No one would want to be a "patient," and therefore "passive," when they can be a "consumer" and take matters into their own hands. By a switch in nomenclature, significant progress appears to have been made.

What makes terms such as this so problematic, to be clear, is not that they do not feel better than "patient"; it is precisely that they do feel better, but via a sleight of hand. People are still subjected to a bogus medical system. Correspondingly, what is happening is still coercive. I am reminded in this regard of feminist icon and survivor Kate Millett (1991) standing in the auditorium of Ontario Institute for Studies in Education, looking everyone in the eye, and stating, "When I consume, I consume scotch. I did not *consume* psychiatric drugs. They were forced down my throat." I am reminded likewise of articles like Weitz's (1994), wherein he argues eloquently that the term "consumer" is a misnomer.

What lies behind these objections is an inconvenient truth that remains true no matter how fervently we may wish to ignore it. That is, by using the term "consumer," we are upholding the regime's pretense that there is real choice in the system. Correspondingly, we are belying a critical part of this community's raison d'être— that choice is not real, that bogus medicine is still the order of the day, that psychiatry is a coercive institution.

However the hybrid initially came about—and I leave this to others to argue about—the problem is compounded when terms like "consumer" mutate into terms like "consumer/survivor." At this point, "consumer/survivor" is employed regularly by governments far and wide, and as such is part of the regime of ruling. Now without question, it looks as if a conundrum were being solved in the very term itself; and so there is no reason to avoid it. Many members of our community like it. Indeed, it has become widely adopted within the community for it looks as though there is something here for everyone, including those who value psychiatric services, whatever their grievances. As such, it appears at once to solve problems between community and the ruling regime and to bridge the differences within our community itself. Additionally—and this clearly is operant—it can open the door to funding. The government in turn likes it, for it enables those with power to appear co-operative, and as every regime knows, one way to defeat a movement is to co-opt its language. What is wrong is that critique has inadvertently slipped away. More accurately, right within the term itself, critique is referenced and annihilated in one fell swoop. Accepting the hybrid "consumer/survivor" is a bit like the feminist movement accepting terms like "lover/rapist." Besides that, the new word has no coherent meaning; the first of the terms effectively neutralizes the second. They enable us to keep the peace all right, but at the expense of forgetting that we are at war.

This last example highlights an additional complexity surrounding the whole use of words. At the same time as names are a response to the state, they are also markers of identity, and even when they are in conformity with the regime of ruling, identities are passionately felt. While the regime of ruling is deeply implicated in the use of the words found in columns one and two—and we forget that to our peril—many people embrace them, make sense of their lives or their friends' lives in and through them. Given their significance to an appreciable number of those who have been through the system, the community as a whole (the antipsychiatry part excepted) uses the hybrid terms. They do so in the interests of being more inclusive, of bridging the divide between survivors who see themselves as having a "disorder" and those who reject the very conceptualization. This effort is to some extent successful. The problems that they present remain fundamental regardless. In other words, despite intentions that are legitimate, indeed laudable, institutional interests are largely being served.

To end by touching on one additional semantic approach that the community takes to accommodate differences in its midst, I would note in passing the strategic use of "and" as in "consumers *and* survivors." Use of such phrases is at once strategic and a heartfelt expression of connection. See, in this regard, the stirring words of Erick Fabris upon attending Mad Pride 2005 (Fabris, in Hook, Goodwin & Fabris, 2005): "I was struck by the continued presence of *both survivors and consumers....* We are proud of who we are, despite what we have been told about ourselves. *Consumers and survivors* continue to rise from the ashes" (emphasis mine).

What is gained by semantic practices such as this is that they place survivors front and centre; they recognize and are respectful of the different ways in which survivors view their experience; and they proudly affirm a common bond. What is sacrificed once again is analysis. What the phrase suggests is that there are two distinct groups—one served well by the system (consumers), one not (survivors). Again the beneficiary is the regime of ruling, for it can easily accommodate a discourse that suggests that it is doing reasonably well but can always improve. Correspondingly, the impression that this phrase creates is that people who *do not theorize themselves as being oppressed* are ipso facto *not being oppressed*. As we all know, however, oppression does not work that way. Using terminology like this, indeed, would be somewhat akin to the early feminists addressing audiences of women by the appellation "women and ladies." However benign their intentions, one has to wonder how feminism would have fared had the early feminists tried to handle semantic/conceptual divisions between women in this fashion.

Closing Remarks and Suggestions

As the foregoing suggests, the community of people who take issue with psychiatry have skillfully crafted new and highly serviceable language. Both the antipsychiatry movement and the Mad movement have put forward and continue to put forward language that provides valuable insight while at the same time displacing and, to varying degrees, unmasking psychiatric discourse. On the other hand, that same community also routinely activates psychiatric language. Even as I write these words, I glance down once again at the poster for Mad Pride, and I am aware that we have work to do. That we do it, I would add, is more important now than ever before, for progressively, psychiatry is pathologizing normative everyday life, and as such, *everyone* is in jeopardy (see Burstow, 2005). This being so, we bear a responsibility here to everyone and not only to current survivors. Correspondingly, it remains the case that psychiatry rules by words. And it remains the case that "the master's tools will never dismantle the master's house."

My hope is that whatever this chapter's limitations, people will emerge from it more word-conscious; moreover, that it will help readers grapple in increasingly reflective ways with "mental health" discourse, whether they be members of the community in question or otherwise thoughtful members of the public at large. In the interest of helping all of us who are critically minded move forward, correspondingly, I end with some tentative meta-level suggestions:

- that we take note of the "the psychiatrist within" as reflected in our language
- that insofar as feasible, we avoid the language of institutional psychiatry, including the governmental terms that prop it up
- that at the same time, we accept that individuals identify differently; and that as sensitive, caring human beings, we diligently respect their right to do so
- that "survivor" not be the sole refusal term in our repertoire
- that overall, we approach language differences in our midst somewhat more from the vantage point of consciousness-raising and somewhat less from the vantage point of accommodation (obviously, the two can connect, and hats off to those who skillfully bring them together)
- that we learn from other movements (for example, if "Mad" is to "antipsychiatry" what "queer" is to "gay," what lessons can be gleaned from the history of gay liberation?)
- that we take care not to subsume the work of all of the constituencies under language that pertains only to one (e.g., that we not call events "antipsychiatry" when they are co-sponsored by Mad organizations; correspondingly, that we not create book titles in which antipsychiatry is assumed/subsumed under "Mad")
- that we look beyond survivors in the here-and-now and ask how our language will affect the larger world, and what type of world it helps create

- that we periodically turn to early critiques of psychiatry by survivors and non-survivors alike, ponder what they are saying, how they are saying it, and why they are using the words that they do
- that we make a point of unpacking any new language by the regime of ruling, including—maybe even *particularly*—language that seems innocuous
- that we take words seriously; that we proceed reflectively, that we stop to consider such questions as: What are the subtext and context of my language? Whose discourse are we adopting? In whose interest is it? What does it make visible, and what does it remove from sight? Who does it touch and how? In the long run, does this terminology lend greater credibility to the medical model and/or institutional psychiatry? Where our words appear to support psychiatry, do we have good reason for using them regardless? A *good enough* reason? Does the trade-off that looked acceptable yesterday still look good today?

PART II

Mad Engagements

Part II theorizes the conflicted relations between psychiatric power and Mad activism by drawing together four chapters that, in various ways, explore the political dilemmas involved in challenging the premises and practices of the contemporary mental health system. The authors showcased here focus, in turn, on the practice of "Mad grief" as a strategy for contesting the medicalization of bereavement; on the experiences of objectification as witnessed in the narratives of Canadian psychiatric survivors; on psychiatrization as a form of epistemic violence that effaces the subjectivities and selves of Madpersons; and on the "double-edged sword" that is the "Mad success" of peer work in the mental "health" system.

In telling their stories of Mad grief, social workers and scholars Jennifer M. Poole and Jennifer Ward (Chapter 6) speak to the colonization of grief by the discourses and practices of modernity and medical science. Their analysis draws variously from Mad Studies, intersectionality theory and method, the social model of disability, Foucauldian notions of knowledge and power, and anti-oppressive social work practice. Poole and Ward observe how a new "science of bereavement" has come to define the conditions and experiences of good, normal grief. Like Mad folk, and *as* Mad folk, grievers who deviate from the accepted script of bereavement—those who express their loss and pain in ways that trespass these clinically and culturally established boundaries—are subject to a host of normalizing strategies. Through the binary, pathologizing lens of medicine, their grieving is construed as inauthentic, maladaptive, inconvenient, dangerous, and sick. A host of labels are devised (among them, "prolonged grief disorder"), assorted forms of "grief work" are assigned, prescriptions are filled, and the transgressive griever is disciplined and enjoined to follow the authorized trajectory back to a functional state of normalcy. As Poole and Ward evocatively show, such a rationalizing model is both oppressive and sanist. It equates with "the minimizing, individualizing, westernizing, professionalizing, categorizing, medicalizing, and sanitizing of grief." In its place, Poole and Ward embrace the practice of Mad grief—a "breaking open the bone"— as a tactic of resistance, of healing and empowerment. To grieve madly, through storytelling and other expressions of lived experience, is to subvert the disciplinary systems that, under modernity, have come to dominate and delimit bereavement. The practice of Mad grief is grounded in a recognition that human suffering comes not from the experience of grief itself, but from the scientific machinery and language that undermine grief and turn it into alienated illness.

In analyzing the autobiographical stories of five Canadian psychiatric survivors, Ji-Eun Lee (Chapter 7) details their experiences of pain and suffering, and their struggles at the hands of psychiatry. In her exposé of the seven themes that emerged from a content analysis of these psychiatric survivor narratives, Lee highlights "the ability of these writings to counter disabling master narratives." These themes include: a) understanding the label of mental illness as deviance rather than illness; b) the feelings of loss of control, freedom, and disempowerment that come with psychiatric involvement; c) the experience of coercion, repression, and punishment within the treatment paradigm; d) developing dependency on the mental health system given that it "facilitates passivity"; e) the movement from initial trust to distrust of caregivers and mental health professionals; f) the development of a stigmatized identity thrust upon patients and the subsequent feelings of self-doubt; and g) the resultant isolation and alienation from the rest of society. Using the framework of symbolic violence throughout her analysis, Lee concludes that although her reading of psychiatric survivor narratives here is concentrated on the "stories of trauma and the experience of powerlessness via the symbolic violence of psychiatry.... Yet, there is another part of this narrative—a story of their/our successful struggle and achievements in identity transformation and community organizing."

Maria Liegghio (Chapter 8) next provides a moving narrative of her mother's treatment at the hands of psychiatry during the days surrounding her death. Through this storying, she connects her personal experiences of caring for her mother with the epistemic violence experienced by psychiatrized people. Liegghio declares: "Humanity is denied not necessarily by the debilitating transformations associated with illness such as the cancer that transformed my mother's body, nor by the prejudices and discrimination associated with being socially constructed as having a 'mental illness,' but rather by a particular type of violence that targets and denies personhood." Her cogent arguments suggest that epistemic violence is inextricably linked to the construction of different forms of madness that serve to deny the legitimacy of the psychiatrized person as a "knower." The professionalized and institutionalized constructions of the psychiatrized person and their experiences, including "the details of their lives become subjugated, disqualified, and ultimately, unrecognizable." In this chapter, Liegghio demonstrates quite powerfully the ways in which family members of psychiatrized people who have passed may embrace a legacy to problematize the relations of power within psychiatry as well as retrieve and (re)assert the humanity, knowledge, experiences, and ways of being of their loved ones.

In Chapter 9, drawing from his experiences as an advocacy facilitator and coordinator at the former Queen Street Mental Health Centre (now CAMH) Patients Council in Toronto, Erick Fabris conducts a narrative-based, first-person inquiry into the politics and ethics of "peer support" in this era of "recovery-based" approaches to mental health intervention. The peer, as Fabris has learned from his years of experience in the role, occupies a fraught and liminal space between the Mad liberation tradition of community engagement and the responsibilizing forces of 21st-century biopsychiatry. In its many forms, the direct entry of survivors into "service" positions, as employees of the system, creates exciting openings for activism, resistance, and empowerment work. At the same time, peer supporters are forever subject to the co-opting forces of mainstream psychiatry, they are readily marginalized and undermined by their professional "colleagues," and what triumphs they are able to wrench from the system are often partial and contingent. Accordingly, a key question is whether "peer services [will] simply augment biomedical approaches that stigmatize ... or will they advance self-help, self-advocacy, mutual aid, and choice?" As Fabris memorably illustrates through his haunting account of a peer/client/friend whose "success" in reducing his medications and leaving hospital turned catastrophic beyond words, this question has no easy answer. Nor, however lacerating they may be, do such tragedies extinguish all hope. Notwithstanding the corrosive effects of "industrial 'necessities,' standards out of scale with human want, [and] best practices in medicine that ignore personal contexts, realities, and complexities," the decades-long history of solidarity, advocacy, and individual and community support among psychiatric survivors (however we/they may self-define) remains a legacy to cherish, and one upon which to build. "The peer movement may not be fully formed," ventures Fabris, "and that's fine. It should not be considered an end in itself, a final merging of patient and doctor, or a final version of the mental patients' liberation front. There is always more we would like to do, a double-edged sword of success, or maybe just a wish to go on."

CHAPTER 6

"Breaking Open the Bone"[1]:
Storying, Sanism, and Mad Grief

Jennifer M. Poole and Jennifer Ward

And then he was gone.

Just a few short months ago, we had been married, a glorious celebration of the life-changing love we had finally found. Just a few short hours ago, we had been out for dinner. We had laughed well, ate well, loved well, and been well. He had wanted to run an errand, so I had headed home alone to finish some work with a smile and a "see you later."

And now here I was, standing in a corner of the emergency room at midnight looking down at his still body. As if in deep repose, his eyes were closed, his hands by his side, and his face warm. And he was alone, the team of doctors and nurses now gone from his side with their machines and monitors.

I stood over him and the words "My beautiful, beautiful man" kept coming out of me. I wanted to curl up close, to wrap myself around him but the "bed" was too small for both of us, so I stood, I touched, I took out the tube in his mouth, I tucked him in carefully, and I talked to him until a cold, stomach-churning, blood-curdling horror started creeping into my bones. A few hours later, the helpful comments began, continuing through the visitations, the funeral, the memorials, the anniversaries, and all the moments since.

"So glad you two didn't have children together," "It'll look bad if you don't spend on the funeral," "You're young and you'll get married again," "He should have taken better care of himself," "You have your work to sustain you," "You should get a pet," "It's been a few months now, I would have thought things would be back to normal," "Now you have so much free time, will you babysit my children?," "I think you're making too much of this," "When can we have you back?," "When my friend lost her partner, she was so stoic, so private about the whole thing," "You should have a baby," "It's been a year, you should try dating," "I think you should talk to someone," "You're so selfish," "Do you want to end up like him?," "Have you considered medication?," "You are clearly not handling this well, perhaps you need to take time off to deal with your

personal issues," "Maybe it's time to take the photos down," "You're not your old happy self," "Take one of these a day," "Call this number," "I want you to see this person," "I want you to come back next week," "I want to introduce you to the other members."

Introduction

In many Western spaces, good grief is quiet, tame, dry, and controlled. It does not make a scene, it does not scream at the attending physician, and it does not soil its pants in shock. It does not sweat, race, wail, smash, and howl. It does not tell the truth about itself, it does not argue or say no to help. It does not resist pathology or naming, it does not resist "expert" information and referral. It knows the difference between "loss" and "bereavement." It defers to those who know best, those who came first, and is always forgiving of those who "can't handle it." It has a time limit and a limit on the range and intensity of moods, behaviours, and emotions that may be displayed. Good grief is gendered, staged, linear, white, and bound by privilege and reason. Good grief is productive, never interfering with the business, the family, or the community. It is graceful and always grateful for expert intervention. It is not angry or selfish. It never goes public. And good grief never makes a list of the caring comments uttered by friends, colleagues, family members, and professionals in the days, weeks, and years that follow its beginnings. Quite simply, good grief never breaks open the bone.

But we are not interested in good grief. In this short chapter, we will be turning our attention to Mad grief instead, a resistance practice that allows, speaks, names, affords, welcomes, and stories the subjugated sense of loss that comes to us all. And in this Mad turn, we seek to start a conversation not about how to progress, recover, and "get over" pain and loss, but how to "get under" it, feel it, and claim it as it comes.

Our interest is born of our own madness and framed by the work of many before us. As we explain in this chapter, it is born of critical/theoretical analyses by scholars such as Foote and Frank (1999) and Ord (2009), our previous work on sanism in the helping professions (Poole et al., 2012), and our critique of Western models of recovery in mental health (Poole, 2011). It is born of a reaction to traditional approaches to grief and to the ongoing encroachment of psychiatry into this sphere of experience. It is also born of our own pain, not so much the pain at the loss but the reactions to our loss including the assessments, the professionals, the concerned friends, the treatments, and the ramifications we encountered while breaking the rules of good grief. Finally it is born of our attention to moments, words, actions, and stories that have become our Mad approach to grief.

Re-theorizing Grief: On Anti-oppression, Intersectionality, Disability, and Sanism

By *Mad* we are referring to a term reclaimed by those who have been pathologized/psychiatrized as "mentally ill," and taking back language that has been used to oppress (Reid, 2008). We are referring to a movement, an identity, a stance, an act of resistance, a theoretical approach, and a burgeoning field of study (Price, 2011). As evidenced by the chapters in this reader, there are many ways to take up a Mad analysis, but because we work out of a school of social work, our particular approach is informed by anti-oppressive social work practice (AOP), intersectionality, and the social model of disability.

AOP has been defined by Dominelli (2002) as a type of social work that "embodies a person-centred philosophy, an egalitarian value system and a focus on process and outcome" (p. 6). An AOP stance assumes that there are multiple forms of oppression, that oppression is tied to unequal power relations, and that critical reflection on these matters is paramount (Healy, 2005). Tied to this approach, intersectionality is concerned with how aspects of social identity—such as race and madness, for example—intersect with oppressions such as sexism and heterosexism (Crenshaw, 1991). With respect to madness, it has been argued that "intersectionality can be thought of as the social, political, and economic processes through which oppression and privilege are experienced by individuals who have the added stigma and discrimination associated with having a mental illness diagnosis" (CGSM, 2010, p. 2).

Despite the increasing use of intersectionality and AOP, however, we are only too aware that helping professions such as ours may often see Mad folk as "in need of [either] treatment, cure or regulation" (Meekosha & Dowse, 2007, p. 170). And so, we also ground our approach in the social model of disability. It locates the difficulties that Mad folk face not simply in our "conditions" but in a "disabling society" permeated by oppressive power relations (Dossa, 2006; Race, Boxall & Carson, 2005), relations that divide, ostracize, individualize, medicalize, and prescribe.

Weaving them together (and with a nod to Foucault), we have already used these three approaches to critique the ubiquitous and popular mental health recovery model/movement/discourse, arguing that while it may not be "bad," at times and in places it is certainly dangerous, exclusive, classist, white, Western, and colonizing (Poole, 2011). Similarly, we have turned the same lens on sanism in the helping professions.

From where we stand, sanism is a devastating form of oppression, often leading to negative stereotyping, discrimination, or arguments that Mad individuals are not fit for professional practice or, indeed, for life (Poole et al., 2012). According to Kalinowski and Risser (2005), sanism also allows for a binary that separates people into a power-up group and a power-down group. The power-up group is assumed to be normal, healthy, and capable. The power-down group is assumed to be sick, disabled, unreliable, and, possibly, violent. This factional splitting ensures a lower standard of service for the power-down group and allows the power-up group to judge, reframe, and belittle the power-down group in pathological terms. It follows that, unlike other intersecting forms of oppression, sanism is rarely spoken of by the power-up group in the academy, even in expressly progressive and anti-oppressive spaces. Histories of the Mad and survivor movements are not regularly taught, pathologizing discourses not deconstructed, and rights work not invoked in favour of courses, theories, and practices that problematize Mad people. Indeed, we have argued that many educators/professionals have been so loyal to medicalizing discourses that sanist aggressions, such as exclusion, dismissal, or labelling (even in the name of "health"), have become "normal" professional practice.

What wakes us in the night is that something similar is happening to those who grieve.

On Traditional Grief Theory

A plethora of material has been written outlining reactions, models, and approaches to grief and loss (Bonanno, 2009; Breen & O'Connor, 2007; Goodkin et al., 2005; Hadad, 2009; Hollander, 2004; Kübler-Ross & Kessler, 2005; Lewis, 1961; Neimeyer, 2005; Parkes, 1996; Rando, 1993; Wolfelt, 2003; Worden, 2009). Most famous perhaps has been Elisabeth Kübler-Ross' staged model (1969). Although she later argued that grief is "not just a series of events, stages or timelines" (Kübler-Ross & Kessler, 2005, p. 203), her work opened the door to a multitude of similar models and frameworks (Hadad, 2009), and scholars continue to present grief in phases, stages, touchstones, and tasks (Kaba et al., 2005; Kübler-Ross & Kessler, 2005; Neimeyer, 2005; O'Hara, 2006; Parkes, 1996; Rando, 1993; Wolfelt, 2003; Worden, 2009). Regardless of type, the central focus of these approaches has always been on moving forward, progressing through, and returning to a state of normalcy and productivity.

Similarly, the traditional grief literature has foregrounded certain themes including individuality, the centrality of the "bond" or attachment the bereaved had with the deceased (Bonanno, 2009; Breen & O'Connor, 2007; Klass, 1996; Kübler-Ross & Kessler, 2005; Hadad, 2009; O'Hara, 2006; Wolfelt, 2003; Worden, 2009) and "making meaning" of the death (Hadad, 2009). Alternatively termed "appreciation of transformation" (Wolfelt, 2003), "meaning-making" is a form of acceptance (Kübler-Ross & Kessler, 2005) and an act of considerable importance if one's grief is to be "uncomplicated," "normal," and "good."

Critiques of the Linear

Yet as central as they are to the "new science of bereavement" (Bonanno, 2009), notions of linearity, progression, individualism, and acceptance have also been critiqued by scholars who work outside the traditional modernist knowledge terrains of psychology, psychiatry, trauma, and loss. Indeed, some critics have charged that in the privileging of progress, "dominant discourses on grief have focused on practices of pathologizing, othering and essentializing those living with loss" (Ord, 2009, p. 197). And these discourses have done this because they and the "epistemologies that underpin them are derived from the modern Enlightenment era" (Kellehear, 2007, cited in Ord, 2009, p. 198).

Such modernist assumptions privilege reason and rational truth, the construction of binaries that separate normal from abnormal (or power-up from power-down), and decide who is allowed to participate in the creation of knowledge in all areas of life, including what we "know" of grief. It follows that grief and madness have, according to Foucault, become sites of disciplinary power in which the grieving (and the Mad) must be "disciplined" by the "normal" for any irrational, unreasonable, or abnormal actions (Foote & Frank, 1999).

> People have these labels attached to them when there is "some disturbance of the normal progress towards resolution" (Rando, 1984, p. 59). *Normal* is defined in terms of *progress*, and abnormal is its opposite, the failure to "accommodate" to the loss (Rando, 1993, pp. 40, 149). Thus abnormal is described variously as absent grief, delayed grief, inhibited grief, distorted or exaggerated grief, conflicted grief, unanticipated grief, chronic or prolonged grief, and either lasts too long (prolonged or chronic) or not long enough (abbreviated). It is either expressed too demonstrably (exaggerated, distorted, conflicted) or not demonstrably enough (absent, inhibited, delayed). What is left over—as normal or "uncomplicated" mourning—becomes difficult to imagine. (Foote & Frank, 1999, p. 164).

Indeed, normal grief, if there ever was such a thing, has been "relegated to the margins" as the criteria for what constitutes "abnormal" or "disenfranchised" grief constantly expand (Foote & Frank, 1999, p. 164). It follows that the medicalization of grief has been on the rise, too, with more and more "types" of abnormal grief finding their way into the psychiatric manual known as the DSM (Breen & O'Connor, 2007; Conway, 2007; Ord, 2009). With inclusion come medical diagnoses and treatments, including "therapeutic" pharmaceuticals meant to ease, numb, and control "symptoms" of grief. Some of the treatments include cognitive behavioural therapy, complicated grief therapy and, of course, a host of antidepressants (Currier, Neimeyer & Berman, 2008; Shear, 2010; Zisook et al., 2001).

For the next version of the DSM, the talk has now turned to "prolonged grief disorder." Replacing "complicated grief," this "disorder"

> may occur when normal grief and loss processes appear to become "stuck" and the symptoms continue unresolved for months and perhaps years. The

nature and closeness of the relationship you had with your loved one (such as the death of a partner, child or parent) and the nature of death (for instance a tragic death) may also prolong the grieving process. If the usual feelings of disbelief, loss, anguish and bitterness over your loss do not go away after six months or more, and if you have difficulty functioning normally, you may have symptoms of Prolonged Grief Disorder. (Grief-Healing-Support.com)

Such a "condition" may become a "disorder" because it defies what Foote and Frank have named the "bereaved role." Inspired by Parsons' "sick role" (1951, cited in Foote & Frank, 1999), a bereaved individual is "excluded" from some forms of "work," but must attend to others such as the "grief work" of seeing a therapist or taking medication. Secondly, the bereaved must allow for and welcome *all* forms of intervention including both "professional" and "lay" forms of help. Finally and most importantly, the bereaved may only occupy this role for a *temporary* period of time such as six months. "The normal expectation is that grief will follow a time-limited linear progression from disorientation to accommodation" (Foote & Frank, 1999, p. 168), and that the bereaved will return to a productive role in society.

For all these reasons, we charge much of the "new science of bereavement" (Bonanno, 2009) not only with modernism but also with sanism. In many Western spaces, the new science of bereavement has separated the normal from the abnormal, the power-up from the power-down, and allowed the proliferation of a multitude of disciplinary micro-aggressions for those who grieve too long, too hard, too loud, or too quietly. Such micro-aggressions have become so common that participation in the minimizing, individualizing, westernizing, professionalizing, categorizing, medicalizing, and sanitizing of grief is "standard" practice. It comes out in a host of different ways—in the kinds of personal comments we list above, in helpful suggestions, in inadequately short bereavement leaves, in the burgeoning fields of grief and bereavement, in psychiatric encroachment, and in a general reluctance to speak, engage in, and feel with grief. We other those who wail in pain, we racialize those who may do it in non-Western ways, and we continue to keep the grievers out of the production of knowledge on and about grief.

Storying Mad Grief

Ruminating on these concerns, in the summer of 2011 we found ourselves at a talk on "how psychiatric survivors can use our stories to change the world" by disability activist, poet, scholar, and author Eli Clare. We also found ourselves riveted by his analyses of storytelling. He thought out loud about the "stories we tell and the stories we don't and the stories that turn over in our bellies." He spoke of their power to be co-opted, to be marketed, and to always transform. He noted that "storytelling is always an act of translation," always a risk, and that we must listen to stories across power, letting ourselves be guided by what we hear. In defence of storytelling and its role in Mad activism and studies, he urged us to tell our stories, to know that one story always begets another, but he also asked us a life-changing, knowledge-shifting question. On the heart of the stories we carry, that question was, "With whom do we break open the bone?"

Curiously, some grief scholars may be in agreement with Clare's focus on breaking open and storying, for a handful have come forward and named formal grief interventions (Bonanno, 2009; Breen & O'Connor, 2007; Hadad, 2009; Hollander, 2004) and professional authority (Bonanno, 2009) as the real "problem" with grief. They suggest that the bereaved and those who aim to assist or "companion" (Wolfelt, 2003) them should turn away from the clinical "grief work" and embrace *storytelling* (Gudmundsdottir, 2009; Hadad, 2009; Hollander, 2004; O'Hara, 2006; Wolfelt, 2003). They argue that the ability to share one's story, without interruption or overt guidance, will enable others to tell their story "without shame, without stigma" (O'Hara, 2006, p. 10). Is this also a practice of Mad grief?

We believe it is and argue that an anti-sanist, non-pathologizing approach to grief has story at its core. This is not the story that, according to Eli Clare, fits with certain criteria of recovery, or "confirms our own frameworks." It simply is. And so we broke open the bone, beginning our chapter with Jennifer M. Poole's grief story—such as it is on this day—and turn now to Jennifer Ward's.

At the age of 17, my friend A was pregnant by a much older man. A had Baby Girl. She also had diabetes, never ate well, and didn't like to cook…. "Unable to care" for her daughter, for the next two years A had an endless cycle of highs and lows, financial difficulties, problems with work, lovers, and friends. Eventually, through a call to a crisis centre, A was placed on a waitlist for "counselling and psychiatric care." During this time, A began to "take out the garbage" in her life…. In my recollection, only her older sister T and I remained. We were constant caregivers. Most often, one of us would care for A's daughter and the other would try to give A reasons to stay alive.

One Friday in March of 2001, A tracked me down at work, demanding that I come to her home. Furious that I wouldn't comply, she hung up on me in rage. It was the last time we ever spoke. I went to her home that night after work…. When I arrived at her home Dido's song "Thank You" played at full volume through the locked door, stubbornly on repeat. I called and called and could hear the phone ringing. I climbed the neighbours' fence into A's backyard, only to find the back door locked and curtains drawn. I ran down the alleyway, tipping over a garbage bin to climb above and peer into her bedroom window…. Through the window and the sheer drapes, I can see her still, still on the bed. My heart sinks, hurts, and I am sure I cried out with all the dread I felt in my body. I tap softly on the window now. No banging, as though I must have known she could not hear me. Down I climb, and walk calmly to the porch, trying that which never occurred to me before. The door is unlocked, was always unlocked, and I think "stupid, stupid, why didn't you check?!" I walked into her unlocked house to find her in bed, dead from an overdose of antidepressants, insulin, and every sugary treat imaginable. Death by chocolate and spoonfuls of strawberry jam.

I was compelled to clean it all up.... Why did I clean it up? ... I was incensed that the emergency personnel walked directly through the flower garden and into her bedroom ... some were out front talking about last night's hockey game and inside I am screaming "my friend is dead!" A hand under my arm leads me to the back of a police cruiser and I think I am being supported. Disappointment being the prevailing theme of the day, I recognize that I am being "questioned," "interrogated" as though I am criminally responsible and not merely failed-friend responsible.... An officer produces several cards that I had given A over the days, weeks, and months. Silly little cards that said "I love you," and "please, please, please stay in this world with me." These cards become proof that I was not criminally responsible for A's death.... It's 11 am and someone hands me a glass of vodka. I drink it and then another, mildly aware of people saying that I should, and should not, have another. I am taken home and put in the shower. Did someone believe that I could wash all this away? ... We planned the funeral, which I can hardly recall and "I got done what I needed to do" (Jamison, 2009, p. 131).

The following month, I arrived in the office of my family doctor to report my "symptoms." Can't sleep, can't eat, terrible flashbacks, easily startled, and experiencing a range of emotions, not all of them "appropriate." Doctor is in over his head and clearly disturbed by my snot- and tear-stained face and my wails of "why?" I am quickly packaged up by his nurse, and escorted down the back stairs—so as not to "disturb" the waiting room full of patients. The nurse puts me in my car and makes sure I buckle up. "Go to the emergency room," she says, "they're expecting you."

And so it began. Quickly, so quickly Doctors 1, 2, and 3 determined I was "suffering" from post-traumatic stress disorder. PTSD, they said, was not uncommon to my experience and I should take the medicine that they could provide, and seek the talk therapy that they could not.... I imagine now, how it could have gone differently. I imagine a circle of family and friends who could sit with me and allow me the space to wail and wonder.

I imagine a doctor willing to listen, instead of writing on a pad. I imagine another doctor who recognized that I didn't want to take the pills that failed to help my friend. I imagine being a person who was "grieving the death of a friend" instead of being the person who (whispered) "found a girl who 'committed'[2] suicide, poor thing."

Discussion: Towards a Practice of Mad Grief

Jennifer Ward's imaginings speak to our need for things to be otherwise. They speak to what may be possible if the grieving were regularly welcomed to teach, write about, and story their pain without clinical assessment, and they speak to our call for more research, discussion, and practice of Mad grief. As we write this, we are reminded that we sit in a place of profound privilege, that we are "safe" enough to ask for these changes when many of our Mad peers are not. We are also mindful of how much our call for storying is indebted not only to disability scholars such as Eli Clare, but also to Indigenous scholars such as Cyndy Baskin, Lynn Lavallee, and Brenda Wastasecoot. As they have taught us over and over again, when we break open the bone and let the stories slip/spew/trip/rage from our lips, we make it possible for others to break out too.

Importantly, we note that our explorations of Mad grief are in the genesis stage, for there are many more things to read, feel, and say out loud together. There is also a growing list of brave hearts and risk-takers who have already broken open the bone. Together we are hoping to begin to change the shape of "grief work" and of "grief science" one Mad moment at a time.

Caveats aside, however, we now "know" something of Mad grief. We know it is a reclaiming of that which has been traditionally used to other, pathologize, and ostracize those who grieve. It may defy categories, binaries of normal or abnormal, may be unstageable, possibly circular, and frequently extended. It may be entirely public. It may tell its truth(s). It may or may not be painful. It may or may not come at appropriate times or in rationally/culturally/socially prescribed and faith-based ways. It may be collective. It may yell. It may not be a problem, not necessarily temporary, Western, and rational. It does not have to be a competition, with awards for deepest attachment, most socially sanctioned love, or most resourced funeral. It does not have to be a science or a market. It does not have to be disciplinary, odd, or a form of bad behaviour to be corrected or rehabilitated. With a nod to AOP and intersectionality, Mad grief does not have to add to someone's existing oppressions, but will always intersect with those oppressions. And so we need to think about how someone's self-identified gender, sexuality, and race, for example, will make it more or less safe to grieve Mad. We need to think about the disciplinary aggressions that kind of griever will already be up against. But with a nod to critical disability studies, we also need to think about what grief gives us, the gifts and knowledge it brings in its wake and how that enables us all. With such a lens, those who are grieving are not the "problem" but society's reactions are when we refuse to make room and time for all that grief brings.

When we envision a practice of Mad grief, we see encouragement for multiple approaches to the pain and an allowance that many forms of healing have a place. A practice of Mad grief would not privilege the pharmaceutical first, for example. It would not necessarily leap to a prescription. Using a Mad grief lens in practice may involve suggesting not that there is something "wrong" or "disordered" with grieving for more than six months, but that this might be exactly the right thing to do. It might suggest that the growing list of grief disorders in the DSM could be traced to neoliberalism and shifting discourses on responsible and productive citizenship. Similarly, a Mad grief lens might suggest political as opposed to clinical "grief work," such as involvement in HIV organizing, suicide prevention and postvention, or in policy change (all of which have helped us much more than the pills we were prescribed). Simply put, using a Mad grief lens might be much more concerned with connecting not individualizing, and rejecting rather than accepting certain forms of intervention and help.

Perhaps it is not so surprising that the only spaces in which we have found such grief liberation practices are those run by people like us—people who have also been constructed as wrong/sick/disordered/anxious/depressed/in need of in-/outpatient care because of how they expressed and communicated the pain. Those folks know what it is to break the rules of good grief, to want to reject help, to want to slap the commentator in anger. They know what it is to break open the bone of grief and story it from down deep. With them, we have sat and listened, nodded and known. For them, we will continue to seek.

Conclusion: The "Raw Importance of the Story"

During his talk, Eli Clare (2011) talked not only of breaking open the bone, but also of showing the "raw importance of the story." With respect to Mad grief, we have endeavoured to do just that, to break open that which has been storying away in our bellies and to show it, however raw. This showing will inevitably make us vulnerable to rebuke and "discipline" from bereavement scientists who know best. However, it is also a matter of grave importance, for we believe that grieving Mad through story is an entirely valid resistance/healing practice. It may demand that we speak to the ugliness that accompanies each empty/complex/contested space left behind by death. In such an embrace of authenticity, it may demand that we break the rules. Such transgressions may extend to "speaking ill of the dead" (Kallos, 2009), for what was imperfect in life remains perfectly imperfect in death and grief. Such transgressions may also mean working to end the commodification of grief and problematizing the inherent power of helping professions in this particular business (McKnight, 1984). In short, we who know Mad grief seek to halt the suffering that comes, not from grieving, but from the subsequent disordering and pathologizing of grief. We seek to allow grief simply to exist. Indeed, as David Reville explains, it does not want someone to "do" it, Mad grief wants someone to sit beside and be with and be in the room as well (Reville, 2011), for as long as it needs to be there.

Something tells us that stories, conversations, and studies of Mad grief may be here for a good long time to come.

Notes

1   With thanks to Eli Clare for this challenge.
2   The Alberta Mental Health Board argues that words such as "commit" add to the suffering felt by those who grieve the suicide death of a loved one. The suffering makes it more difficult for people to reach out for help or for others to reach in to assist them (www.albertahealthservices. ca/MentalHealthWellness/hi-mhw-sps-language-of-suicide-1p.pdf).

CHAPTER 7

Mad as Hell: The Objectifying Experience of Symbolic Violence

Ji-Eun Lee

Locating Myself in Canadian Mad Studies and the World of Mad Narratives

What do Canadian Mad Studies have to do with someone like me who lives in Canada as an international student from Korea? While I am usually hesitant to be so "out there" with this part of my identity, I am, indeed, a psychiatric survivor who survived the Westernized Korean mental health system. Locating myself this way, it is certainly not a surprise that because of my own lived experience, I have become passionate about Mad Studies by and for Mad people, which led me to write my undergraduate dissertation on which this chapter is based. Basically, reading people's stories about their painful struggles and sense of powerlessness in the face of powerful political actors, such as psychiatrists and the medical establishment, was one way to make sense of my own traumatic experience. Furthermore, it is interesting how, regardless of the variance in health care in different countries, there is much similarity. So I analyzed the stories of my peer survivors, and my own story is much implicated in them.

As we all know, there are extensive accounts written from the perspective of mental health professionals about patients/consumers/survivors.[1] They include case studies and educational books. And yet, there are relatively few stories about the suffering of service users from their own perspectives. Thus, one may sadly conclude that "the tendency endemic in psychiatry [is] to neglect the personal and subjective aspects of an individual's experience" (Roberts, 2000, p. 433; see also Whitwell, 2005). This exclusion of human suffering is reproduced continuously by biomedical science—a discipline that manufactures and perpetuates disorders of all kinds (Kleinman, 1988; Miller, 2004). In this chapter, I engage with the suffering of people as they become recipients of care in psychiatric hospitals, using five written autobiographical accounts of Canadian psychiatric survivors. These stories constitute valuable sources of information, telling us where the traditional system often fails.

Method

These survivor narratives were selected from a review of Canadian survivor literature since the 1970s. It was during that decade that the antipsychiatry movement came to the fore and the psychiatric survivor movement formally emerged, becoming increasingly active through the 1970s and 1980s. These narratives are found in books, and on the Internet. With one exception, all of the survivors included here are women. The stories of "outspoken leaders" in the survivor movement, as well as "ordinary" people's stories, are included in order to increase representativeness. Selections were based on the ability of these writings to counter disabling master narratives (Baldwin, 2005). The writing and re-authoring of life stories by survivors often works to contest prevailing psychiatric narratives whereby experts retell the stories of patients/consumers through professional interpretation.

Content analysis is used to identify seven major underlying themes emerging in these survivor narratives. Whereas such an approach cannot provide a holistic analysis of people's life stories (Lieblich et al., 1998), it has the advantage of revealing the consistent patterns that emerge from analyzing the stories. For the purpose of examining people's experience of powerlessness upon their entry to a psychiatric ward, the following information was collected and organized in a chart (see Appendix 7.1): whether or not they mention the experience of being silenced; if they have been hospitalized involuntarily and/or received forced treatments; whether or not they continue to use the service; and if and when they stopped treatment. This information is important because it demonstrates the range of situations that reinforce or promote people's sense of powerlessness and distress.

Bourdieu's Concept of Symbolic Violence

Coined by sociologist Pierre Bourdieu as a way of critiquing domination, symbolic violence refers to "the subtle imposition of systems of meaning that legitimize and thus solidify structures of inequality" (Wacquant, 2006, p. 3). Symbolic violence is difficult to recognize because its practices are deeply ingrained in everyday activities. The benefit of using this concept is that it shows the subtlety of violence, its possibility of occurrence without actors' intentions and/or realization (Schubert, 2002), and its systemic nature as an institutionalized form of violence.

According to Crossley (2004), "one of the key injuries which both psychiatry and the wider society might be said to inflict upon [psychiatric patients] is the symbolic violence of disqualification and stigmatization" (p. 172). Because the power of psychiatry and the mental health system depends on symbolic power to define reality and to categorize the distress people experience, the violence and other harm it can cause are also symbolic by nature. Especially nowadays, "[m]ental distress is pre-defined in [W]estern culture by the discourses of psychiatry, whose reach has extended beyond the realms of a professional clique into the domain of everyday discourse" (Crossley, 2004, p. 162). For this reason, we need to consider the broad and diverse forms of symbolic violence experienced by patients in the mental health system across a range of interventions, including psychotherapy, community intervention, involuntary hospitalization, and other forced treatments.

Major Themes Underlying the Survivor Narratives
Mental Illness as Deviance

In comparing psychiatric survivors' accounts with other mainstream literature that is largely written by academics and/or practising clinicians, one encounters contrasting explanations of their suffering. While the biomedical model of mental illness[2] focuses on the abnormality of brain chemistry or pathological causes (Johnstone, 2000), many psychiatric survivors' accounts talk about the external circumstances that have led them to be emotionally distressed and/or temporarily behaviourally out of control.

Attributing mental illness to genetic causes does not necessarily reduce stigmatization, but rather may increase stigma in some cases with its beliefs of persistence and transmissibility (Phelan, 2005, p. 319). Although not explicitly stated, many survivors seem to have the insight that framing their distress as a disorder or sickness does not take away their pain of social isolation. Shimrat (1997), for instance, asserts:

> For years the community mental health industry has been putting out literature that tries to alleviate prejudice against crazy people. But these educational efforts have been based on the notion that crazy people are sick and that it's okay to be sick. This approach doesn't work…. In any case, "the public" does not think that crazy people are okay, any more than it ever has. And we crazies are in no way helped by the belief, used to justify dubious treatments, that craziness is an illness. (pp. 26–27)

Supeene (1990) expresses a similar sentiment:

> No explanation of psychiatric suffering prevents blaming. A compassionate view of mental and emotional distress is as the outcome of hardship: craziness is just another way of suffering. But someone whom hardship has driven crazy can be told she is the author of her own hardship, or that she must have been unstable to begin with, or that she doesn't handle stress well. (p. 164)

Alternatively, survivors tend to view themselves as nonconformists who are arbitrarily labelled as mentally ill by those who are in positions of power and who have a vested interest in the mental health industry. Weitz chronicles how his nonconformity and rebellion were perceived by his parents to signify that there was something wrong with him: "I suppose I said what might be interpreted as some impulsive or insulting things to my parents. They didn't know what to do with me…. I wasn't the good, middle-class Jewish son that I had been. I was acting weird. I said I wanted to join the Marines during the Korean war. All this convinced my parents that I needed treatment" (Weitz, in Shimrat, 1997, p. 46).

Shimrat (1997) also starts her narration with this notion of nonconformity: "All my life, people have been telling me that I'm weird" (p. 11). She goes on to say that "[she] was crazy when [she] got locked up, but not sick" (p. 16), signalling that her acknowledgment of nonconformity was not the same thing as the admission of illness. In another account, Weitz (1988) recalls a psychiatrist's refusal to understand him on his own terms, and the latter's inclination instead to engage with his parents' understanding: "I was angry at my parents and with good reason.... The shrink refused to understand that. According to them, I was 'mentally ill' or 'schizophrenic'— not angry" (p. 287).

In line with the above survivors' accounts, a compliant patient is generally seen as less ill and is treated better than a non-compliant patient by the hospital staff. Patients in a locked ward, through many trials and errors, learn this lesson over time. It is these patients who are seen as recovered and who get discharged quickly. Shimrat (1997) was given an injection of sedatives and placed in a seclusion room where she felt sheer humiliation and terror. Coming to a realization that there was no one to protect her but herself and that she could be there forever, and because all kinds of horrible things were done to her for the purpose of "treatment" and behavioural change, she started to "behave." "After a long time, I hit upon the magic words that would actually open the door: I told them I understood that I was sick, and I was willing to take their pills. They let me out into the ward" (pp. 14–15). These kinds of incidents are commonplace, because there seems to be little or no understanding of the distinction between refusing help and non-compliance. Whereas patients in a locked ward are exercising their rights, hospital staff tend to paint all with the brush of non-compliance. This distinction is conflated with the prevailing view that associates resistance to treatment with people's "lack of insight," taking it as the very evidence of one's mental illness.

Loss of Control and Freedom, and Disempowerment

Although "powerlessness" originated as a psychological construct (Baistow, 2000), people's experiences of feeling powerless and helpless have a social basis. What could be more disempowering than being committed to a psychiatric ward?[3] From the moment of committal, the person loses the freedom to make basic daily life decisions and to exercise choice over all the things (i.e., movement, diet, activity, social contact) that most people take for granted. Although the patient who comes to the hospital voluntarily may be treated better and be given more freedom than their involuntary counterparts, their status can shift abruptly. There is also the question of what is "truly" voluntary. Recalling her experiences with institutionalization, Findlay (1975) suggests that if fear and manipulation are used to make one "voluntarily" go into the hospital, one's admission is not voluntary in any meaningful sense. "Dr. Young and Dr. Duggan," she writes, "put me in psychiatric hospitals. They didn't commit me; they merely threatened to commit me if I didn't sign myself in. I went" (p. 65).

Powerlessness is further heightened as the newly admitted patient becomes aware of how little choice she has in coping with the hospital environment and in the direction of treatment:

> I was surprised when the nurse stopped to give me my morning drugs. He must have the wrong person, because I wasn't here for pills.... When I asked what the pills were for, the nurse replied, "The doctor ordered them. Take them, they are good for you!" (Pratt, 1988, p. 61)
>
> As I wondered how much longer I could tolerate this situation, the psychiatrist suddenly informed me that, starting the next day, he was going to give me shock treatments.... When I had to sign a release form for the shock treatments, I didn't realize that I had signed away all my rights and power. (pp. 62–63)

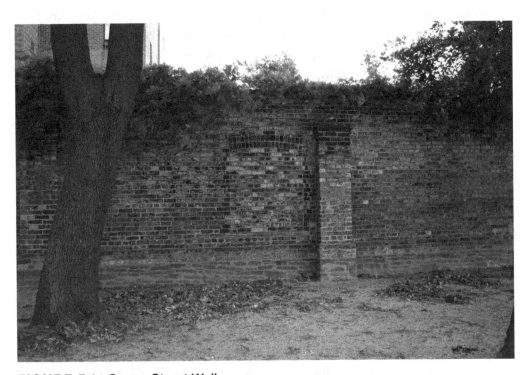

FIGURE 7.1: Queen Street Wall

South boundary wall built by unpaid patient labourers in 1860 at the then Provincial Lunatic Asylum, now the Centre for Addiction and Mental Health in Toronto.

Source: Geoffrey Reaume

Don Weitz recalls his experience of loss of control and feelings of disempowerment as a result of insulin shock treatment:

> My insulin-induced hunger or forced starvation was intense and excruciatingly painful. It went to the core of my very being.... Subcoma shock, also called hypoglycaemic shock, was extremely debilitating and torturous.... As [insulin] dose increases, you lose considerable emotional and physical control.... 110 insulin shocks later, I felt wasted physically-emotionally-intellectually, I was totally wiped out from this so-called "safe and effective treatment" for "schizophrenia." (Weitz, 2003)

Moreover, people feel disempowerment not only in the face of a drastic treatment but also in the everyday life of a psychiatric ward. In such an insulated place with much restriction over freedom of movement, people have to rely on the hospital staff for such basic things as getting medication for a headache. Supeene (1990) talks of the frustration of waiting for the hospital staff to take action on a request: "Patients were expected to be available whenever their doctors wanted them. So if you wanted a weekend pass or change in medications or whatever, you couldn't leave the ward until your doctor found time for you. We were always waiting for something" (p. 27).

In studying patients' feelings of safety and threat on an acute mental health ward, Wood and Pistrang (2004), through semi-structured interviews with both hospital staff and in-patients, found that patients' complaints are routinely silenced by the staff's repeated inaction, inappropriate responses, and unavailability (see also Robins, Sauvageot, Cusack, Suffoletta-Maierle & Frueh, 2005). These experiences, along with other normalized practices such as forcible administration of medication and restraints, inevitably result in increased feelings of helplessness, and loss of trust and safety (Wood & Pistrang, 2004).

Additionally, not knowing what is being recorded about his/her behaviour in the chart and the feeling of being "on public display" can be an utterly disempowering experience, as the following two narratives testify:

> Since I was suicidal they put me on "constant observation" which meant that I was watched 24 hours a day by a ward aide who sat at the foot of my bed and read *True Confessions*. Every move that I made was "symptomatic"— a feature of my disease. They searched my belongings.... I was naked and there was nowhere to go to escape their eyes.... My self no longer resided in my body ... but in a file folder accessible to everyone in the hospital but me. I had no way of knowing what was in the folder, whether it was true or false, compiled by a series of doctor's remarks and nurse's shift notes. (Findlay, 1975, pp. 69–70)

[M]y problems and emotions were in the public domain but theirs were their own. (Supeene, 1990, p. 38)

Coercion, Repression, and the Feeling of Being Punished

From the clinician's point of view, one condition of treatment is that patients comply with the plans and goals. In fact, when other treatments fail and the patient is difficult to manage, there remain only four options: "seclude them, restrain them, medicate them or pass the problem to someone else" (Mason, as cited in Hoekstra, Lendemeijer & Jansen, 2004, p. 277). However, mental health service users and psychiatric survivors argue that the use of force should be permitted only as a last resort with strict criteria attached, because it is traumatic and results in the loss of trust in the service and in the professionals (see O'Hagan, 2004a).

Hoekstra et al.'s (2004) research on psychiatric patients who have been secluded (locked in a small room alone) for a period of time vividly sketches people's acute feelings of losing power and autonomy when going through such an experience. In particular, they feared the absolute power of the nurse and the reoccurrence of seclusion. Being unable to talk about their experiences with others also gave them no option but to rely on themselves in order to cope with the traumatic effects of seclusion (Hoekstra et al., 2004).

In a psychiatric ward, the possibility of coercive intervention is often unspoken; nevertheless, it exists to strike fear in patients and to control their behaviours. When co-operation becomes difficult to come by, however, the clinical staff creates a context of coercion tacitly, knowing that patients are unaware of their rights and of the mental health legislation, by simply telling them that they *have to* (Sjöström, 2006). As a result, patients believe that they do not have a choice and that if they do not comply, they will be coerced. Some of the experiences of coercion shared by the survivors selected for this analysis are evident in the following narratives. Supeene (1990) confirms the implicit nature of coercive power in psychiatry:

[Y]ou assume threats are there even though they're not stated.... [C]onscious coercive intent is not required for every instance of coercion. On the contrary. Conscious effort would be required to refrain from coercion. Staff would have to state explicitly that the patient was free to make decisions of treatment and it would have to be spelled out that there weren't any strings.... No one could be certified or involuntarily discharged in retribution for non-violent non-co-operation. There could be no screaming in the bubble room, and no drugged zombies in the halls. (pp. 35–36)

Other common incidents where patients may get "punished" occur when they refuse to take medication. As an example, a young man who was in the same psychiatric ward as Pratt (1988) was given electroshock the day following his refusal to take medication (p. 69). In another account, a patient who simply desired to go for a walk was seen as deliberately disobeying, and thus directly challenging the authority of her psychiatrist. All of sudden, four men appeared and

> each took an arm or leg and half-dragged, half-carried me back to the isolation room.... They threw me on a cot in the isolation room where my coat and jeans were forcibly removed. I tried to bury myself in the blankets, not knowing what other clothing was to be removed or what was to happen to me next. I felt violated by four men who watched me as my jeans were stripped. A needle was jammed into my hip, a sedative I believe. The psychiatrist warned me that if I ever went for a walk again I would be transferred to a locked ward in a large city hospital. He also informed me that shock treatments would start the next day. They left me thoroughly humiliated, with wounded pride and a sore hip. (Pratt, 1988, pp. 66–67)

These kinds of repeated exposures to the experience of being "crushed" (Chamberlin, 1995) will, in time, lead to what is called "spirit breaking." According to Deegan (2000), this breaking of spirit "occurs as a result of those cumulative experiences in which [they] are humiliated and made to feel less than human, in which [their] will to live is deeply shaken or broken, in which [their] hopes are shattered and in which 'giving up,' apathy and indifference become a way of surviving and protecting the last vestiges of the wounded self" (p. 200).

Ultimately, patients give up fighting against the institution and surrender in exhaustion. For it is only when they are seen as "getting better" and, hence complying with treatment and behavioural norms, that they are able to speed up their release from the hospital. Weitz (1988) mentions how this "recovery" process induces a patient to conform—first, becoming compliant with a treatment, and then, saying things that the psychiatrists like to hear:

> [The two months of subcoma insulin shock treatment] succeeded in making me conform and stop saying things conventional people might think were outlandish. (in Shimrat, 1997, p. 46)

> I persuaded the shrinks to let me out by telling them I planned to go back to university—a nice conventional, middle-class thing to do, and be a "good boy." (Weitz, 1988, p. 288)

If one behaves better or pretends to feel better for fear of being punished and/or detained longer, is this really an improvement?

Although some of the hospital staff may well be aware of the harmful effects of these treatments and the spurious changes that the fear produces, they may still use force and other methods that are terrifying to already confused patients. One possible reason for the continuing use of force is that, through their professional training and occupational socialization, staff are encouraged to distance themselves from patients. By empathizing with patients, professional mental health workers may not be able to maintain the necessary emotional distance required to carry out unpleasant duties like restraining patients (Wood & Pistrang, 2004).

Dependency on the Mental Health System

In many survivors' experiences, the system facilitates passivity (see Roe & Ronen, 2003) and dependency (Marsh, 2000, p. 1452). One example is the reliance on medication to manage symptoms, as Shimrat (1997) recounts: "They had me on a drug called Haldol, which I later found out was a neuroleptic. It made my muscles spasm. It hurt to move, but I couldn't keep still. My hands and feet twitched. My face convulsed. I drooled when I lay down. My skin was so dry it was coming off in flakes. I was horribly constipated. The Haldol didn't touch my craziness, though" (p. 15). Supeene (1990) adds: "It is much more helpful to learn to change what you see ... than to resign yourself to taking strong psychotropic drugs which dull all your power of perception" (p. 46). Another example is electroshock therapy, which erases one's memories and induces passivity and compliance. While Shimrat (1997) was able to escape electroshock treatment due to her mother's resistance, her "roommate" patient was given shocks for her "impulsive" buying and "inappropriate" dressing behaviour, which were considered signs of "manic-depressive" illness (pp. 20–21).

Broadly speaking, for almost all psychiatric survivors, human agency has been compromised by the denial of self-determination in traditional mental health care, even though it is essential for recovery (see Kumar, 2000). In Supeene's (1990) words: "Psychiatry contradicts itself. It asserts that the patient is an autonomous person worthy of respect who must be helped to become more autonomous. But patients are helped as the doctor thinks best. So much for autonomy" (p. 38; see also Findlay, 1975).

Nowadays, we observe a shift in official and public images of psychiatrized people. People who were once seen as passive patients are now considered active consumers (Lupton, 1997). Influenced by the incursion of consumerism into health care, people are "empowered" to be in charge of their own health and to make the decisions that are best for them. Whereas this liberal humanist rhetoric of empowerment may sound promising, it has been criticized for its vagueness and failure to produce results (Masterson & Owen, 2006; McCubbin & Cohen, 1998). Whatever the rhetoric of self-empowerment informing the mental health system, society continues to believe that "mental patients" are not rational and do not know what is best for themselves (see McCubbin & Cohen, 1998). This belief strengthens the paternalistic attitudes of mental health professionals, as evidenced by the fact that "informed consent" requirements are often ignored and inadequately explained to patients. The seemingly contradictory empowerment rhetoric and paternalistic practices help psychiatry to maintain the denial that many who seek help are ordinary people (Johnstone, 2000), and to monopolize their classification into different psychiatric disorders. One undesired and paradoxical effect for those who come in contact with the psychiatric system is that their seeking help is both encouraged and pathologized at the same time.

As revealed in the sample survivor narratives, patients also become dependent on the mental health system and workers, due largely to the fact that the hospital environment bears little resemblance to the outside world. Without sufficient preparation prior to discharge, patients are not ready to deal with the daily demands that exist outside of mental hospitals. As a result, if newly discharged patients are unable to access the assistance they need, they may fail to cope and accordingly be readmitted to the hospital. This will reaffirm the mental health workers' beliefs that the patients are severely ill, while confirming the patients' fear that they cannot make it without help from the system, no matter how hard they try. The following excerpts from the survivor narratives illustrate the initial terror of returning home from hospital and this hard-to-break cycle of readmission:

> They let me go. Needless to say, none of the problems that had driven me crazy in the first place had been addressed by the professionals in charge of me. (Shimrat, 1997, p. 17)

> When the psychiatrist agreed to let me go home, he said that I should make an appointment to see him in two weeks. I panicked. It was the same as before—going from total dependence to total independence. (Pratt, 1988, p. 67)

> There were more hospitalizations. Each time I was admitted, it only confirmed my belief that I was really crazy and needed psychiatric help.... [D]epression due to the belief that I was incurably crazy, admittance to the mental health centre, increased depression because this only confirmed my suspicions, shock treatments, release—starting the circle again.... If you committed suicide, they said you went to hell. I had hell on earth. (Pratt, 1988, p. 65)

Movement from Trust to Distrust (of Caregivers and Professionals)

It is a mistake to think that psychiatric survivors are unusually skeptical people. On the contrary, the narratives of the survivors canvassed in this study showed that they did not have such an attitude when they first sought help. Indeed, these psychiatric survivors' testimonies illustrate a process whereby trust is lost; a movement from naiveté to suspicion. Their growing sense of disappointment and betrayal was directed not only towards the mental health professionals and the system that hurts in the name of help, but also towards those caregivers (i.e., family, friends) who, rather than choosing other methods of helping or questioning the experts, decided to entrust their loved ones to the hands of psychiatrists. Although not as explicitly mentioned as the sense of disappointment and betrayal they felt towards mental health professionals and the system, this sentiment exists in most of the sample narratives. Not being able to trust those to whom one is closest, in and of itself, causes an extremely painful sense of grief and loss; it can be dangerous to one's sense of self. Pratt's (1988) depression may then be understood as a perfectly normal outcome: "I was sure these people would know what was needed to help me. After all, they were the ones who had admitted me, diagnosed me, prescribed drugs and wrote reports about me. So here I was, deciding to make my life an open book, but no one was turning the pages. I became more and more depressed" (p. 62).

Unfortunately, the loss of trust is too great for some patients/consumers, and they permanently withdraw from the system:

> There should be a way to explain how I got from there to here. I will never go back to psychiatrists.... I don't really know what made me change. My fervent faith in the psychiatric version of my life just eroded slowly away, until I could no longer sustain the effort necessary to live in that made-up world. (Findlay, 1975, p. 71)

> I left [the psychiatrist's] office and the [mental health] centre, promising that I'd never see him, the centre or any other "mental hospital" again. I have kept my promise. (Pratt, 1988, p. 69)

Stigmatized Identity and Self-Doubt

Across cultures and in various languages, there are negative perceptions towards those who have a so-called mental illness. Community responses often show a polarity between pity and rejection. These responses are common not only among the general public, but also in the perspectives of mental health professionals. The psychiatric stigma, whether visible or not, will have repercussions for other aspects of people's lives, such as divorce and child custody or employment prospects. This is the case even for individuals who live in relatively progressive communities. Further, even those who are emotionally resilient are said to struggle with the discrimination and the social consequences associated with being labelled as "mentally ill" (Johnstone, 2000; see also Herman & Musolf, 1998). As Pratt (1988) recalls, it was her fear of being crazy that paralyzed her: "I had only jokingly used the word 'crazy' before, but now its full meaning hit home, hard. The words seemed to grow louder and louder inside my brain, echoing off the walls of my head.... This feeling of being crazy and being seen to be crazy would last forever" (p. 64).

Johnstone (2000) explains the process of internalizing stigmatized identities among populations with "mental illness": "Instead of being enabled to locate a significant portion of their problems where they belong, in externally imposed conditions and expectations, they adopt and impose those same conditions on themselves, and the messages they receive about being inadequate, defective, abnormal and inferior are translated into actually *experiencing themselves* as inadequate, defective, abnormal and inferior" (p. 209, original emphasis).

Since their perceptions of reality have been repeatedly taken by others as unreal, pathological and unreliable, people with psychiatric labels begin to doubt themselves and learn not to trust their feelings and judgment (see Roe & Ronen, 2003). The narratives of Findlay (1975) and Supeene (1990) describe this process of losing self-conviction:

> The shrinks had a corner on my reality.... Because I was mentally ill I had no credibility: they could believe my answers or not, as they chose. If my answers were wrong, I was denying the problem; if I disagreed with them I was hostile and/or experiencing resistance to treatment.... If I refused to answer their questions I was resistant; if I told them it didn't matter I was denying. There was no way to convince them otherwise.... *They* got to decide what was true and real for me. And their job was to convince, persuade, seduce or threaten me to accept that reality as my own. At the time, I did not see their version as wrong, but my version as wrong.... I *believed* that I was merely hostile to, resisting, denying, my "true" problems. (Findlay, 1975, pp. 62–63, original emphasis)

> It was in hospital that I lost my determination, my courage.... It was also while in hospital that I began really to dislike and to distrust myself.... It isn't even very surprising that people who are deprived of autonomy and who are told that it is because they are incompetent to care for themselves come to believe it and to doubt their own strength and distrust their own perceptions and decisions. (Supeene, 1990, p. 59)

Also, patients can easily notice when other patients go through this process of losing faith in themselves. Shimrat (1997) provides an explanation for this sad phenomenon:

> Every day I talked with Penny and other women patients who were convinced that they were bad people. All of them were perfectly nice people, but had been persuaded otherwise. I think it was often some combination of growing up female, being screwed around by their families and by men, and what happened once they were in the hands of the "helping" professionals that made them so mixed up. (p. 22)

Isolation/Alienation

Human suffering has the potential to isolate the sufferer from the rest of society. When a person experiences a disability, unemployment, loss of a loved one, or a personal crisis, the pain of living may intensify to the point where he/she withdraws from others. Similarly, people who experience emotional distress often retreat from social encounters despite their need for social companionship. Yet ironically, sometimes in mental hospitals a patient's friendship with another patient is viewed suspiciously, even if the relationship is reciprocal. For example, Pratt's (1988) first day at a psychiatric ward was overwhelmingly scary, but the fellow patients comforted her. That "[patients] were better than the trained staff at helping each other" (p. 60) seemed strange to her. For Shimrat (1997), likewise, friendship with other patients "kept [her] going" (p. 16). Despite the importance of friendships, staff are often reluctant to facilitate them among patients and ex-patients. As Supeene (1990) recollects, "[o]n the ward, friendship was very important. Unfortunately, former patients were prohibited from visiting the ward.... This rule prevented or hindered friendships from developing among patients, thus cutting off important mutual support, and reinforcing patients' dependence on professionals" (p. 29).

A nagging sense of needing to be out of the hospital, combined with the isolating experience of hospitalization, has also recurrently alienated patients from their social networks outside the hospital. Consider the anguish of Pratt (1988): "I was lonely for parents and friends. I was so far away from home and had no way of getting in touch with them" (p. 61). A patient may feel isolated due to emotional distance as much as geographical distance. An effect of her hospitalization, Irit Shimrat (1997) now realizes, is that her world and that of her family and friends who visited her grew miles apart. This estrangement was made clear by some awkward visits by Shimrat's father and mother. They were not sure what kind of face to put on when visiting their daughter in a "loony bin," and so they dealt with this stressful situation in two completely opposite ways: "[My father's] visits were terrible. He'd hold my hand and gaze into my eyes, obviously scared and miserable. I'd sit silently and wait for him to leave. When my mother came ... it was completely different. She'd put on music and dance with me. She made a huge effort to act cheerfully and normally" (p. 15). No matter how well-intended they were, while Shimrat's father's response did not help because he seemed to be immersed in his own grief, her mother's response was equally unhelpful in that she was acting as if nothing had happened—in a way, denying Shimrat's reality of being in a mental hospital. This was the moment when Shimrat realized that the communication between her and her parents had broken down; she consequently felt emotional distance from them both.

Survivors' experiences of isolation/alienation do not necessarily end with getting out of the hospital. On the contrary, for some patients, it is a lifelong struggle to cope with these disempowering experiences, especially if there are few "Others" around them who can validate their experience of the world.

Conclusion: An Insane System and a Sane Response

As we have seen, psychiatric survivors' narratives differ greatly from that of the predominant biomedical narrative in their experiences of suffering and of the mental health system. Compared to the biomedical narrative, the accounts of survivors are much more personal and immediate; there is an elaboration of contextual factors that led them to problems in living, and how treatment that is supposed to help has actually exacerbated their suffering. Accordingly, survivors' stories go beyond their symptoms—those on which psychiatry extensively focuses—and show that their lives have meaning and purpose. By now, it also should be clear that while people commit themselves or are committed by family and friends with the hope of going to a place where they can rest and take refuge from all the problems of living in the outside world, the reality of a psychiatric hospital is not conducive to such. Furthermore, the very experience of being treated like naughty children—during the admission process and throughout the hospitalization—and having an official hospital record causes shame and humiliation, adding many more difficulties in coping with life.

My motivation for writing this chapter has not been to portray them/us as passive victims. Stories of trauma and the experience of powerlessness via the symbolic violence of psychiatry represent one important part of survivor narratives. Yet, there is another part of this narrative—a story of their/our successful struggle and achievements in identity transformation and community organizing—which can be found in the writings of other contributors to this book. Given what they/we have been through and the long-lasting impact this experience has on their/our lives, the only natural response is to be angry[4] at a system that frequently perpetuates harm in the name of help, and to direct their/our anger towards changing the system. If they/we are traumatized by the system that is purporting to help, who is there to help them/us heal from these experiences? This is why psychiatric survivors are angry.

Notes

1 There are many different ways in which a person identifies herself as someone who previously used and/or is currently using mental health services. Because terminology is very important, there is much discussion and debate about the terminology of madness. To represent this diversity in how people see themselves in relation to mental health services and how they have been treated, the term *consumer/survivor/ex-patient* is often used in the literature (see Burstow, Chapter 5). In this chapter, I mainly use "patient" and "survivor." While my natural inclination is to favour "psychiatric survivor," in some places I use "patient" instead to connote unwanted captivity in a psychiatric ward.

2 The biomedical model of mental illness considers people's biological makeup as the main cause; all others, including family upbringing and life experiences, are only *precipitating* factors. This model heavily emphasizes biological intervention such as pharmaceuticals as a treatment of

choice, and its dominance in the mental health system precludes imagining other alternatives (Boyle, 2006; Johnstone, 2000).

3   Hospitalization may be a life-defining moment for those who are institutionalized. In an excellent study by Roe and Ronen (2003) on people's understanding of hospitalization, the authors observed that the majority of mental patients seem to suffer from many troublesome effects of hospitalization, including passivity, painful confrontation with the personal meaning of hospitalization, loss of one's previous public image, loss of real-life skills, and loss of self-esteem. Their findings suggest that "hospitalization is probably one of the most challenging experiences in the course of illness and recovery" (Roe & Ronen, 2003, p. 329).

4   Nowadays, anger is a demonized human emotion in our society that must to be "managed" with the help of an expert (i.e., therapist) and constant self-monitoring. For psychiatric survivors, however, being able to feel angry and to freely show its expression (in a nonviolent way, of course) without repression has another level of meaning. Since their emotional expressions in a psychiatric ward have been translated into the symptoms of their illnesses and thus must be repressed with medication and so forth, they/we find much significance in being able to do so without fearsome consequences; after all, those who do not feel angry in an appropriate circumstance cannot be "normal" either. Moreover, anger is often the starting point of recognizing the injustice around us as a precondition for taking action. This is evident in many different kinds of social movements, whether the issue is gender, poverty, or the environment. Anger, too, occupies an important place in the psychiatric survivor movement, as well as in individual survivors' healing journeys. It is the force that motivates survivors to speak out, to connect with others in solidarity, to make one realize one's strength, to step out of one's individual experience of suffering, and to take on the bigger cause of changing the mental health system to better serve people in distress.

Acknowledgment

I would like to thank each of my survivor peers before me who, by their courageous acts, have removed some of the tough obstacles to accessing our own stories. In my mind, you all are the heroes of Canadian Mad Studies.

Appendix 7.1: Powerlessness of a "Mental Patient" in a Psychiatric Ward

	Experience of Being Silenced	Involuntary Hospitalization and/or Forced Treatments	Length and Continuity of Services
Findlay, B. (F)	Implicitly assumed by the psychiatrists' interpretations that ignored her version of reality	Hospitalizations, medication, (psychotherapy)	Not clear
Pratt, M. (F)	Implicitly assumed in the experience of being given limited choices and being put into an isolation room instead of being able to explain to her psychiatrist why she wanted another option	(Counselling), drugs, 40 shock treatments, forced injection, isolation room	1978–1980? (More than 2 years)
Shimrat, I. (F)	Implicitly assumed in being ignored when yelling for help from a seclusion room, being restrained	Restraints, solitary confinement, forced injection, medication, involuntary hospitalization	Not clear
Supeene, S.L. (F)	Explicitly mentioned and implicitly assumed throughout	Medication, hospitalizations	1979–1981? (A couple of years of being in and out of hospitals + one and a half years of taking medications after the last hospitalization)
Weitz, D. (M)	Implicitly assumed in receiving insulin shock treatments without informed consent	Involuntary hospitalization, forced starvation followed by insulin coma treatments	1951–1953? ("psychiatric abuse started in 1951 when I was locked up for over a year")

Counselling and psychotherapy are included here (in brackets) under "Involuntary Hospitalization and/or Forced Treatments" because some survivors' stories included them as part of their mental health system experience (because contact with a counsellor/psychotherapist led them or others to conclude that they needed to be hospitalized, or because they received "talking therapy" during their stay as in-patients in the hospitals). However, I have found that the difference between psychotherapy/counselling and psychiatry is taken for granted by many (Western) people (feminist professors, radical thinkers, and even some survivors). Inherent in this "split" is the belief that psychiatric practices, more often than not, harm people, but that psychotherapy/counselling does not.

I have included them here to show that psychotherapy/counselling is not inherently good, and that it can be as dangerous and oppressive as psychiatric practices. In my view, these are not two distinct practices of the mental health system; rather, they are both found on a continuum, where a survivor can travel back and forth easily, with one leading to another. Placing these two terms in brackets connotes the indirect/less explicit relevance to involuntary hospitalization.

CHAPTER 8

A Denial of Being:
Psychiatrization as Epistemic Violence

Maria Liegghio

Introduction: Positioning Myself

> *I am so angry! Today on this cold, Canadian winter day I am accompanying my mother, dying of cancer, living with physical pain, and struggling with mental confusion to the palliative care unit at the hospital after spending six months caring for her at home. All her in-home nursing and personal care support has been withdrawn and we have no other choice but to consider a hospitalization against my mother's wishes. And why—because someone in their position as helping authority decided she was a risk of harm to the visiting staff because of her history of "mental illness." The mental confusion and agitation was the evidence that the "mental illness" was active. But why can't they see that the confusion and agitation is not about her diagnosis of "bipolar disorder" but rather because the liver cancer has taken over her body's ability to process the toxins. The confusion and agitation come from the accumulation of those toxins. What risk of harm could this woman, too physically withered and weak to sit up, possibly pose to herself or others?*

As I considered a beginning for this chapter and contemplated the ideas I plan to discuss, at the back of my mind sit the memories of my mother and her life with "mental illness," as defined under dominant psy discourses and practices (Rose, 1998). From the start, I cannot help but declare that at the core of this chapter are my personal experiences of the ways psychiatrized people are denied their voices and, ultimately, their very existence as legitimate knowers. Based on my experiences, I propose that madness refers to a range of experiences—thoughts, moods, behaviours—that are different from and challenge, resist, or do not conform to dominant, psychiatric constructions of "normal" versus "disordered" or "ill" mental health. Rather than adopting dominant psy constructions of mental health as a negative condition to alter, control, or repair, I view madness as a social category among other categories like race, class, gender, sexuality, age, or ability that define our identities and experiences.

Our experiences of madness inform and construct the ways we see, feel, think, interpret, and make meaning of ourselves, of others, and of the physical and social worlds around us. In addition, our "mental health" is constituted by the ways certain experiences, subjectivities, and subjects are privileged over others within society at the level of social relations, structures, and discourses. Under dominant psy discourses and practices, psychiatrized people are disadvantaged against constructions of "normal mental health" and experience their identities as pathologized and devalued, and their humanity is denied. From my experience, humanity is denied not necessarily by the debilitating transformations associated with illness such as the cancer that transformed my mother's body, nor by the prejudices and discrimination associated with being socially constructed as having a "mental illness," but rather by a particular type of violence that targets and denies personhood. This type of violence is epistemic (Spivak, 2005).

The purpose of this chapter is to explore the notion of epistemic violence and its relevance to the lives of psychiatrized people.[1] I begin by defining the concept of epistemic violence, explain its relevance, and then end with a discussion about the potential for social justice that can come from action inspired by a commitment to end epistemic violence. I propose that justice becomes possible by adopting a commitment and then practices that bring back into existence the knowledge, ways of knowing, and ways of being of people who have been psychiatrized due to nonconforming thoughts and behaviours.

Epistemic Violence and "Mental Illness": Being Disqualified as a Legitimate Knower

> *And in my anger, I look out the window at the approaching horizon and see the hospital, and I ask, what is going on? Is this really just a misunderstanding about a failing liver versus a mental illness? How is it possible that the knowledge of her impending death no longer exists and instead, the knowledge of "mental illness" and all the prejudices associated with it have taken over and are used to justify such action, as to deny the necessary services and to deny the wishes of a dying woman?*

Epistemic violence refers to the ways certain persons or groups within society are disqualified as legitimate knowers at a structural level through various institutional processes and practices (Spivak, 2005). A concept originating from postcolonial studies, epistemic violence describes and explains the institutional processes and practices committed against persons or groups, such as Aboriginal peoples, that deny their worldviews, knowledge, and ways of knowing and, consequently, efface their ways of being. For Aboriginal peoples, this includes the historical construction of their very beings as less than human—as "primitive" or "savage" (Marker, 2003). Epistemic violence does not only render the person or group invisible within society, but it is also a form of silencing that renders certain persons and groups unable to speak and to be heard (Dotson, 2011).

I propose that this type of violence has relevance to the experiences of psychiatrized people. It has relevance because of the structural ways persons deemed to have a "mental illness" are made out of existence primarily through localized psy discourses (Rose, 1998), mandates, and practices. Applied to the experiences of psychiatrized people, epistemic violence is the treatment of their knowledge and ways of knowing as something other than knowledge and other than legitimate. It is more than being silenced or dehumanized by stigmatizing and sanist practices, such as diagnosis and classification. Rather, the violence occurs when different forms of madness are constructed in particular ways and then used to diminish and deny the legitimacy of the knower. It is the very denial of a person's legitimacy as a knower—their knowledge and their ways of knowing—that renders that person out of existence, unable to be heard and to have their interests count.

Epistemic violence begins at the very place where people and their experiences intersect with the apparatuses of psychiatry. Prominent sociologist and feminist thinker Dorothy Smith (1990) asserts that "mental illness represents a recycled reality" (p. 130). She explains that "mental illness" is a social construction formed at the place where people's experiences intersect with psychiatry—its structures and practices. When individuals come into contact with professional and institutional processes, they share details about their lives (their moods, thoughts, behaviours, fears, distress, struggles, responses, and hopes). Those details are reinterpreted and re-storied into professionalized formulations. In the professionalized and institutionalized descriptions, the person, their experiences, and the details of their lives become subjugated, disqualified, and ultimately, unrecognizable (Habermas, 1971; Harding, 1987, 2006; Smith, 1990). For instance, psychiatric tools like the *Diagnostic and Statistical Manual of Mental Disorders* (DSM) (American Psychiatric Association, 2000) represent an institutional text that marks the place where psychiatry and individual knowledge and ways of knowing intersect and join. Through the process of diagnosis, the DSM is applied to a person to identify, label, and mark certain nonconforming people as different against normative psychiatric standards (Morley, 2003; Rusch, Angermeyer & Corrigan, 2005). The process renders the individual and their subjective experiences into a sort of *non-existence* and what is left are the professionalized constructions, the labels that are supposed to represent an illness.

Some argue that the person becomes invisible and is silenced against the psychiatric classifications (Crowe & Alavi, 1999; Marker, 2003; Vanheule, 2011), but in my opinion these critiques do not go far enough. In my mind, the person is still visible, but is visible in a particular kind of way, as a person deemed *ill* or *disordered*. Consequently, she is treated accordingly, as a person with an undesirable illness that needs to be changed, controlled, repaired, or altered. When the details of people's lives are reinterpreted into professional explanations and formulations (Habermas, 1971; Harding, 1987, 2006; Rose, 1998), epistemic violence has occurred. Epistemic violence has occurred as the person is rendered out of existence by the assertion that their experiences are "disordered," or the symptoms of a "mental illness" (Baldwin, 2005). The effect is the social denial and removal of psychiatrized people from legitimate social positions as legitimate knowers. Instead, the DSM categories become the social texts that speak for, on behalf of, and in place of the individual. Stigmatizing constructions, specifically the negative social meanings associated with "mental illness," become the rationale for the disqualification of psychiatrized people as legitimate knowers. These constructions, including the stereotypes of being incompetent, disordered, unpredictable, or dangerous (Corrigan, 2007; Corrigan, Kerr & Knudsen, 2005; Corrigan et al., 2003), become the mechanisms used to diminish and deny psychiatrized people their social legitimacy as knowers. In the next section, I explore the ways that being constructed as incompetent and dangerous are central to the epistemic disqualification of psychiatrized people.

Epistemic Violence: Being Disqualified as Incompetent and Dangerous

> And why all my anger?—because at the end of the day, my mother is being coerced and forced to die the way the health care system believes a woman diagnosed with a "mental illness" should die—in hospital—away from her home, family, and community! In her near 20-year history of living with a diagnosis that carried strong stigmatizing reactions, my mother never actually harmed nor threatened to harm herself or others, and yet at the moment of her death, the potential for harm was used as the rationale for the removal of the in-home services necessary for her to live and die at home. She was disqualified as a legitimate knower because she was constructed as dangerous. The knowledge—ultimately her knowledge—of her impending death was dismissed and other interventions were activated. The withdrawal of home care services forced a hospitalization against her wishes and against our wishes as family members.

For an individual to be disqualified as a legitimate knower, certain constructions become necessary in order to justify the disqualification. For psychiatrized people, being constructed as "incompetent" and "dangerous" becomes a powerful mechanism leading to their disqualification as legitimate knowers. Each construction forms a rationale for disqualifying and denying the person's knowledge and ways of knowing. The disqualification corresponds to a particular form of prejudice and discrimination faced by individuals deemed "mentally ill." This intolerance is known as sanism (LeFrançois, 2013; Perlin, 2003; Poole et al., 2012). It becomes the rationale for particular interventions, including the use of coercion and force.

Being Disqualified as Incompetent

A prejudice associated with being psychiatrized is the belief that the person has a flawed or disordered way of seeing, perceiving, judging, and thus, knowing reality (Vanheule, 2011). Constructed as disordered, the psychiatrized person is disqualified as a legitimate knower and deemed incompetent. Constructions of incompetence include beliefs that the person is incapable of making appropriate decisions and of caring for herself or others (Corrigan, Kerr & Knudsen, 2005; Link et al., 1987; Overton & Medina, 2008; Piner & Kahle, 1984). For instance, under dominant psy discourses and practices a person who has alternative experiences of reality, often pathologized as being "psychotic" or as having "hallucinations," is disqualified as a legitimate knower because their experiences are interpreted within a modernist framework as a break from reality, a break from what is considered to be real or true (Baldwin, 2005; Vanheule, 2011).

As mentioned, some suggest that persons constructed as incompetent become invisible within the mental health system (Crowe & Alavi, 1999), while others argue that a person with an alternative experience of reality is silenced from voicing their distress in their own narrative styles (Crowe & Alavi, 1999; Vanheule, 2011) and perhaps within their own framework of understanding reality; however, this critique does not go far enough to name and explain the violence committed against these psychiatrized people. Ultimately, the person is not truly invisible to those who treat her as incompetent, ill, or disordered. The epistemic violence is not the dismissing of the person, voice, or perspective as disordered. It is rather the denial of the person as a legitimate knower. Dismissed as incompetent, the psychiatrized person cannot get their knowledge, the content of their experiences, or their ways of knowing recognized and heard as legitimate. Alternative experiences of reality—defined as "psychosis" or "hallucinations"—become the rationale for the denial of their legitimacy as a knower. Rendered incompetent, persons are disqualified as legitimate knowers and lose their epistemic agency, specifically losing their ability to speak on their own behalf and to be heard on their own terms and in their own styles (Dotson, 2011).

Being Disqualified as Dangerous

A second prejudice associated with being diagnosed with "mental illness" consists of beliefs that the person is *dangerous* or *potentially dangerous* (Corrigan, Kerr & Knudsen, 2005). Being constructed as dangerous is a powerful mechanism that sets the stage for epistemic violence. Under psy discourses, a dangerous person is someone who is unpredictable, who cannot be trusted, who threatens the public order, and who, consequently, needs to be controlled. Protecting public order, which represents the well-being of many at the risk of abrogating the rights of the individual, becomes central to the justification for the use of such interventions as forced hospitalization, observation, medication, and restraint (Pescosolido, Monahan, Link, Stueve & Kikuzawa, 1999). At the centre of this intervention is fear.

Psychiatrized people come to embody the social fear held about "mental illness" and about persons deemed to have a "mental illness." Any claims a person labelled as dangerous or potentially dangerous makes about their life, distress, and needs are overshadowed by fears of that person. It is the fear that fuels the justification of the separation and removal of psychiatrized people from positions of legitimate social standing, including their position as legitimate knowers. Under dominant psy discourses the disqualification does not necessarily depend on actual harm, but rather begins with beliefs about the person's potential for harm (Pescosolido et al. 1999; see also Warme, Chapter 15). In other words, in order for danger to be seen, there need not be any history of actual harm committed. A mere perception that harm is possible may suffice.

Possibilities for Social Justice: Bringing Persons Back into Existence

And why all my anger—because at the end of the day, I was forced to witness and coerced to participate in an unjust process that denied my mother, a woman I loved, her dignity and her humanity as a whole and valued person.

If epistemic violence is to deny being, then the response to the violence is to construct ways that bring psychiatrized people back into existence. Restoring a person's epistemic existence requires conscious acts that construct, support, and give legitimacy to the person as someone with legitimate ways of knowing and, ultimately, legitimate ways of being. If epistemic violence is understood as the non-recognition of being, then resistance to epistemic violence would mean bringing into being that which is denied existence. However, given that non-recognition occurs in structural and institutional ways, resistance to epistemic violence means not changing the individual, but rather, changing the structures and institutional processes and practices that, in various forms, deny particular forms of existence (Spivak, 2005). Resistance to epistemic violence should denounce the institutional assaults enacted through localized practices against one's being—assaults against nonconforming narratives, knowledges, and ways of knowing.

It is not enough to give voice but one must think of voice in different ways—in ways that recognize difference as legitimate rather than measuring differences against a standard of *normal* (Goldenberg, 2007). An interesting approach is suggested by Crowe and Alavi (1999) who propose that dominant psy practice for dealing with "mad talk"—the talk associated with alternative experiences of reality labelled as "delusions" and "psychosis"—is to dismiss it as "disordered" and wrong. By dismissing the talk as "disordered," its content, metaphors, and messages of distress are also dismissed. The person, their knowledge and ways of knowing, are de-centred and marginalized, while the social meanings attached to the label of "disorder" become the organizing experience for understanding and treating the person. On the other hand, if the style and content of a person's talk were understood and treated as the only safe means of communicating distress, then the person, their experiences, knowledge and ways of knowing could be re-centred as important (Crowe & Alavi, 1999). The person is reinstated as a legitimate knower with legitimate knowledge, and is valued rather than diminished. Humanity is restored, rather than denied, through the recognition that certain expressions, such as "mad talk," are legitimate ways for some people to narrate their knowledge, including their experiences of distress, euphoria, and/or confusion.

Perhaps the same can be argued about expressions and actions that evoke fear and concerns about risk of harm and dangerousness. If expressions of threat and harm are also seen as legitimate ways of knowing and experiencing distress, then psychiatrized people can be repositioned as legitimate knowers, and the potential for their humanity restored. Social justice is possible if interventions are aimed at restoring humanity rather than removing the person. I am not suggesting that harm be allowed to occur or that the risks of harm are not to be taken seriously, but I am suggesting that we rethink our dominant practices of isolating and controlling threat. I am suggesting that we replace fear with a commitment that centres the person's humanity through the recognition that expressions of madness—even dangerous ones, however rare— are a way of knowing.

Conclusion: Bestowed with a Legacy

According to philosopher Thomas Attig (2004), I am bestowed with a legacy:

> Those we grieve have given us their legacies to have and to hold after they have died.... We in turn give their legacies places in our hearts, in the vital centers of our lives. We can experience and express our continuing love for not only as we miss them but as we cherish their memories and life stories and open ourselves to and embrace what we find valuable in their practical, soulful, and spiritual legacies. (p. 356)

After a week in the hospital, the palliative care doctor used his authority to veto the decisions made by the home care providers and discharged my mother once again to our family's care. Within a two-week period my mother died as she wanted, in her own home among family and friends—her personhood recognized and loved. My mother is missed and the telling of her story has become the telling of my story as a witness and steward of her knowledge—as her daughter, a social worker, and now an emerging academic.

To write this chapter is my way of embracing the legacy I am left and to bring back into existence my mother's humanity, her knowledge, experiences, and ways of being. I write to denounce the injustice that occurred in those final days and to claim justice for my mother and all other psychiatrized people. But my mother alone did not experience the social injustice of having her knowledge and personhood denied. I too, as her daughter, the witness and steward of those experiences, need justice because of the harm I experienced in those days from the epistemic violence committed against my mother. As a socially and academically sanctioned space, social justice becomes possible through the writing of this chapter, and the production of other such critical texts, which offer a forum for naming, describing, and denouncing forms of violence committed against psychiatrized people. In my experience, such violence is committed not as a misunderstanding about a failing liver or as another example of the stigma of "mental illness," but as epistemic violence—the disqualification of psychiatrized people as legitimate knowers with legitimate knowledge and ways of being.

Note

1 I want to acknowledge and thank Dr. Shoshana Pollack, a professor in the Faculty of Social Work at Wilfrid Laurier University and one of my early mentors in my doctoral studies, who was instrumental in introducing me to the concept of epistemic violence and its potential applications to madness.

CHAPTER 9

Mad Success: What Could Go Wrong When Psychiatry Employs Us as "Peers"?

Erick Fabris

Success is a double-edged sword, I was telling my friend today as we lounged in a tub. While we sat back, minus champagne and caviar, we felt rich inside because we appreciate each other's friendship. We joked about some of the rich characters in our midst, and came around to our respective jobs, quipping about identity politics. Whereas my friend talked about relationships between broader identifications (in sexuality, race, gender, and disability), lamenting a common lack of class analysis and pitting identities against one another, my thoughts skipped over how people are classified "mad" or "ill" (I was once made a mental patient), and set upon how some of us Mad[1] folk are considered more "functional" than others. Without attention to how some people are disabled by treatments, we are then employed in the social service industry as "peers." I tried working in this industry as an "advocate" before the peer identity was widely adopted.

My chapter uses narrative inquiry (Conle, 1999) to explore the political question of class and identity underpinning individual and collective success in mad-conceived peoples' movements. Narrative inquiry is a method that allows for a description of lived experiences relating to social structures, institutions, and theories. This kind of storytelling is an ethnography, one that bridges academic and personal knowledges. I will introduce my stories with a bit of background from the literature. I will not draw conclusions, though I will describe my own thoughts within these stories.

I was told, while being institutionalized, that I would likely never work again. Yet we now witness institutions such as Yale University in the USA training users of psychiatric services in "peer support" work: "These services are intended to train and employ consumers of the mental health system to function as peer supports and assist other consumers in coping with the sometimes frightening and chaotic environments of urgent access centers and emergency rooms" (Yale School of Medicine, n.d.). Such a prestigious offering shows how rapidly the concept and business of mutual aid have spread, and not without some of their critical and empowering language. In my own psychiatric jurisdiction of Ontario, a "career track" website on "community mental health" identifies "peer specialists" trained in "information and referral, skills training, emotional support, goal setting and attainment, *advocacy*, role modeling, and interpersonal skills" (Ontario Ministry of Health and Long-Term Care, n.d.). I've italicized the term "advocacy" because dedicated advocacy services that are funded "at arm's length" from the provincial health ministry are currently being divested in Ontario. They have been the only Canadian services of this kind, so peer workers and others will be expected to take up the slack. Contesting existing commercial "help" systems has most often been done for free.

Peer work is considered a part of the new and controversial "recovery-based approach" to mental health service delivery. This approach promotes the social basis for achieving health, even for people given biomedical diagnoses of the "psychotic disorder" variety. Recovery-based approaches value patients' choices and the need for risk-taking in social life. Peer workers would amplify this self-healing by the example of their own success. Certainly, the case has been made for peer work (Daniels et al., 2010; O'Hagan, Cyr, McKee & Priest, 2010), but when peer support is conceived as yet another brand of mental health product that is "still early in its development," rather than as a tacit knowledge about the experience of advocating for and "healing" the social self, no quantitative differences in service outcomes are found (Davidson, Chinman, Sells & Rowe, 2006).

The issue of implementation shows the fissure between self-help and industrial work. Frost, Heinz, and Bach (2011) say, "many [professional] service providers are unsure of how to include peer specialists in their organizations and may be skeptical of their value," though White et al. (2003) reported from their survey results that, in Ontario in 2003, many peer workers were "integrated" into Assertive Community Treatment teams and they enjoyed "equal and better job satisfaction" than their professional coworkers. Other researchers have found that service providers are often slow to welcome peer support workers into the field (Richard, Jongbloed & MacFarlane, 2009). Professionals have shown stigmatizing prejudice towards people labelled with mental illnesses (Peris et al., 2008), even more so than the general public, which continues to hold beliefs that psychosocial rather than biomedical events cause "madness" (Read et al., 2006). That is, lay folk think distress arises from situational problems, not an inborn condition linked to dangerousness, as evidenced in commonplace "mental health" legislation. When one considers how some professionals intend to instruct patients in their own consumer-based recovery erstwhile reinforcing the medical services they deliver (Bielavitz, Wisdom & Pollack, 2011), we might understand how peer workers perceive clinicians to be discriminating against patients and themselves (Stromwall, Holley & Bashor, 2011).

The question remains, will peer services simply augment biomedical approaches that stigmatize, as Read et al. (2006) have argued, or will they advance self-help, self-advocacy, mutual aid, and choice? In practice, the latter need not mean an all-or-nothing approach: "take risks or you will not be helped." But will the peer "movement" have any functions beyond psychiatry?

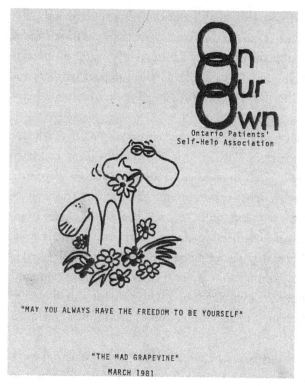

FIGURE 9.1: On Our Own

This image reproduces the cover of the March 1981 edition of the newsletter the *Mad Grapevine*, published by the Ontario Patients' Self-Help Association in Toronto. The phrase "On our own" has special meaning for the psychiatric survivor community. Among other references, it was the title of the late activist Judi Chamberlin's 1978 book.

Source: Psychiatric Survivor Archives of Toronto, 1981.

The question might be addressed by considering the term "peer" itself. As a highly friendly moniker outside the context of psychiatry, "peer" has none of the competitive tension commonly associated with modern industry. Applied to the mental illness industry, however, the term "peer" suggests no affiliation with the more contentious identities brought by patients over the last few decades, like "consumer," "user," or "survivor" of psychiatry. "Peer" suggests an equal partnership between provider and patient because the provider in this case is still a patient. Yet the term obscures the fact that a peer worker is paid, whereas the patient is not. On the other hand, the peer worker is not paid as much as the professional worker, nor does she have the administrative privileges, licensed affiliations, and authoritative influences in decisions affecting the patient's life. By naming ourselves peers, will we never be regarded as professionals? Likewise, by cleaving to psychiatry, will we paradoxically cleave ourselves away from the lay people's distresses and supports? Surely, after a long hard day of enforcing "compliance," visiting disgruntled recipients of mandatory care, or any other work required of psychiatric employees, will we be unable or unwilling to freely help others? In my own experiences, I have found psychiatry to discourage me from freely giving away my social self.

"Free" help was the foundation of mental patients' movements leading to the peer phenomenon. But peer terminology makes no allusion to collective powers advocated for and won by psychiatric patients collectively since the 1960s, in the form of the "mental patients' liberation movement," the "psychiatric survivor movement" (Chamberlin, 1978; Morrison, 2005), or their offshoots in the "user," "consumer," and more recently "mad"[2] movements, to name a few. These identifications, which have been used by some of us in our work "within" the psychiatric system, such as through "consumer/survivor" initiatives in Ontario (Church, 1995; see also Church, Chapter 13), may be reduced to the "client/provider" dichotomy of psychiatric pamphlets. "Peer" work tries to bridge that divide, as the word "prosumer" did in the 1990s and still today (Dorsey, 2008). By doing so, "peer" presents an occultation of grassroots resistance and the appearance of a politics-free psychiatry. It also harkens back to a time when patient labour was taken for granted and patients operated much of the asylum, all in the name of therapy, providing for an image of psychiatry as progressive and productive (Reaume, 2000).

Some readers may dispute the idea that psychiatry is a very powerful force in Western society, unless perhaps they have read Ethan Watters (2010) on the Americanization of "crazy" around the world (see also McCubbin, 1998; Pilgrim & Rogers, 2005; Scull, 2010; Sharfstein, 2005, to name a few). It could be argued that psychiatric workers face stigmas like those imposed on patients, leading to lost revenues and opportunity (while the stigma of labels may spill onto professionals, the "stigma" of iatrogenic impairments is simply a lack of public confidence in psychiatry). If White et al. (2003) are right, and peers benefit in ways professionals do not, it may be because they are not responsible for the treatments imposed, but hope to help people get through psychiatrization (of course, it could also be because they disprove prognostications that they will never work).

I, for one, seem to be making a return on my academic writing, digging up psychiatry's misadventures, lost aims, and pokey practices. My book *Tranquil Prisons* took four years to write and edit, and it was well worth it (Fabris, 2011). As an ethnographer of the psychiatric industry, having no reason to frame my efforts in terms of searching for "best practices," I have felt quite free to call attention to some of psychiatry's more glaring problems, not because I enjoy crying foul, but because I feel it's right to decry foul treatment of others. I consider my refusal to shut up about it a success, emotionally and professionally. My success is not unique I think; many psychiatric survivors have increased their social capital through activism and advocacy in some vein. I hope more people will work to examine and contest psychiatric force instead of becoming caught up in coercive practices once imposed on them.

As I lounged and chatted with my friend today, I thought back to the night before. Walking around in my neighbourhood, I noticed an old acquaintance (I will call him "Prem"). He was someone I used to see on a regular basis at the local institution, the Queen Street Mental Health Centre (which is now part of Toronto's Centre for Addiction and Mental Health). I worked there in the 1990s as a consumer/survivor advocate. My title was "advocacy facilitator" and later "coordinator," and there was no pretense about my "mental" politics: the Queen Street Patients Council did a lot of complaining about "systemic abuses," and drew both admiration and disdain for seeking less use of restraints, the creation of a psychiatric drug detoxification program, safe wards for female patients, and so on. I saw myself not as less than a professional advocate (they rarely made demands on a systemic level), but certainly as less financed (though no advocacy service is well-resourced). One might wonder why advocates even bother; the most transparent institutions seldom keep records of restraints use, electroshock, chemical interventions, and so on. Advocates have to do everything from scratch, often with contemptuous or threatened workers who refuse to be interrupted in their interventions.

Last night Prem was still being intervened upon as an outpatient. He walked back and forth along the street, gazing above the horizon with an expression of yearning, never turning his head to notice where he was or who was around him. Knowing him, I wanted to introduce myself and say, "have a fiver," or "hey, what's up?" As I told my friend, however, I was rushing and I decided not to go through with what could be a long encounter. I wanted to help out a fellow traveller on the road out of bedlam. Why didn't I? Where was my Mad pride? Where was my psychiatric survivor solidarity?

I have actually seen Prem in the neighbourhood many times before.

"Prem!" I once called to him on a streetcar. He looked around, feigning ease, wondering who was shouting. When he located me, a half-smile and slight frown came over his face, slowly, before he looked away again. I assumed he couldn't remember me because he was a bit dazed from "his meds." I approached and said I was from the patient council, "at Queen Street." He nodded without looking embarrassed about being linked to the asylum at all, but after a few words, he had little to say. It felt as if he couldn't really recognize me. Soon I took my leave, smiling, complimenting, and wondering what had I really accomplished, if anything, working at the asylum for a decade? As I told my friend, instead of saying hello and handing him a few dollars last night, I stayed out of his way. It was a classic avoidance of the mental patient, I said. It might also be considered a classic white guy avoidance of people of colour. I wondered about our separate fates; I with my published book and professorial duties, he with his disability cheque and wandering gaze.

Success comes with disappointments. Some say it comes on the backs of others, given the competitive systems of exchange we use. There are only so many spots available. Others insist that all things being equal, we do well to better our lot while others ne'er do well. But how can anyone who is being tranquilized by overzealous clinicians with a self-interested faith in psychopharmacology, who seldom reflect on their professional powers, ever be able to compete? The focus required for success, and the continuity of struggle from day to day, are difficult enough for anyone, and especially for minorities of race, gender, sexuality, and disability in any given context. How about people imposed upon with "neuroleptic" tranquilizers? Neuroleptics (meaning "nerve seizers" in Greek) are known to inhibit cognitive and affective brain functions, rendering a person more compliant through a process of blocking dopamine receptor cells. While this may seem a good idea to those who think mental patients are a constant danger to themselves or others—perhaps a better idea than locking them in cages—drugs do decrease life expectancy by an average of 25 years when researchers account for lifestyle and other factors (Whitaker, 2010). So it seems to me that the bootstrap-pulling expected of the psychiatrically disabled (and by this I mean those impaired by psychiatric drugs and electroshock) is an absurd and insulting demand. Success can be sweet, I said to my friend, but not if some people never get a chance to pursue it.

Looking back, there were indeed successes in my work as an advocate. These successes were few, given the prevailing concern of clinicians for the functioning of the ward, leaving patients' needs second. One success was greater than the rest, and I want to write about it, but it has an unhappy, tragic ending. I want to tell you about it in part to get it off my chest, but also to give you an idea of the life and death struggles involved when we try to help people who are being intervened upon.

For many of us who wiggle out of coercive interventions and are lucky enough to find work, it may be said that we are fortunate because we have enough support to carry us through such an emergency. As a white boy with no visible disabilities, all I had to do to succeed as a child was apply myself at school. I did so as a welcome diversion from the storms at home. I excelled and was recognized for it, but I noticed so many others dropping behind. Girls did not seem to be rewarded like the boys at times, and some of the more angry boys were browbeaten into thinking they would never "do better in school." One kid was told he would end up in jail by a teacher. "I just know I'll be reading it in the papers," she declared. As for me, I wished I could be more like those who refused to do well, or who simply had lost interest by the middle grades. My success may have been secured because it was expected of me in a working-class school, amongst Italian Canadians, with traditional heterosexist values. Someone like Prem would not have such a system behind him as he tried to navigate Toronto and Canadian culture.

"Ranji," an East Indian man I tried to advocate for, was one of the nicest people I've met in the asylum. He walked into the council office one day and told me that he was sick to his stomach every morning, vomiting with pain, shaking at times. His tongue would spasm in embarrassing ways—due to the "side" effects of his "medication," he insisted, despite his workers telling him otherwise. I started asking questions on his unit and got the usual runaround. But I talked about Ranji with the head psychiatrist, and he became interested, which was a game changer for us. One summer day on the grounds of the asylum, we chanced upon this doctor, tanned and buff, looking almost golden from vacationing.

"Hello!" I motioned to him. His face contracted when he saw me. We'd sparred in several meetings over patients' rights, so he was at pains to hear me out. "You seem well rested," I said. I introduced him to Ranji.

"I just got back from canoeing up north," he smiled with that kid-like charm. "It was just amazing."

"You've got quite a tan too," I rejoined.

"Yes!" He looked at Ranji. "So ... tell me, um ..."

"Ranji," offered my ... "client"? What was our relationship exactly? The both of us were far lower on the ladder than our esteemed doctor. "Peer"? I was bringing in $24,000 per year, gross, and I spoke fluent English. I had years of experience and connections in Canadian settler culture. Ranji, on the other hand, was a divorced, unemployed South Asian male who spoke only a bit of English. What he had going for him was enthusiasm, a recognition of other people, and a wish to survive. My advocacy relationship to Ranji was at the least unexpected, a stroke of good luck for most mental patients, given the lack of individual advocacy on the wards. His health was declining daily and he was quite desperate to get help. The doctors on his ward seemed to have no insight into what ailed him. Having no luck with the asylum's professional advocates, he sought out the patient council, and, well, there I was.

The head doctor finally said, "Ranji ... you're having some stomach upset. I get that." Ranji's tongue darted in and out of his mouth involuntarily as he frowned to focus. "How old are you, anyway?"

"I'm 26, sir," he said blandly.

The doctor's eyes opened wide with hope. "I'm in my sixties! You're still a young man. Compared to me, you're healthy as an ox!"

Ranji and I stood nonplussed. Here was a lead man, the top of his field (whatever his mistakes). He'd had the good life for decades. His body was built up bigger than mine, and nearly twice the size of Ranji's. He was larger than life, single-handedly directing strategic planning at the centre. I remember his signature on our request forms; bold and easy circles. And what a masterful conversationalist; here he was complimenting Ranji on his health when Ranji had so desperately sought it for weeks.

"Well," I broke in, "he's vomiting a lot, and he's got the shakes." That last word unsettled the psychiatrist a bit. "And he's not sleeping well, a symptom you folks try to deal with, right?"

"Certainly," the psychiatrist came back to earth again. "Not to worry. I'll look into this and I'll get back to you." Then with spirit he bounded off. "I better run if I'm going to make my appointment!" And so the man who had once been heard to argue that he was a survivor himself because he had once suffered "depression" now moved like a quarterback to the institution's main entrance, through heavy doors that patients struggled to open, if they weren't locked. Yet his was the most spirited response I've ever received regarding patients' complaints.

In a few days, I was asked to meet with Ranji's workers—without Ranji, of course. I would have none of that tactic, and I insisted he be present. I asked them if they'd heard of tardive dyskinesia, and they replied that they had not (this was the mid-1990s, when such terms were still being introduced by critical psychiatrists who challenged the profession from within) (Breggin, 1991). They asked me incredulously, as though

I'd found the term on a cereal box, "Are you a doctor?" I provided them with some readings, and the facts of Ranji's complaints. I obligingly led them through questions they could not simply ignore without being sarcastic or dismissive. Psychiatrists did not like funny patients. Ranji sat silent and attentive, "playing the game" as survivors say.

Within a week came the incredible news. Ranji told me his doctors had significantly reduced his dosage. That made me worry. I had reduced my own dosage very slowly to avoid withdrawal reactions a few years earlier. A sharp reduction would likely result in withdrawal. I worried also that they and Ranji would assume this withdrawal was a "relapse" of his assumed illness, proving again that the medical model was sound. He would then be administered antipsychotics more aggressively, and I would be to blame for insisting on interfering with their intervention.

But thankfully none of that happened. In a week, his worst "side" effects subsided. After a couple of weeks, he felt better physically and seemed genuinely happy, as if his life was finally working out. I secretly worried that it was all too soon, and the withdrawal would sneak in later. But I could only marvel at the immediate positive outcome. The lack of treatment was working! Imagine if more patients were given a chance to reduce their dosages to a manageable level, I thought. Could this be a success that might encourage more clinicians to follow suit?

Ranji was soon discharged to a boarding home up the street. He visited and continued to participate in our council's activities when he could. He also seemed to get some of his more relaxed personality back, as he took more control over his life. But in only a few days, I received news from one of his doctors that Ranji was in hospital!

"He relapsed?" I asked, using terminology the doctor could understand.

"No," he said, "I mean, he's at a general hospital. He's got third-degree burns all over his body."

"What?" I sometimes wondered if staff always lied, the way they had lied to me as an in-patient. Then I felt an immediate sense of guilt, that this was my fault somehow.

"A fire broke out in his room, probably a cigarette. He's in intensive care. You might want to see him, but it's not a pretty sight." At least the doctor was concerned, and even kind enough to tell me—without laying any blame. Maybe he too felt he'd made a mistake.

I still couldn't believe it. From guilt I moved to blame. Had Ranji started the fire or had someone else? Was it an accident? What kind of building was it—was it up to code? Did it have any fire preventions? So many mental patients have died in tinderbox fires, like Zelda Fitzgerald, famous wife of *The Great Gatsby's* author, I thought.

Before I had the stomach to go visit him, a few days later I was told that Ranji had succumbed to his injuries. There was simply too much damage to his body. I wished I had at least gone to see him and faced my feelings more honestly. As I think of him now, I wonder at my thoughts then. I considered all of the problems the system had brought him, and finally all the other systems that allowed for that boarding home to go up in flames so quickly that he could not escape. I suspected system workers would have liked to blame me for "getting his hopes up." But what hurt, really, was that I cared about the guy. He was a worthy friend. Maybe he could have worked for the council someday. I didn't reflect on that and it may have caused me to shut down a bit; I had "crossed the boundary" that many clinicians never cross.

Success came and went in an instant. With Ranji's loss, I wondered if advocacy was merely adding more confusion to a disorderly system. I wondered if any of the changes the council demanded would ever be taken up seriously, or be taken up piecemeal to thwart change. I continued to provide patients with information, suggesting alternatives as though they were simply choices while treatments were being imposed. Rarely did I push with the passion required for success. Of course, most patients did not take up the alternatives given the intensive management of their everyday lives, down to the neuron. The council continued to protest, to no avail.

The reason I tell this terrible story is that those of us who stick around to work in the psychiatric system need to remember that there is death in this system. Even psychiatrists and administrators will admit that services are not always "under control," so getting people out of one danger may lead them into others. This is not to say we should let things be; this story shows how dismal things are. Critics say there will be tragedies in any system that is underfunded, that tries to respond to public fears of "psychotic" violence, that issues treatments as if they were vitamins when there is reason to suspect they are dangerous. There will be tragedies in which one's hope for a more humane, kind, personal response, to use those hackneyed old terms, will be thwarted by industrial "necessities," standards out of scale with human want, best practices in medicine that ignore personal contexts, realities, and complexities. Also, there will be tragedies when we, as minor players, manage to interrupt the interveners. But how can we pretend to set ourselves apart from the system when the system has encroached on us so?

One perspective that keeps me going, despite the overwhelming odds against Mad people, is our history. Yes, survivors fight each other, and consumers too. We often dismiss our own work, and sometimes instead of noticing it is being hemmed in by professionals who take shortcuts, we speak of their successes over ours. How often have we worked hard to help someone out, finding them a place to eat or to sleep, and when it's all over they credit the "medication" for their success, or the kindness of someone in authority? I feel we must celebrate the work of psychiatric patients in helping each other, and the collective work of psychiatric survivors especially. Peer employment is based on that work of solidarity, mutual aid, and self-advocacy. What is important about this history is the recognition that we cannot simply empower someone else; we can only work together for change, even if we cannot share the same experiences.

If peers forget to stand up for themselves and for patients, they will absolve themselves of responsibility and lose their raison d'être. The more success I enjoy, the more responsibility I seem to have. But maybe the balance is found through believing in ourselves, and thinking of "success" not as "responsibility," but rather as the joy of pursuing our dreams. There is no simple story when psychiatric patients are at risk of iatrogenic impairments and related accidents. We know from the pretensions and double standards of many interventionists that winning is always contingent. The peer movement may not be fully formed, and that's fine. It should not be considered an end in itself, a final merging of patient and doctor, or a final version of the mental patients' liberation front. There is always more we would like to do, a double-edged sword of success, or maybe just a wish to go on.

My friend and I parted a few hours later. I had waited to write this chapter for some time, and it seems like a dream that our conversation inspired it. A story is sometimes told before it can be written.

A postscript: The next day I see a third man I used to know at Queen Street. He used to work there. He is also South Asian, but this man's eyes are not heavy, and his walk is not stiff. When he passes he notices me looking at him with a bit of a smile. He nods to me. I think to myself, recognition is better than success.

Notes

1 For me "madness" is just "sound mind" (i.e., these divisive terms are false, and if anyone wishes to they could rationalize or understand any other person). I propose the proper noun "Mad" to mean the group of us considered crazy or deemed ill by sanists (who create these categories through an interpreting "stare": Fabris, 2011) and are politically conscious of this. Thus, "Mad" is a historical rather than a descriptive or essential category, proposed for political action and discussion. This term does not depend on critical psychiatrists' ideas about the construction of mental disorder, or language-conscious historians' discussions on the rationalism behind legal "sanity."

2 Unlike my term "Mad," this word in lower case is used by many activists and writers, often as a more general or social term (and therefore a claimable word, as in "queer" or "Queer" theory) to describe or reclaim experiences that clinicians dubiously identify as symptoms of a theoretical "mental illness" or "mental disorder" (see Dr. Allen Frances, 2009, for a discussion of the vagaries of designing the medical labels in the *Diagnostic and Statistical Manual*).

PART III   Critiques of Psychiatry: Practice and Pedagogy

In Part III, four of Canada's leading Mad activists and scholars explore some of the pressing concerns presently being addressed by people and organizations involved in the critique of psychiatry and the pursuit of human justice by and for Mad people. Each of these chapters considers, in various ways, the methods and strategies through which critical thinking about psychiatry and mental health rights can be converted into radical engagement and transformative practice. The issues canvassed by these authors include the catastrophic human toll of the community mental "health" movement; the ongoing travesty of abuse, camouflaged as treatment, that is electroshock; and the challenges faced by those involved in bringing Mad-centred teaching and learning curricula into the nation's schools and universities.

In "The Tragic Farce of 'Community Mental Health Care'" (Chapter 10), Irit Shimrat pulls back the façade of the community mental health (CMH) paradigm to expose the devastating realities of community-based psychiatric intervention in this present era of "deinstitutionalization" and the alleged "end of the asylum." Harnessing transcripts of client records compiled by an anonymous team of Canadian mental health workers, Shimrat chronicles a contemporary CMH apparatus that eerily reproduces the worst features of the snake pits and cuckoo's nests of yesteryear—a system that "as currently practised promotes neither community nor mental health." Framed by Shimrat's own experiences as a survivor of multiple psychiatric incarcerations, these transcripts make for explosive reading. We witness professional hubris at its very worst: clients being drugged and electroshocked into resentful docility (all in the name of compassion and therapy); health care workers seemingly incapable of recognizing the failure of their vaunted treatments and the damage they inflict; expert-"patient" encounters in which any efforts by the latter to express autonomy or (even worse) resistance are viewed as markers of "mental illness"; medical power structures that disproportionately disadvantage the elderly (in particular, senior women), children, teenagers, and Aboriginal Canadians—in short, a system that perpetuates powerlessness, social isolation, humiliation, self-loathing, and despair among the very people it is mandated to help. Yet, as Shimrat perceptively observes, the "tragic farce" depicted in this chapter is far from being an inevitability. Investing her narrative with an affecting message of hope, Shimrat cites examples of genuine community involvement in peer support and recovery such as the celebrated Mental Patients Association (MPA) and Vancouver Emotional Emergency Centre (VEEC)—projects which, for a time, succeeded famously while fending off the alienating and co-opting forces of institutional psychiatry, Big Pharma, and the neoliberal state. In stark contrast to the travesties that we observe throughout this chapter, such visions of community and care are still worth struggling for, now more than ever. "I dream of a society brave and moral enough," concludes Shimrat, "to eschew the whole paradigm of mental health and illness, replacing it with the creation of real community, and real help, of the kind and quality briefly achieved in Vancouver in the early 1970s."

The contribution by antipsychiatry activist Don Weitz (Chapter 11) provides a radical critique of electroshock, known officially as "electroconvulsive therapy" or "ECT," which is denounced as a form of torture under the guise of therapy. The way in which ECT is administered, the rationale for its use by psychiatrists, and its impact on people who undergo electroshock are discussed within the context of activist work by the Coalition Against Psychiatric Assault who have long protested this "treatment." The reasons why ECT should be banned are detailed, with reference to its sexist and ageist implementation, along with studies that report how it causes memory loss. Weitz also provides statistical evidence from Ontario to support his arguments and notes how mental health professionals who criticize ECT are rare (particularly in Canada) and, in one case at least, led to a doctor being fired. This is all powerful enough, but his article's most memorable words come from the testimonies of individual Canadian electroshock survivors convened by the Coalition Against Psychiatric Assault in 2005. Weitz concludes with a series of recommendations by a panel from this gathering that provides reasons for abolishing ECT and providing alternative forms of humane supports for people experiencing madness. That the Ontario Minister of Health and Long-Term Care never responded to these recommendations makes it all the more imperative that this vital information be published in this collection.

In his reflections on eight years of teaching in the School of Disability Studies at Ryerson University in Toronto (Chapter 12), David Reville weighs the trials and triumphs of teaching Mad People's History and A History of Madness from the perspectives of people who have lived this topic to students from across the university.

In doing so, he raises issues about how to integrate Mad people as active participants and shapers of the university curriculum whilst also enabling Mad Studies to take root, grow, and flourish inside and outside the academy. Reville also notes how the challenges of teaching this topic, both in the classroom and on the World Wide Web, were addressed with innovative approaches that broadened its appeal and made it more accessible to people with a psychiatric history. Underlying this chapter is how these course offerings led to further creative scholarly and artistic endeavors by students and faculty alike whilst involving people beyond campus in cultural and learned productions about what it means to be "Mad." Given all of this activity, the answer to Reville's question in the title of his article, "Is Mad Studies Emerging as a New Field of Inquiry?", appears to be "yes." By outlining various options for transforming educational possibilities into realities, it is clear from this chapter that developing a curriculum from Mad-people-positive perspectives is both attainable and abundantly fruitful for all concerned.

In Chapter 13, Kathryn Church takes the reader through the journey towards incorporating madness as a substantive part of the curriculum at Ryerson University's School of Disability Studies. This is a parallel narrative, from her perspective, that complements David Reville's chapter, which highlights this process from his perspective. Specifically, the chapter describes the process of bringing experiential knowledge to the teaching of madness by involving psychiatric survivors as guest lecturers, co-teaching an entire course with a Mad-positive academic and a Mad-identified sessional instructor, and supporting a Mad-identified person as a core instructor and obtaining adjunct professor status for him. Church underscores the importance of Reville's involvement in the program given his ability to "use his personal story to pursue social change," the "emphasis on political autobiography," and the recognition that "the lived experience of madness [is] a fundamental form of expertise that fuels people's resistance to psychiatric definition and oppression." In analyzing her relationship in this process, Church discusses the contradictions in needing to "relinquish the pedagogical centre" at a time when gendered relations in the academy have meant that "as a woman making [her] way in an institution that is still surprised [women] are here—seizing that centre has been essential." Understanding the complicated array of privileged and disadvantaged relations, Church impresses the importance of political-minded engagement as both an academic and activist. "The hidden syllabus lay in the absolute respect we gave each other as we taught across these differences."

CHAPTER 10

The Tragic Farce of "Community Mental Health Care"

Irit Shimrat

Since the advent of deinstitutionalization, the mental health industry has been obliged to create an increasing number and variety of services within the community. There has, for instance, been a proliferation of so-called Mental Health Clubhouses. These provide a haven for people who have nowhere else to be, and who are often too heavily medicated to function in mainstream society. At those I've visited, Clubhouse members generally spend their days drinking bad (but free) coffee; eating cheap, starchy food; staring at the walls or watching television; or, at best, playing cards or board games in a desultory manner. Meanwhile, staff who get paid—never enough, apparently—to supervise them can frequently be found closeted away, chatting in their offices (just like the nurses on every psych ward I've been locked up on). Of course, if anyone misbehaves, staff are quick to intervene, with disciplinary measures ranging from banning to re-hospitalization.

Then there is supportive housing within the community: i.e., for-profit residential settings such as long-term care facilities and psychiatric rooming houses and boarding homes. Here medications are generally doled out by staff, residents sit and twitch or aimlessly pace, and restrictive rules are enforced. Again, the threat of hospitalization is ever-present if anyone gets out of line.

Many Clubhouse members and supportive-housing dwellers spend long, dull years being shunted back and forth between such venues, community crisis facilities (mini-hospitals offering short-term treatment), and hospital wards, their identities and activities revolving around diagnosis and medication.

Most pernicious, in my view, is the Community Mental Health Care Team. Upon release from hospital, mental patients are often encouraged—and sometimes legally obliged—to attend their local Care Team on a regular basis. Here they are seen by social workers, nurses, psychologists and, of course, psychiatrists. The latter group strives to ensure that service recipients stay on their psychiatric medications—medications that can cause grave damage to body, brain, and mind, often precipitating the very problems they purport to solve (see Whitaker, 2010).

Community mental health service providers, like their institutional counterparts, genuinely want to help, and believe they are helping, their clients/patients. Their inability to perceive the deleterious effects of what they do is natural, given our society's fear of difference and its need to relieve families of their disruptive members, coupled with the huge volume of pharmaceutical company propaganda that informs mass media and influences medical education (see Szasz, 2001).

Likewise, Community Mental Health (CMH) service recipients may speak highly of their Care Team—sometimes because they otherwise receive no attention whatsoever. And many feel that the drugs are doing more good than harm. I attribute this in some measure to the placebo effect, but it is also the case that the stimulating/tranquilizing effects of some of these drugs can bring relief from depression/agitation—and that for some people neuroleptics do reduce distressing thoughts/perceptions/feelings. The problem, besides the other deleterious effects discussed below, is that *psychiatric drugs reduce people's ability to think and feel at all.* Thus they impede those who take them from dealing with underlying problems. Furthermore, many of these drugs are extremely addictive (see Moncrieff, 2008).

Some years ago, a young man living in a major Canadian city got a job transcribing Care Team records. His transcriptions were added to the files kept on recipients of the agency's services. Horrified by what he was reading and typing, he secretly made copies. Some time later, he gave these to me.

Please note that although these records are not current, I have good reason to believe—based on writings from and about, and discussions with, people presently attending Care Teams—that nothing has changed. The administration of psychiatric drug cocktails is even more extensive today than when these records were transcribed. It is not unusual for someone to be simultaneously dosed with neuroleptics (see Martensson, 1998),[1] benzodiazepines,[2] antidepressants (see Glenmullen, 2000; Healy, 2004),[3] and "mood stabilizers."[4] (The *Compendium of Pharmaceuticals and Specialties* [CPS][5] and other pharmaceutical literature warn that many of these drugs should not be used concurrently.) All of these drugs are used on people of all ages, although the literature cautions against giving them to children and to the elderly. In fact, one of their major uses is controlling the behaviour of both age groups, for the convenience of caregivers within family, institutional, and CMH settings. Children, and even babies, are increasingly given diagnoses—and consequently treatments—that used to be reserved only for adults (bipolar disorder, schizophrenia, etc.). In addition to any or all of the kinds of drugs listed above, children are likely to be given methylphenidate (Ritalin) and other psychostimulants if labelled with attention deficit disorder.[6]

Patients who do not respond to drug treatment may well be treated with electroshock (ECT).[7] Furthermore, Health Canada having recently acknowledged, in the face of increased evidence, that these drugs cause damage to unborn babies, ECT has now become the treatment of choice for pregnant women.[8]

In the following excerpts, I have replaced the names of specific neuroleptics with the designation "[neuroleptic]." These drugs are virtually interchangeable in terms of their effects (regardless of psychiatry's contention that the newer so-called atypicals are less harmful than the older phenothiazines. The atypicals in fact cause alarming new problems, such as diabetes, in addition to most of those for which the older drugs are notorious). Likewise, I have used "[antidepressant]," etc., rather than employing specific drug names.

Why Do People Go Mad?

Psychiatry attributes the onset of insanity to genetic predisposition and/or imbalanced brain chemicals. This explanation, never scientifically proven, lays the foundation for the view that mental diversity—extreme/unusual thoughts and emotions—constitutes illness, and therefore falls into the purview of medicine. Thus theorists, policy-makers, and practitioners can conveniently ignore the impact of the real-life experiences (see, e.g., Horwitz & Wakefield, 2007) that actually cause what used to be called nervous breakdowns.

In the course of my work over the years[9] (and in hospitals where I've been incarcerated and CMH facilities I've visited, beginning in 1978), I have spoken and corresponded with numerous recipients of psychiatric treatment. In all this time, I have yet to find a single person who did not enter the system after some precipitating trauma.

The Care Team's records contain heartbreaking examples:

- A man with a history of "multiple hospitalizations due to paranoid feelings after his father was charged with the murder of his mother" is diagnosed with "chronic paranoid schizophrenia," for which he is treated with three different neuroleptics—to which, the writer notes, he "has had bad reactions.... He comes here for regular injections.[10] He has been somewhat anxious about his father's trial and conviction."
- A woman's "first psychotic episode was after an accident where a boat capsized.... She was admitted four days later and hospitalized for four months," during which time she was given 10 ECTs and high doses of two neuroleptics. Further hospitalizations occurred after a parent died and after a boyfriend left her. An empathic listener might have been helpful on any of these occasions. Instead, she was diagnosed with "chronic undifferentiated schizophrenia" and continued to be treated with ECT and neuroleptics. The writer notes, "There was a silly quality to her presentation and she was incoherent and often disconnected"—ignoring the fact that the treatments administered are well known to cause incoherence and feelings of disconnection.

What Happens When Madness Is Treated Medically?

In the war against mental illness, the main weapons in psychiatry's arsenal (and the military terminology is appropriate here, given the casualties resulting from treatment) are diagnosis, drugs, and ECT. The practice of stigmatizing human beings with psychiatric labels is responsible for immense social and psychological damage (see Caplan, 1996). Far more serious, however, is the debilitation engendered by the actual treatments (see Bentall, 2009; Moncrieff, 2008). One of the worst and most common of these is tardive dyskinesia (TD).[11]

According to the CPS, "It is suggested that all antipsychotic agents be discontinued if [TD symptoms] appear." The stiffness, shuffling gait, and involuntary movements that characterize TD are unmistakable. Yet clinicians often seem unable to distinguish TD effects from the symptoms of so-called mental illness. Even when they recognize TD, they generally continue neuroleptic treatment.

Psychiatric jargon obfuscates the fact that no scientific truth underlies the profession's interpretations of human behaviour. We find a blatant instance of this, and of the conflation of mental illness symptoms with iatrogenic damage, in the case of a man described as having "many years of clearly schizoid functioning, with an apparent deterioration from general paranoid personality demeanour into a frank mixed grandiose and persecutory paranoid delusional state presenting with both anticholinergic and extrapyramidal features."[12] Describing this man's observed tremor and bradykinesia (slowed or decreased movement—a TD symptom), the writer proclaims that "it is difficult to sort out between his illness and possible medication side-effects."

Another man, consigned to a psychiatric ward on the Care Team's say-so, "is possibly developing Parkinson's disorder, as a tremor is significant and noted by staff.... Apparently he does a lot of walking"—a symptom of akathisia[13]—"and they have been trying to get him to walk less.... He is also noted to have oral-buccal [mouth and cheek] tardive dyskinesia. At this time I'm planning to leave his medications as they are."

In another striking instance of wrongly continued treatment, the writer declares, "If patient's parkinsonian features continue to increase, it would be because the patient has an underlying Parkinson's Disease. Or it could be due to the [neuroleptic]. Meanwhile, we have continued with [neuroleptic]." He goes on to describe such well-known TD effects as "shuffling gait, mask-like facial expression, poverty of movement, tremor in the hands and cogwheel rigidity in the upper limbs," and adds, "she also continues to show evidence of significant cognitive impairment. Clinical Impression: Subcortical dementia." Cognitive impairment, including dementia, can be brought on by neuroleptics.

One of the ways in which mental health professionals judge patients' progress, or lack thereof, is by determining their degree of "insight"—which seems to be defined as willingness to agree with the practitioner's assessment of, and prescription for, the problem:

- "He was very preoccupied by the previous dystonic reactions of his tongue, and fearful that it [*sic*] could happen again … he showed no insight into his preoccupation with his tongue and it seemed all his anxiety was displaced onto this. He was superficially compliant and had insight into the need for continuing [neuroleptic]."
- "She has clearly stated that she does not wish follow-up with us … she is both delusional and without insight."

Sometimes, the Care Team's descriptions of the situations in which they have inadvertently placed their wards would be funny, if they weren't so sad: "She has some involuntary movements of her legs but this did not seem to bother her significantly and may provide some kind of exercise for her leg muscles—she does not walk very much."

Treatment Failure

One cannot overestimate the capacity of CMH service providers to ignore the failure of their ongoing treatments.

- A man who "is on the highest amount of medication he has been on in the last 10 years" continues to experience auditory hallucinations. "It may be that a lot of these delusions are so ingrained that they just don't respond to the [neuroleptic], but we'll have to judge that … so we'll go ahead and further increase his [neuroleptic]."
- A woman described as "notoriously noncompliant with medications," admitted to hospital on the Care Team's recommendation, "has been unstable for years and has been tried on many medications. She has apparently had no significant help from these. When asked what was most helpful to her, she describes 'love and kindness.' Plan: Increase [neuroleptic], with a plan for ECT if she continues to fail to respond to medications."

A common but rarely recognized paradoxical effect of neuroleptics is the exacerbation of psychosis. I myself have experienced this over and over again, and always the clinician's response is to up the dose. For me this has taken place only in hospitals, since I always go off the drugs as soon as they let me go. But the most terrifying thing about community mental health is that it *never* lets you go.

A woman experiencing "increasing auditory hallucinations even while on medications" says, "I've felt people trying to rape me spiritually." The clinician carps, "An ongoing issue was the patient's angry bitterness regarding her prescribed medication."

And it cannot be overemphasized that, when the Care Team fails you badly enough, they will throw you back into the bin. A woman who "remains delusional and continues to experience hallucinations, despite being administered [neuroleptic] daily," is hospitalized on the Care Team's recommendation. They continue to keep tabs on her via reports from hospital staff, who "suspect she is continuing to experience hallucinations." She is expected to use hospital passes to attend the Care Team. A mystified Care Team psychiatrist writes, "She cancelled her visit because she was angry at writer for reasons unknown. It was decided to switch her to [injectable neuroleptic]. She hides much of her psychotic thinking, as she continues to believe staff are not to be trusted." Why, one wonders, would she believe otherwise?

Care Team members never appear to worry when patients fail to thank them for their services. Rather, they congratulate themselves on the basis of assurances from relatives with, as it were, keener insight: "Her sister gave writer a call today, just to express her appreciation re our care of the patient. The sister had apparently received a call in recent days from the patient, indicating she did not wish to continue with our Team."

Death Wish as Treatment Outcome

It is not unusual for the despair engendered by the attenuation of people's lives at the hands of community (and other) mental health experts to make them want to die. One recipient of the Care Team's care is noted to have said, "The doctor never said a word to me, but just gave me pills.... I feel I am a complete failure. I feel I am being punished.... I hate myself. I would kill myself if I had the chance." Another "stated that she's been having thoughts and dreams of suicide, and fears that people will take her to the hospital." A third, in her sixties, had lost her secretarial position and was anxious and depressed about having to take computer upgrading courses. She "has consequently required ongoing supportive treatment and medications. She says that in spite of [nine different] present medications she feels depressed as ever." However, all is well, as far as the writer is concerned: "She has settled in adequately at [psychiatric boarding home].... She describes herself as stumbling along and sitting around waiting to die."

A male patient "was averse to coming into the crisis facility and in the end I convinced him to take some extra [neuroleptic] and that he go each day to the drop-in to pick it up, which he really didn't like but I told him it was either that or the facility. He told me that if he got another injection he would kill himself." Another "was suicidal as a result" of the fact that "he was salivating excessively from the [neuroleptic]. Emergency Psychiatric Services had to be called."

Intrusion

The administration of unwanted services is not confined to the office. Care Team members have, and use, the power to intrude upon people in their own homes—a key feature of CMH. In one striking example, Care Team members arrive, unannounced, at the home of an elderly woman who has for several decades been on three neuroleptics, two antidepressants, and a benzodiazepine, and is diagnosed with "dementia, of the Alzheimer's type, with delusions" (caused, perhaps, by the neuroleptics?). "Impression: A lady dressed in her housecoat, obviously just out of the shower because she was not expecting any visitors.... Affect is mostly anxiety and irritation. Mental status exam showed a gross disorientation in time, [and she was not] able to tell the date, day, month or year. The interview was rather difficult, as she obviously resented our being there. She was quite irate with our enquiries ... [and showed] some signs of mild depression with sad affect and some feelings of resignation about life soon being over for her, though no immediate suicidal intention."

Though this woman "denied suicidal ideation," the writer continues, she "just wishes she was dead." Two paragraphs later, he notes, "I have been in touch with Public Trustee, who want [sic] to sell her furniture, as she won't be needing it anymore."

Besides the other kinds of coercion and intrusion at their disposal, Care Teams can and do make use of police force to get people hospitalized. I know what it's like to have the police called on me by people who didn't like the way I was behaving (though in every instance I was being a nuisance, not a danger to self or others). Too many times, I have been apprehended by armed and uniformed officers who then transported me, in handcuffs, to the nearest hospital for psychiatric care. Upon arrival, I've been stripped naked, shot up with a neuroleptic, tied to a bed, and, redundantly, locked into an isolation cell. (This procedure has not changed at all between 1978, when it first happened to me, and the present.) So I empathize with the woman of whom the Care Team notes, "Patient appeared to have little insight into her illness and stated, 'I am not ill. I was kidnapped by the police and sent to hospital.'"

Oppression and Denigration of Specific Population Groups
Elderly Women

Psychiatry is often used particularly harshly against older women.[14] More women than men are electroshocked, and most of these women are old. The routine abuse that takes place on geriatric psychiatry wards includes tying people into chairs all day to keep them from "wandering," and quieting them with massive doses of neuroleptics and, if that fails, ECT. Long-term CMH care facilities are no better:

- A very old woman is placed in a community (for-profit) care home on the Care Team's recommendation. After several ECT treatments, "the nurse commented that she seemed to be 'too demented to be depressed now.' Before, she was quite a self-effacing person and now she consistently interrupts people with questions such as, 'What do I do now? Where am I? Help me.'"

- Another senior citizen in a similar situation was a thorn in her caregivers' collective side: "Staff were becoming exhausted by her demanding, importuning, somatizing and perseverative behaviour, and requested [the Care Team's] help.... Grief counselling was attempted but unsuccessful because of her memory loss.... An admission to the [provincial psychiatric hospital] was arranged, where she was treated with ECT and psychotropic medications"—both of which, of course, cause memory loss. "An effort was made to arrange outpatient ECT at a general hospital but the administrator rejected this idea with the argument that the gain from the previous ECT was not sufficient to spend more effort and taxpayers' money for, in effect, diminishing returns." Nevertheless, "a referral was made to [provincial psychiatric hospital], where she received eight ECT treatments.... Her cognitive impairment appears to be increasing, and this may be contributing to making her behaviour more manageable."

In one notable instance, the Care Team uses a method other than drugging and electroshock to control behaviour. A woman in her seventies who has been placed in residential care at the Care Team's behest "has talked to other residents about us when she's been angry with us. I suggested that she might not want to do that, reinforcing to her the importance of keeping boundaries. She has also been using the technique [suggested by the writer] of talking to her doll. I encouraged her to continue that." This is a classic example not only of psychiatry's infantilization of adults, but of how community mental health as currently practised promotes neither community nor mental health, in this case by keeping a patient from communicating with her fellow residents and from working through her problems in a rational, viable manner. It is also, of course, a startling instance of psychiatric ass-covering.

Children

The psychiatric drugging of children and even infants is increasing exponentially as more and more childhood behaviours are pathologized.[15] Consequently, CMH and other practitioners are inflicting more and more physical damage on growing brains and bodies, in the process crushing young minds, spirits, and personalities before they can fully develop. Psychiatrized children have voiced many of the same concerns about medication as their adult counterparts, with particular emphasis on forced compliance, adverse effects, and rebound effects. (The latter term refers to the extremely common phenomenon of going off the drugs only to find that the original problem recurs, often in a more severe form than it originally took.)

I do not know at what age a child can begin to be subjected to the ministrations of CMH practitioners, but young children certainly appear in the Care Team's records. I will limit myself to one example, from which I quote at length. The subject is a child who shows evidence of high intelligence: "Mother was pleased with his academic development in that he learned to read at the age of four." Yet he is first pathologized before starting school, on the grounds of developmental difficulties. Once in school, he is bullied by, and aggressive towards, other children, though "preoccupied with 'doing the right thing' and, with guidance and discussion, becomes in fact rigid and obsessed about appropriate behaviour."

In notations regarding family history, some bizarre details are seen as "quite relevant to this patient's difficulty.... Mother's brother has a son who is left-handed.... On the father's side, there is a history of asthma and one nephew who is in jail."

In the pre-school years, the boy "was noted to have delayed speech and poor articulation, poor hand-eye coordination and received speech therapy. He will bring up his own misbehaviours from the past at night before bed and repeatedly ask questions about what he did or should have done. When he is anxious about something he perseverates ... going over and over the possible outcomes and all the possible situations related to that topic."

Might it not be that his mother's insistence that something was wrong with him, and her requirement that he attend the Care Team, affect how this child feels and behaves?

The writer goes on to say, "The fact that he is quite rigid should make it easier to train him regarding socially appropriate behaviour." He then notes that "a child with his mixed difficulties is not likely to have a dramatic response to any specific medication. Nevertheless, certain symptoms may be targeted. For example, if significant attentional problems are present, a trial of methylphenidate should be considered for improved classroom attendance. If the obsessional features persist, an antidepressant could potentially be helpful. If impulsive behaviours predominate, a medication such as clonidine[16] could be considered."

Teenagers and Young Adults

Many people go mad or become depressed in their teens as the result of existential crises and/or trauma arising from family, romantic, or academic misfortunes, or from past or present bullying. It has been argued, and I certainly believe, that empathic support in going through such crises without psychiatric intervention is likely to help young people emerge not only unscathed but strengthened, and to grow up to be sound, creative, engaged, and well-socialized community members (see Breggin, 1998a, 2008b; Laing, 1971; Laing & Esterson, 1964; Whitaker, 2002, 2010). The psychiatric labelling, humiliation, and treatment of this population has resulted in widespread suffering among nonconforming (i.e., our best and brightest) teens and young adults, drugged—often against their will, and never with their fully informed consent, as the necessary information is simply not provided—with substances far worse than any recreational drug they might actually *want* to take. These unfortunate young people, like psychiatrized children, are likely to be a drain on the public purse—and, more to the point, debilitated and miserable—for the rest of their lives.

- A teenager whom the Care Team has diagnosed with "parent/child problem, conduct disorder with histrionic traits, pervasive development disorder, developmental coordination disorder, attitude problems, obsessional traits and impulsivity," heavily medicated, is noted to be engaging in "inappropriate conversation" characterized by "disjointed topics." The writer adds, "Of course her request for a reduction in medications may have some very significant elements of denial around the illness.... If symptoms persist, I would recommend [three neuroleptics, in combination]."
- Another teen "shows an oppositional defiance style and a temperament with emotional reactivity.... Should she show any signs of accelerated mood, grandiosity, disinhibition, decreased sleep, etc., her [neuroleptic] should be stepped up promptly." Again, please bear in mind that all the symptoms listed can be exacerbated, or even caused, by neuroleptics.
- A third teen is "still quite preoccupied with her creative abilities, and her concern is that she hasn't had this [*sic*] in quite a period of time. I wonder if some of her creative bursts weren't actually when she was psychotic and she is confusing that with creative ability. Plan: Increase [neuroleptic]."

Aboriginal Canadians

Native Canadians make up a disproportionate percentage of our society's homeless, impoverished, and imprisoned populations. Their all-too-common psychiatrization must be viewed in light of the genocide—considered by many to be ongoing—perpetrated by the dominant, colonizing white race (see Smith, 2006). Team members write about their Aboriginal service recipients with even more arrogance and contempt than they generally display:

- A man assessed as a "totally dependent personality type with seeming inability to achieve motivation," whose "primary concern is the acquisition of medications," is diagnosed with "alcohol abuse and delusional disorder, persecutory type" and treated with [benzodiazepines] and [injectible neuroleptics]. "Mental status exam revealed a young Native man of solid build. He volunteered no information but would respond with one-word answers." (Might one not speculate that he was attending the Care Team because he would otherwise be put back in hospital, and was justifiably suspicious and miserable and therefore not forthcoming?) "He spoke in a low voice and there is great poverty of content.... He appeared to have little insight into his difficulties and did not appear to be too bright. It was difficult to settle him down and he had to be given [neuroleptic] twice before he began to be calmed down. There was also a highly dependent quality and a slightly manipulative quality to the anxiety attack, as if to elicit attention. Diagnostic Impression: He's developed a severe tardive dyskinesia over the last two years and has been treated with botulinum toxin for severe blepharospasm[17] ... he complains of several somatic complaints. Plan: His medication may need to be reduced eventually."

- A Métis woman, noted to have been abused as a child and later by her husband, has had all of her children taken from her and put into foster homes. "She was irritable with my questions and complained that I'd given her the pills that made her crazy when she first came to this city.... She has responded briefly to ECT, which oblates the hallucinations, but these return reasonably rapidly. Generally she has been medication-resistant, noncompliant, and even in long-term hospitalizations has shown little improvement. She has mild oral-buccal tardive dyskinesia. A seizure following use of [antidepressant] was noted. The primary issue here is to try to build some therapeutic alliance with this chronically suspicious woman."

- An Aboriginal woman on three neuroleptics, one recently increased, has a long history of involuntary hospital admissions: "Many of her delusions persist; however, she's less troubled by them.... In mini mental status exam, she wrote: 'I want to go home.' It was noted that her lower right arm and hand are edematous and held in a fixed, pendant position with fingers straight"—a classic dystonia symptom. "The patient's speech is only partially coherent." The writer does not see high-dose neuroleptics as causing or contributing to any of these problems, and ends her report with the telling statement, "she has the reputation of being a difficult boarder."

Conclusion

Community mental health praxis results in a vast number of human lives primarily characterized by cognitive impairment, chronic illness and, most ironically, social isolation far more severe than that suffered in the bad old days of long-term institutionalization.

Awful as it is to be locked up on a psych ward, at least we patients have each other. When I've been inside, I have always experienced a sense of belonging. Many of us were able and willing to listen to each other's stories with the patience, gentleness, humour, and empathy lacking in our keepers. Ironically, we got a real sense of community from—and were helped to regain our ability to function by—other "sick" people.

On the other hand, institutionalization—becoming habituated to and dependent on absolute routine, constant companionship, and being enclosed in a small space—sets in very quickly. Back in my apartment after even the briefest of psychiatric incarcerations, I have felt lost, disoriented, and hideously lonely. I have also been plagued by withdrawal effects such as insomnia, anxiety, and loss of mental acuity, though drugged for only a few days. Always, when released, I am instructed to hook up with my local Community Mental Health Care Team. Always, I say that I will do so. I then go home, get over the effects of what the hospital has done to me, and get on with my life—a life, I might add, both enjoyable and useful, despite the fact that I go nuts now and again.

As I write this, a dear friend who was locked up on a suburban psych ward earlier this year is being coerced to attend her local Care Team. The Care Team injects her with an atypical neuroleptic that is already causing dystonic and cognitive difficulties, and tests her blood to ensure that she is maintaining what they call therapeutic levels of several other psychiatric drugs they make her take.

Her outpatient committal order—euphemistically called "extended leave" in British Columbia's Mental Health Act—obliges her to subject herself to this ongoing damage and humiliation, on pain of reincarceration if she fails to comply. She and far too many others are receiving community mental health services because they have no choice (Fabris, 2011). And too many of those who could otherwise choose have had the will to do so knocked out of them by years of brain-damaging, soul-destroying treatment—and by trusting their caregivers' judgment that this is what's best for them.

There are so many alternatives to community mental health care as it currently exists. If people could be socialized from an early age to be aware of, and take care of, themselves and each other, much of what is construed as mental illness would never come to pass in the first place. Good nutrition, exercise, sleep, yoga, meditation, tai chi, and/or countless other practices stemming from many different cultures (including those of our country's Aboriginal peoples) could replace psychiatric treatment, with better results, and improve the lives of those it has already harmed. So could various creative, intellectual, social, political, and other pursuits.

In the early 1970s, in Vancouver, Lanny Beckman founded the Mental Patients Association (MPA) (see Beckman & Davies, Chapter 3). Governed and operated by its members, MPA gave them a safe place in which to live and socialize. In its current incarnation, as the Motivation, Power and Achievement Society, it is a mainstream CMH organization with a huge professional staff. But the original MPA helped damaged people regain stability, volition, creativity, and improved quality of life, by providing actual community.

As for dealing with emotional crisis, in 1974 a group of people that included some MPA members—and no mental health professionals—founded the groundbreaking Vancouver Emotional Emergency Centre (VEEC).[18] Wildly successful, VEEC lost its funding two years later; it was too much of a threat to the mental health establishment. Ellen Frank, a VEEC co-founder and early staff member, points out that "when you're in a crisis, you need a safe place. It's just logical. Of course people lose their minds, because the world's crazy. Rich people lose their minds all the time, but can cover it. Most people who come to VEEC had nowhere to live, no money, no job—no purpose. People need a reason to get up in the morning. That's why many of them later became volunteers there" (quoted in Shimrat, 2011, p. 13). Lanny calls psychiatry "the medicalization of prejudice. People who 'go crazy' can either be given over to psychiatric care, or somehow live in a society that is uncaring and lacks love. MPA tried to say that the real choice is to have a place to go where you're loved when you're crazy. The question of craziness would disappear if we lived in a humane world. If someone was in a state of incredible pain, the issue would not be one of diagnosis. Instead, it would be saying, 'What can we do to help you?'" (quoted in Shimrat, 1997, p. 57).

I dream of a society brave and moral enough to eschew the whole paradigm of mental health and illness, replacing it with the creation of real community, and real help, of the kind and quality briefly achieved in Vancouver in the early 1970s.

Notes

1   Also called antipsychotics, neuroleptics are generally accompanied by drugs meant to minimize their adverse effects, which of course have adverse effects of their own. Among many other diseases and conditions, neuroleptics can cause pancreatitis, heart disease, agranulocytosis, and neuroleptic malignant syndrome (NMS), in which temperature regulation centres fail, causing temperature to increase suddenly. NMS can be fatal. Sudden death is also listed as a possible adverse effect. Withdrawal psychosis is common. See the work of Peter Breggin (1998c, 2008b) and Robert Whitaker (2002, 2010) to read more about the harm caused by these and other psychiatric drugs.

2   These are highly addictive drugs of the Valium family, given to counteract anxiety. See www.non-benzodiazepines.org.uk/books.html.

3   Antidepressants can cause heart disease, sexual dysfunction, increased seizure risk, agitation, insomnia, nausea, vomiting, diarrhea, weight gain, and suicidal/homicidal ideation. As is the case with most psychiatric drugs, withdrawal can be a nightmare, and can result in extreme exacerbation of the condition for which the drugs were prescribed.

4   This class of drugs is best exemplified by lithium, which can cause damage to, and ultimately failure of, the liver and kidneys. People on lithium must have their blood tested frequently, as the so-called therapeutic dose is dangerously close to a lethal one.

5   See http://twu.ca/library/ecps.htm. The CPS is the primary source of information about medications for Canadian doctors. Of course, they are also flooded with promotions from drug companies.

6   Ritalin and similar drugs, chemically related to methamphetamine (speed), cause untold long-term damage in an ever-increasing number of children, and are used even on babies (see, for example, Breggin, 1998c; LeFrançois, 2006, 2008).

7   In so-called electroshock therapy, electricity is applied to the brain, resulting in a period of unconsciousness from which the patient may emerge in a state of euphoria similar to that

caused by other traumatic brain injuries. ECT use is on the rise, as it is much cheaper than drugs, resulting in a higher profit margin for practitioners. Whereas it used to be used almost exclusively on people diagnosed with depression, it is now used much more broadly. In Canada doctors get paid for each shock administered. ECT causes memory loss, cognitive impairment, and other common effects of brain damage. I have met mothers who emerged from a course of treatments unable to remember or recognize their own children. For more information, see Andre (2009), the website www.madnessradio.net/madness-radio-electroshock-deception-linda-andre, and Weitz (Chapter 11).

8   See www.hc-sc.gc.ca/ahcasc/media/advisories-avis/_2011/2011_78-eng.php.

9   This has included conducting interviews for two CBC *Ideas* radio programs (Shimrat, 1990, 1991) and for my book *Call Me Crazy: Stories from the Mad Movement* (1997); coordinating and editing the newsletter of the Ontario Psychiatric Survivors' Alliance (1990–1992); and editing *Phoenix Rising: The Voice of the Psychiatrized* (see www.psychiatricsurvivorarchives.com/phoenix.html) in the late 1980s, *Second Opinion* (newsletter of SOS—the Second Opinion Society—Whitehorse, Yukon) in the early 1990s, and, since 2009, the *Networker* (formerly the *Bulletin*, newsletter of the West Coast Mental Health Network—see www.wcmhn.org for back issues).

10   Intramuscular injections of neuroleptic drugs (often given in the buttocks) are routinely used on hospital patients who are non-compliant in regard to medication (i.e., if you won't swallow the pills, a nurse will jab you by force—backed up by, if you struggle, a posse of orderlies to hold you down). Depot (long-acting) injections are used on non-compliant patients in community settings.

11   Tardive dyskinesia (TD) is a painful, disfiguring, and sometimes incapacitating neurological syndrome resulting primarily from the use of neuroleptics, though other psychiatric drugs also cause it. TD causes tremors, tics, spasms, twitches, and other involuntary movements, especially of the face, tongue, and limbs. Some of its effects are similar to those of Parkinson's disease, and these are collectively referred to as "parkinsonism." Due to the widespread and increasing use of neuroleptic drugs, the incidence of TD has reached epidemic proportions. See Breggin (2008b), Breggin & Cohen (1999), and Whitaker (2002, 2010).

12   Extrapyramidal effects, which typify TD, include constipation, dry eyes and mouth, slowing of urination, blurred vision, dizziness, tremor, slurred speech, akathisia, dystonia (abnormal muscle tone resulting in muscular spasms and bizarre postures), anxiety, distress, and paranoia.

13   Akathisia is a movement disorder that often accompanies TD. It is characterized by muscular quivering, restlessness, and the inability to sit still.

14   See Rob Wipond at http://robwipond.com/?cat=35 and Don Weitz at www.ect.org/resources/elderly.html.

15   On the subject of drugging children, see the work of Breggin (1998a,c), LeFrançois (2006, 2008), and Whitaker (2002, 2010).

16   A drug developed for the treatment of high blood pressure, clonidine is now also used on children considered to have attention deficit disorder.

17   Blepharospasm involves spasmodic winking caused by the involuntary contraction of an eyelid muscle, commonly seen in TD.

18   See Judi Chamberlin at http://goo.gl/38HHO, where the chapter on VEEC in her book *On Our Own* (1978) is reproduced.

CHAPTER 11

Electroshock: Torture as "Treatment"

Don Weitz[1]

First Do No Harm—The Hippocratic Oath

Electroshock is violence.

—Ramsey Clark, human rights advocate, former US Attorney General
Invited address at Annual Meeting, American Psychiatric Association,
New York City (1983)

A part of me has been wiped away—ECT should be banned absolutely, no question.

—Paivi, electroshock survivor, testimony during public hearings,
Toronto (2005)

I am a proud antipsychiatry activist, survivor of forced insulin shock treatments, and member of the Coordinating Committee of the Coalition Against Psychiatric Assault (CAPA). CAPA is a grassroots, human rights organization founded in 2003 in Toronto. It takes nonviolent strategic political actions and is committed to building a humane world that does not pathologize, marginalize, stigmatize, discriminate against, and oppress people. Strategizing against electroshock ("electroconvulsive therapy" or "ECT") is one of CAPA's two priority issues. Our other priority is strategizing against psychiatric drugs—public educational campaigns, community outreach initiatives, and nonviolent protests are major aspects of our work. Psychiatric drugs such as antidepressants and neuroleptics ("antipsychotics") are extremely harmful. These neurotoxins frequently cause serious medical and psychological conditions including trauma, memory loss, disability, neurological disorders including brain damage, and sometimes death. They also violate our human rights (Breggin, 2008a; Frank, 2006a,b; Weitz, 2008).

I want to focus on the psychiatric procedure of electroshock, arguably psychiatry's most controversial treatment. This is a serious understatement. Electroshock is an unethical, if not criminal, assault on people's brains, health, and lives, particularly when administered without informed consent, against a person's will. Many shock survivors and activists call ECT torture.

The Electroshock Procedure

- No food or drink 8–10 hours before ECT.
- A tranquilizer, sedative, and muscle relaxant are administered before the electric current is turned on; they raise the brain's seizure threshold, so much higher voltages are necessary to trigger the seizure.
- The muscle relaxant, a derivative of curare, is so powerful that it paralyzes all muscles in the body including the diaphragm, so the person can't breathe and oxygen must be administered.
- The person is asleep or unconscious during the treatment.
- Two electrodes with electricity-conducting jelly or gel are placed on the head over the temporal lobes (seat of memory function)—they are placed on one side ("unilateral ECT") or more commonly on both sides ("bilateral ECT").
- An average of 200 volts of electricity is delivered to the brain—today's ECT machines can deliver up to 450 volts (Cameron, 1994).
- The electric current usually lasts 1–2 seconds, frequently longer.

Immediate/Temporary Effects

- Grand mal epileptic-type seizure and convulsion lasting approximately 60 seconds—shock promoters called this seizure *therapeutic*.
- Sudden increase in heart rate and blood pressure.
- Coma lasting 10–20 minutes.
- Upon awakening, the person immediately experiences a severe, migraine-type headache that lasts a few hours, disorientation (e.g., not knowing your name, where you are), confusion, muscle and physical weakness, nausea, and memory loss.

Long-Term/Permanent Effects

- Brain damage: nerve cell death and small hemorrhages in blood vessels (Breggin, 1998b; Frank, 1990; Friedberg, 1977).
- Memory loss for personal experiences and events occurring months or years *before* ECT (retrograde amnesia) (Janis, 1950; Janis & Astrachan, 1951; Squire & Slater, 1983).
- Memory loss of recently learned information, knowledge, or new experiences *after* ECT (anterograde amnesia).
- Difficulty concentrating, reading, and retaining new information.

- Reduced or impaired intelligence.
- Loss of creativity.

These very serious, health-threatening effects—particularly brain damage, blood vessel hemorrhages, permanent memory loss, and death—have been known and documented in the medical literature for many years (Breggin, 2008a; Frank, 2006a,b). However, they are consistently and unethically minimized or denied by Canadian and American psychiatric organizations and the mainstream media. For example, in its 2009 position paper on ECT, the Canadian Psychiatric Association inaccurately and irresponsibly claims there is "[no] credible evidence that ECT causes structural brain damage," yet cites only one review (not a study) to support its sweeping conclusion (Enns et al., 2009). Nevertheless, there is conclusive scientific evidence of ECT-caused brain damage (Breggin, 1998b; Calloway et al., 1981; Dolan, 2009; Frank, 1998; Friedberg, 1977; Read & Bentall, 2010; Sterling, 2002).

On March 1, 2009, the CAPA Executive wrote a letter to Health Minister David Caplan urging the government to "ban the practice of electroshock in Ontario" and "declare an immediate moratorium on electroshock administered to women and the elderly." In our letter, we also asked Caplan to invite government officials to attend our Mother's Day protest entitled "Stop Shocking Our Mothers and Grandmothers." However, neither Caplan nor any government official replied, and no government officials came to our rally and protest in Queen's Park, which attracted over 100 citizens. CAPA strongly recommends a total and immediate ban on electroshock. Specifically, we strongly recommend this legislative committee (Select Committee on Mental Health and Addictions) ban or at least call a moratorium on electroshock in Ontario (Coalition Against Psychiatric Assault, 2009).

Women and elderly citizens are the prime targets of electroshock. There are two main reasons for urging a total ban or moratorium on electroshock:

1. Electroshock is a serious violation of human rights and medical ethics.
2. It has caused and continues to cause serious harm including trauma, permanent memory loss, brain damage, and sometimes death (Breggin, 1997, 1998b; Frank, 1990). In 2007, Dr. Harold Sackeim, a widely known shock promoter, published the largest scientific study to date in which he and other researchers conclusively proved that electroshock causes massive and permanent memory loss and brain damage, with women and the elderly suffering the most damage. The Sackeim study also clearly showed that brain damage occurred whether ECT was administered on one side (unilateral) or both sides of the head (bilateral) (Coalition Against Psychiatric Assault, 2007; Sackeim et al., 2007).

Dr. Bonnie Burstow, chair of CAPA, antipsychiatry activist, and widely respected feminist and faculty member at Ontario Institute for Studies in Education/University of Toronto, asserts that electroshock is "a form of violence against women" and must end. All CAPA members agree with Dr. Burstow's analysis and conclusion, as do many other psychiatric survivors and antipsychiatry activists. Since electroshock is a form of "violence against women," feminists and women's organizations should become more involved in the struggle to abolish shock (Burstow, 2006a,b).

According to ECT statistics I have obtained from the Ontario government's Ministry of Health and Long-Term Care, approximately 1,500–2,000 people have been shocked annually for many years in the province; the prime targets are women and the elderly (Ontario Ministry of Health and Long-Term Care, 2000–2004). Two to three times more women than men undergo electroshock; elderly women and young mothers diagnosed with postpartum depression are at great risk of being electroshocked. In short, sexist and ageist factors influence the practice of electroshock in Ontario, as well as other provinces and states in the United States (Weitz, 1997). So far, no Canadian psychiatrist or neurologist has publicly criticized electroshock; not one has called for a ban or moratorium. Their shameful silence speaks volumes and is a stain on the medical profession. However, several psychiatrists, neurologists, and psychologists in the United States, New Zealand, the United Kingdom, Ireland, and a few other European countries have spoken out; they have publicly denounced electroshock as harmful and unethical and called for a ban (Breggin, 1997, 2008a; Corry, 2008; Friedberg, 1977; Sterling, 2002).

Since the dramatic shock scene in the 1975 film *One Flew Over the Cuckoo's Nest*, the public and even many health professionals wrongly assume that electroshock is no longer administered. Except for 41 days in 1982 in Berkeley, California, electroshock has never been banned (Frank, 2006a,b; Quigley, 1983). In fact, electroshock has been increasingly administered during the last 10 to 15 years and administered in virtually all general and psychiatric hospitals in Ontario. Unfortunately, ECT is covered by the Ontario Health Insurance Plan (OHIP) as a medical procedure and currently costs Ontario taxpayers approximately $2 million each year.

Ontario ECT Statistics

Shock statistics I've obtained from the Ontario government's Ministry of Health and Long-Term Care, as well as California and Texas in the United States, clearly show that large numbers of ECTs have been administered during the last 5 to 10 years (Ontario Ministry of Health and Long-Term Care, 2000–2004). It's worth emphasizing that women and elderly people, especially women 60 years and older, are its main targets. For example, in 2001–2002 in Ontario, a total of 14,034 ECTs were administered to 1,656 citizens—roughly nine ECTs per person. Over two-thirds, 68 percent, were women. Elderly women 65 years and older were shocked about three times more often than elderly men. Electroshock is not only "a form of violence against women," as

Dr. Bonnie Burstow asserts, but a form of elder abuse (Burstow, 2006a,b). A similar gender and age pattern is obvious in the ECT statistics during the next two years. For example, in 2002–2003, a total of 15,507 shocks were administered to approximately 1,700 people in Ontario's general and psychiatric hospitals. Sixty-three percent of all electroshock was administered to women, and 41 percent of these women were 60 years and older. In 2003–2004, 14,238 ECTs were administered to approximately 1,600 people, 62 percent were administered to women, and 43 percent of these women were 60 years and older. Statistics for other years report that 68–70 percent of shock survivors are women, clearly revealing that two to three times more women than men are electroshocked (Ontario Ministry of Health and Long-Term Care, 2000–2004). These statistics are underestimates, incomplete, and unreliable since many hospitals do not keep accurate and complete records; they're not legally required to report all ECTs to the Ministry. Nevertheless, the gender and age pattern is significant. In the United States, at least 100,000 people are electroshocked each year—probably more. There are no accurate and reliable national "ECT" figures for Canada. That's mainly because Statistics Canada stopped collecting them in 1979; in 1994, the Canadian Institute for Health Information assumed from Statistics Canada responsibility for data collection and dissemination for hospital morbidity and surgical procedures.

Ten years ago in BC, psychiatrist Jaime Paredes was fired shortly after filing a complaint with Health Minister Corky Evans in which he criticized the shocking of disproportionately large numbers of elderly patients in Vancouver's Riverview Hospital (Fong & Mulgrew, 2001). Recent shock statistics for British Columbia document this fact, particularly regarding women 60 years and older (BC ECT Statistics, 2008). A few years earlier in the 1990s in Madison, Wisconsin, psychiatric nurse Stacie Neldaughter was also fired and lost her nursing license for speaking out against the shocking of elderly women patients in St. Mary's Hospital—she was accused of "coercing" patients to refuse consent (LeClaire, 2011). Unfortunately, there is still no whistle-blowing law in Canada to protect the jobs of health professionals when they expose psychiatric or medical abuses as human rights violations. Fear of losing their job is one major reason why the vast majority of doctors and nurses remain silent; consequently, they allow this elder abuse to continue.

There are also no mandatory ECT reporting laws or regulations in Canada that require hospitals to report all shock procedures, medical complications, and ECT-related deaths to provincial ministries of health or Health Canada. So far, hospital reporting of electroshock has been discretionary or voluntary in every province in Canada, and every state in the United States except two (Texas and California). Given that electroshock is controversial and harmful, this patchwork of ECT statistics is inexcusable, irresponsible, and incompetent. The public and researchers have a right to this information; it should be consolidated, and easily and freely accessible. After I applied in 2005 to the "Access to Information" department of the Ontario government's Ministry of Health and Long-Term Care and appealed its unjust and unreasonable refusals of my request, I waited almost two years to receive eight pages of essentially useless ECT statistics for 2002–2004. For this information, the Ministry initially charged me an outrageous fee of over $5,000(!), which I refused to pay. After two successful appeals, the fee was finally waived after Ontario's Information and Privacy Commissioner supported my appeals (Cribb, 2007).

> That the Ministry of Health require mandatory reporting by hospitals of data on the use of ECT to a central data bank. These data should be used to monitor the use of ECT and to identify and deal with any unusual or unacceptable practices. These data should be published annually and should be available to the public and to researchers.

This is one of many major recommendations in the Ontario government's 1985 *Report of the Electro-Convulsive Therapy Review Committee*; the vast majority have never been implemented—a good reason to *discontinue* ECT, according to lawyer and chairman Charles J. Clarke (Ontario Ministry of Health, 1985).

Wendy Funk, Wayne Lax, Sue Clark-Wittenberg, and Carla McKague are four Canadian shock survivors who have publicly and courageously spoken out against electroshock and want it banned— so have many other shock survivors, activists and critics in Canada, the United States, and other countries. Wendy is an author and a good friend. Twenty years after she was forcibly electroshocked over 40 times in Alberta in 1989, she has no memory of approximately 30 years of her life, and has no memory of raising her children. The electroshocks totally and indiscriminately erased these precious memories; they also ruined her promising social work career and dashed her hope of going to law

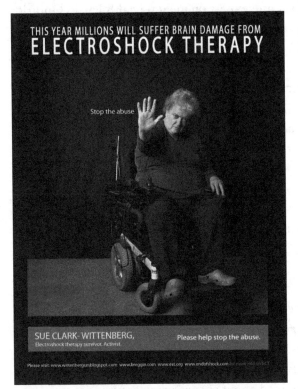

FIGURE 11.1: Sue Clark-Wittenberg

A survivor of involuntary institutionalization and electroshock, Ottawa resident Sue Clark-Wittenberg is an important figure in the Canadian psychiatric survivor community.

Source: Photographed by Crila for crimomedia.com, 2008.

school. These facts, her horrific hospital experiences, and courageous resistance are documented in her outstanding book *"What Difference Does It Make?": The Journey of a Soul Survivor* (Funk, 1998).

In Kenora, Ontario, Wayne Lax was subjected to at least 80 electroshocks and countless doses of psychiatric drugs over a 20-year period, against his will, as treatments for his alcoholism. Ever since his hospital release in 1992, Wayne has had major memory problems; he doesn't remember several old friends he met in hospital. Sue Clark-Wittenberg was 17 in 1973 when she was forcibly electroshocked five times in the former Brockville Psychiatric Hospital in Ontario. She was severely traumatized while the nurses and attendants physically dragged her screaming and resisting to the ECT room. During one *treatment*, her heart stopped and she had to be revived. Today, 36 years later, Sue still has problems remembering, concentrating, and learning, yet she has become a courageous activist by speaking out and is co-founder of the International Campaign to Ban Electroshock (ICBE, 2009).

Carla McKague is my very close friend. For many years she was widely respected and consulted as an outstanding lawyer and expert on mental health law in Ontario and Canada; she is co-author of *Mental Health Law in Canada* (1987). Carla also successfully advocated for "Mrs. T," a woman locked up in Hamilton Psychiatric Hospital where her psychiatrist threatened to electroshock her against her will and that of her family. Although the legal case was lost, Carla helped "Mrs. T" escape electroshock (Weitz, 1984). In 1963, while depressed, Carla consulted a psychiatrist in the community who admitted her to Henderson General Hospital. After a 20-minute interview, he prescribed 15 ECTs; as a result of the shocks, Carla suffered permanent memory loss as well as major losses in her awesome intelligence and musical ability.

In April 2005, CAPA organized four days of public hearings on electroshock and psychiatric drugs entitled "Enquiry into Psychiatry"; two days of hearings on electroshock were held in the Council Chamber of Toronto City Hall. These hearings, as well as previous hearings in October 1984, organized by the Ontario Coalition to Stop Electroshock were prompted by the Ontario government's consistent refusal to call public hearings on electroshock, and its refusal to act on its own recommendations in the 1985 *Report of the Electro-Convulsive Therapy Review Committee*. CAPA's public hearings in 2005 were facilitated by an independent panel that later wrote a report titled *Electroshock Is Not a Healing Option*. Several psychiatric survivors courageously testified about some of their traumatic, memory-destroying shock experiences; most advocated a total ban. Unfortunately, there was no media coverage of their riveting and powerful testimony in these historic hearings; no government officials attended. Fortunately, there is a DVD of this important educational and public event (Myers & Burstow, 2006; Report of the Panel on Electroshock, 2005).

Shock Survivor Testimony

What follows is a very small sample of this shock survivor testimony delivered during two days of public hearings held in Toronto City Hall organized by CAPA in April 2005. In graphic and moving detail, these survivors courageously describe how electroshock destroyed years of memories, damaged some of their intellectual and creative abilities, and traumatized them; these so-called "transient" or "temporary" effects are still felt 10 to 30 years later. All were shocked against their will, without informed consent—they were denied basic information about the effects of ECT, told nothing about alternatives, and denied a second opinion; all were coerced, humiliated, abused, and partly disabled. Informed consent for ECT is a sham, a sick joke (Report of the Panel on Electroshock, 2005). The following survivor excerpts are from the 2005 hearings, noted above:

Jacqueline: [I can't recall experiences] between 1995 and 1999.... Pre-1995 has been wiped out for me by ECT.... When I woke up after the first treatment, I didn't know the year or what country I was in.

Wayne: As a result of the shock treatments, I am missing large portions of my memory. When I walk down the halls of Lakehead Psychiatric Hospital, patients come up to me and say "Hi," they know me, but I have no idea who they are. I have no memory. A part of me is missing forever.

Wendy: After 14 months locked up in a psychiatric unit, I returned home to a family I have no memory of. My social work career and law aspirations vanished. The intent of ECT is to kill brain cells.

Maynard: Once after I had shock treatment, when my mother and my aunt came to visit me, I couldn't tell one from the other. When I woke up after the first treatment, I didn't know the year or what country I was in.

Paivi: [Electroshock caused an] excruciating headache. I thought my head was about to explode; it was so bad I was unable to eat for the next 2 days. [Electroshock] stunted my creativity, my imagination.... I used to be able to use my imagination to paint ... this extreme treatment has numbed my emotions. The numbed emotions continue today. I've never been able to connect. It's as if I'm looking through a window watching.... I had to relearn how to write a sentence, how to write a paragraph, how to calculate multiplication tables, I'm not as quick or smart as I used to be ... a part of my being has been wiped away. ECT should be banned absolutely, no question.

Carla: I couldn't memorize music anymore. I played the piano. I would spend hours trying to memorize one page of music. I kept waiting for them to come back and they didn't ... huge chunks of my life are

	still missing.... I had no idea what I was getting into. Nobody told me anything.
Mel:	Chunks of my memory are still missing.
Wayne:	They [psychiatrists] treated us like guinea pigs ... why would delivering electricity through a brain be anything less than destructive and damaging?
Jerry:	The scoline [Ed.: muscle relaxant succinycholine] felt like somebody pouring ice cubes into your lungs.... It was almost like I died 36 times.
Chris:	[Electroshock is] a blunt forced trauma to the brain. Electroshock should be banned. In no way is it a healing option.
Mel:	Shock should be banned.
Sue:	It was a traumatizing experience for me that still haunts me to this day.... Electroshock is barbaric, unethical, torture. ECT must be stopped, [it's] a crime against humanity.

At least two survivors testified that the psychiatrists had threatened them with electroshock and/or hospitalization. For example:

Paivi:	"Change your lifestyle or I am bringing you in [to the hospital]" [Ed.: her psychiatrist's sexist threat].

Although Anik (pseudonym) was not electroshocked, she testified that she was "threatened with electroshock" after a psychiatrist discovered she had suffered sexual abuse and trauma.

The disastrous, brain-damaging effects of electroshock have been well documented in studies published in medical and psychiatric journals for approximately 60 years. In the 1950s, approximately 10 years after ECT was introduced as a psychiatric treatment in the United States, Canada, and Europe, animal and human autopsy and neurological studies were published that clearly revealed brain damage. CT-scan studies in the 1980s and similar studies in subsequent years have also documented brain damage (Breggin, 1998b; Calloway et al., 1981; Frank, 1990). Psychiatric researchers have rarely conducted *effectiveness* studies of long-term effects lasting more than eight weeks. In the early 1950s, Yale psychologist Irving Janis conducted the first long-term scientific study of memory loss; it clearly showed that if memory loss from electroshock persisted for one year or longer, it was permanent; however, 60 years later, other researchers have never tried to replicate this study (Janis, 1948, 1950; Janis & Astrachan, 1951). Many shock researchers and promoters have been exposed as lying about ECT's alleged *safety and effectiveness*, and covering up the brain damage caused by the shock machines (Andre,

2009; Cameron, 1994). Health Canada officials and the Food and Drug Administration (FDA) in the United States have acknowledged that they have never tested shock machines for their *medical safety* (Lyons, 2002). Although the FDA has classified shock machines as class-III or *high risk* since 1978, it planned to reclassify them as class-II, or *low risk*, mainly because of pro-shock lobbying by the American Psychiatric Association (Andre, 2009). However, during public hearings in January 2011, powerful testimony from many shock survivors, activists, several psychiatrists and psychologists convinced the FDA panel to continue classifying ECT in class-III as high risk; the FDA also recommended pre-market approval assessments of the machines' alleged safety and effectiveness (Breeding, 2011; Coalition Against Psychiatric Assault, 2011a,b; MedPage, 2011). Health Canada currently, but weakly, classifies the machines as *potentially hazardous*. The advocacy/human rights organization MindFreedom International, which represents approximately 100 survivor/human rights organizations in 14 countries, recently launched a public campaign to stop the FDA's deregulation of this allegedly safe and effective medical device (MindFreedom, 2009).

Recommendations

In its 2005 report, *Electroshock Is Not a Healing Option*, the shock panel made four major recommendations addressed to the Ontario government's Ministry of Health and Long-Term Care. The Minister (George Smitherman at the time) never replied and never addressed these recommendations:

1. Ban Electroshock

   The panel unanimously recommends that the Minister ban electroshock throughout Ontario. This key recommendation supports the shock ban urged by most people who testified. We call attention to a major conclusion written twenty years ago by Charles J. Clark, Q.C., former chairperson of the Ontario government's 1985 Report of the Electro-Convulsive Therapy Review Committee: "The recommendations of the Review Committee place particularly heavy responsibilities upon the medical profession, the hospitals where ECT is administered, and the Ministry of Health. The chairman holds the view that unless those responsibilities are accepted and fulfilled, there is a *strong argument for the discontinuance of ECT as a treatment*" [Emphasis original]. Since virtually none of the Committee's 39 recommendations have been implemented in the last 24 years, this fact alone justifies a ban on electroshock.

2. Draft Shock Ban Law

   We urge the Minister to draft a law to ban electroshock in Ontario. More specifically, we recommend an amendment to section 49(1) in Ontario's

Mental Health Act, which will prohibit administering electroshock to any patient or person. The Section currently prohibits psychosurgery for involuntary patients.

3.   Public Hearings

The Ministry should call and hold public hearings across Ontario on electroshock as soon as possible. These hearings should focus on current ECT practice, adverse effects, risks, alternatives, and human rights violations. Citizens who undergo electroshock and/or have been threatened with electroshock should be encouraged to testify and given priority when making oral or written submissions. To date, no government in Ontario or Canada has held public hearings on electroshock. Before the Ministry of Health released the *Report of the Electro-Convulsive Therapy Review Committee* in December 1985, it requested written submissions only from the public; the Ministry refused citizen requests for public hearings. We believe this refusal was unreasonable, discriminatory, and undemocratic.

4.   A Healing House

As a pilot project, the Minister in consultation with the Minister of Community and Social Services, the Citizen's Working Committee on Electroshock, and the Toronto Disaster Relief Committee should facilitate the establishment of a Healing House for psychiatric survivors trying to recover from electroshock. (Report of the Panel on Electroshock, 2005)

Several other major recommendations in the report are addressed to the Toronto Board of Health and Health Canada. A major recommendation to establish an "Adverse Electroshock Reaction Program-Databank" was specifically addressed to Health Canada: "It should be modeled after its Adverse Drug Reaction Program." Although CAPA sent these government agencies a copy of the report four years ago, none have replied; none have shown any interest or political will in implementing any recommendation. It is CAPA's hope that the Ontario government will at last act on these recommendations.

Finally, I call attention to the growing international resistance to electroshock, which started in California in the early 1980s (Frank, 1983; Quigley, 1983). During the last three years, public protests have also been held in Toronto, Ottawa, Montreal; Cork, Ireland; and Austin, Texas. At the initiative and leadership of CAPA, the Canadian protests were held on or close to Mother's Day to publicize the fact that it is mainly young mothers and elderly women who are being targeted, traumatized, and damaged by electroshock. The theme of these protests is "Stop Shocking Our Mothers and Grandmothers." Protests were held in Toronto on May 10, 2010, during an international conference titled PsychOUT: A Conference for Organizing Resistance Against Psychiatry, and a few days later in Montreal and Ireland.

We urged the Ontario government's Select Committee on Mental Health and Addictions and then Ontario Health Minister David Caplan to act on our recommendations, particularly the recommendation to ban electroshock, or at least call for a moratorium and public hearings (CAPA, 2009). Ontario could be the first province that bans electroshock, the first province that protects thousands of vulnerable citizens, particularly women and the elderly, from this psychiatric assault on their health, lives, and human rights. If not now, when?

Note

1 This chapter is an edited and revised version of an oral presentation delivered on behalf of the Coalition Against Psychiatric Assault before the Ontario government's Select Committee on Mental Health and Addictions at a public hearing in Toronto on September 23, 2009.

CHAPTER 12

Is Mad Studies Emerging as a New Field of Inquiry?

David Reville

Introduction

> *I have seen/the new gods come/and the old gods go.*
> —Carl Sandburg (1914)

My career as a mental patient began in 1965, before deinstitutionalization, before the Mental Health Act,[1] before community mental health, before Laing,[2] before the mental patients' liberation movement,[3] before "consumer participation,"[4] and years before "recovery." From an entry point in the School of Disability Studies at Ryerson University, I am eight years into a project aimed at creating space for Mad Studies in the university. For some time now, I have been wondering if Mad Studies is emerging as a new field of inquiry. I'm going to tell the story about madness at Ryerson not just because it's a good story and one dear to my heart, but also because I hope it is a moral tale as well, one that might be used for blueprint copying and/or idea diffusion. Are there lessons for practice that might be used by Mad activists and scholars who want to create spaces for Mad Studies at other universities and in other communities?

A Few Words on Words

For *Mad Matters*, I don't need to explain why I write about "madness," not "mental illness." Perhaps I do need to explain how I refer to Mad people and why I refer to them that way. Counting down 40-plus years, I have referred to myself as: a manic-depressive, a barely employable person, an ex-inmate, a consumer, a consumer/survivor, a (psychiatric) survivor, and a Mad person. I shall be using the last two terms to describe people like me in this chapter. However, even readers of this book may not be familiar with two other terms that I may have coined: "Mad positive" and "high-knowledge crazies." "Mad positive" is a bookend to "Mad identified." A "Mad-positive" person does not identify as Mad but supports the goals of those who do. "High-knowledge crazies" are Mad-identified people who are doing or have done post-graduate work. Tip: you can spot a high-knowledge crazy this way—in the room they come and go/talking of Michel Foucault.[5] I am pleased to see that there are more and more "high-knowledge crazies" all the time. Using the terms in a sentence, Kathryn Church is Mad positive and Jiji Voronka is a high-knowledge crazy. Both Kathryn and Jiji have contributed to this volume.

The Emergence of "Mad Studies"

I've been talking about Mad Studies since the winter of 2010. I know that because the last module of my Mad People's History course is entitled "Whither the Mad Movement, Whither Mad Studies?" I learned, just recently, that Richard Ingram[6] has been talking about Mad Studies since May 3, 2008, when he gave a talk at a disability studies student conference at Syracuse University. Here's what his abstract says:

> The "psychiatric survivor" or "Mad pride" movement has ... given birth to what I suggest should henceforth be referred to as "Mad studies" perspectives based on a transformative re-evaluation of the category of "Madness."

My entry point, though, came not in the form of an invitation to speak at a conference but in a telephone call that I received in the spring of 2004 from an old friend.[7] Would I be interested in coming to Ryerson to teach A History of Madness? The call was unexpected but timely. After I left public service in 1996,[8] I set up a consulting practice—David Reville & Associates (DRA). DRA does social research and community development for consumer/survivor initiatives, governments, and, often, the Centre for Addiction and Mental Health, Canada's largest mental health and addiction teaching hospital. By 2004, I was ready for a new challenge. This is the story about what happened after I said yes.

Jumping into the Deep End

When I arrived at the School of Disability Studies in the fall of 2004, there was already a course called Mad People's History (DST 504). Geoffrey Reaume had taught it three times at Ryerson University in 2002–2003.[9] In addition, Geoffrey had developed an outline for a course called A History of Madness (DST 500) shortly before being hired elsewhere. The Faculty of Arts accepted DST 500 as an upper-level liberal arts elective but, as of the summer of 2004, it had not yet been offered in the course calendar. I had jumped into the deep end. In a couple of months, I'd be teaching a brand-new course developed by someone else and, within two weeks of getting the marks in for that one, I'd be teaching another course developed and taught by a Mad professor with a serious PhD.

I spent the summer fretting over Geoff's outline for A History of Madness and reading and rereading the reader he'd put together for Mad People's History. I was in despair; I didn't know most of Geoff's material. I called Kathryn Church and asked for help; she told me to teach to what I knew. So I taught to some of what I knew for A History of Madness and some of what I knew for Mad People's History. I had 43 and 16 students respectively in the first two semesters. I learned a lot from those first students. I also learned a lot from Jiji Voronka, then a research associate for the Ryerson-RBC Institute for Disability Studies Research and Education; I had hired her to be my TA for that first semester. I had a lot to learn. Except for some guest lectures, I'd not set foot in a university for over 30 years; I had no clue how today's universities worked.

A History of Madness Takes Off

Something happened between the fall of 2004 and the fall of 2005. The Faculty of Arts called the School of Disability Studies: Would we offer a second section[10] of A History of Madness? Yes, we would. I asked the School of Disability Studies to bring in Jim Ward. Jim and I had been friends since the early 1980s; what's more, Jim was a proper sociologist. As consultants, we had worked together on homelessness and mental health issues many, many times. Jim and I reworked the course and set out to team-teach it. The *Ryersonian* described us as "the schizophrenic team" (*Ryersonian*, 2006); Jim described us as "two old white buggers with mustaches." The next year we taught four sections of DST 500 and the year after that six sections. Erick Fabris joined the team for the fall of 2010 and Jiji Voronka for the winter of 2011. Erick and Jiji are high-knowledge crazies, Mad-identified scholars working on PhDs at the University of Toronto. More than 330 students from all five faculties at Ryerson take A History of Madness each year.

Mad People's History Heads for Cyberspace

I taught Mad People's History for three semesters on Thursday evenings. I remember with special fondness the winter semester of 2008. That year Ruth Ruth Stackhouse[11] was in my class and Ruth Ruth, as always, had an idea. She planned to develop a play about three of the patient labourers Geoff Reaume had written about (Reaume, 2000) and she was going to use my class as a place to workshop her play. So, every Thursday evening, Ruth Ruth's players would drift into the class and, once the class was over, we'd rehearse. My role was to run the PowerPoint that Ruth Ruth was creating as part of the backdrop for the play. The next spring Ruth Ruth and a psychiatric survivor named Myrna Schacherl travelled to Vancouver to present the play at Bob Menzies' madness conference.[12] Once there, Ruth Ruth recruited some more actors, among them, Richard Ingram and Jiji Voronka.

After the 2008 winter semester, Melanie Panitch, then director of the School of Disability Studies, suggested that Mad People's History become an online course.

She got in touch with the director of Digital Education Strategies at the G. Raymond Chang School of Continuing Education and persuaded him to hire me to develop an online version. It was to be a "tied" course, that is, one offered jointly by the School of Disability Studies and the Chang School of Continuing Education. The advantage for the School of Disability Studies was obvious: most of our students do not live in Toronto so an online version of the course would mean an increase in the number of electives available to them.

The G. Raymond Chang School of Continuing Education is Canada's largest continuing education program with approximately 70,000 enrollments a year. It offers over 1,400 courses and 77 certificate programs for adult learners. It has developed over 350 distance education courses including over 300 degree-credit courses in various formats: Internet, classroom/Internet (hybrids), videoconference/Internet, and print based. Had I known all that before my first meeting with the instructional designers, I might not have been as surprised as I was by what happened next. For my new role as a subject matter expert, I had put all my lecture notes, PowerPoints, reading lists, rock and roll playlists, and movie titles into a big, fat binder and walked it over to the Chang School of Continuing Education.

Then I waited for the email that said it was all terrific. Hah! What arrived instead was a template with lots of boxes with names like "Learning Objectives" and "Learning Outcomes" and other mysterious things. I was then introduced to two young instructional designers who said they would tell me if and when I had the boxes filled in correctly. When I was in the mental hospital, my outgoing mail was read before it was sent. If some hospital official didn't like what I wrote, the letter would come back with a stamp on it reading "Return to Patient for Correction." I soon learned to smuggle letters out.

Now it was happening again. Only this time, the stamp was being applied by the two instructional designers. I was writing a module about madness and gender, and I had what I thought was the perfect moral tale: The Holy Maid of Kent was irritating Henry VIII by predicting that he would die if he broke with Rome so that he could marry Anne Boleyn. So all the king's men put about the "nuts and sluts" rumours about the Holy Maid of Kent and, once demonized, she could be hanged. And she was on the Tyburn gallows in 1534 (Shagan, 2003). My module was returned to me, a big red circle around "nuts and sluts." I went to see the two designers. "This," I said, "has been returned to patient for correction." They looked at me blankly.

It went on like that for months and months. I was particularly dense about learning objectives. I would say that I hoped that students would realize there was more than one story to be told about madness. No, I was told, that's not a proper learning objective. Eventually, in despair, I gave the job over to Dr. Church. She read the many pages of instructions about learning objectives and put together the acceptable words. "Knowing," "understanding," and "getting a glimmer of" were not among them.

A year or so into the process, Kathryn got a call from one of the managers of the Digital Education Strategies department. Not long after her meeting, I was called into a very peculiar meeting at which the two young instructional designers were replaced by another young woman whose background was in cultural studies. Suddenly, we were on the fast track and my folk narratives—"nuts and sluts" and all—were just fine, thank you very much. Moreover, there appeared a young Russian filmmaker who was eager to work with me on developing webdocs. Everything went swimmingly until the librarian advised, at the eleventh hour, that my reading list contained too many books for which copyright permission was required and, alas, the library had no money to purchase copyrights. In a panic, I began to search the net for free digital equivalents. Kathryn pulled a research assistant off another project and she helped me round up enough readings. Otherwise, my goose would have been cooked.

Online instruction has drawbacks. Because Mad people's history is happening all the time, my habit had been to incorporate breaking news into my lectures. That's a problem if the entire course has to be online on day one. Now I have learned to break the news in announcements, messages, and a blog. In the fall of 2011, I'm into my fourth online semester. I'm getting the hang of it. In fact, I have become addicted to the discussion board. I discuss things in the middle of the night with other night owls. I shall die at the keyboard.

If You Do Stuff, Stuff Happens: This Is Madness!

In her leadership facilitation work, Pat Capponi, a Toronto-based Mad activist, used to tell participants "If you do stuff, stuff happens." It's an aphorism I like and I use it often. If you start a history of madness course, stuff happens. One day a student approached us (at the time Jim Ward and I were the History of Madness team) and asked if she could do an artistic project as a final assignment. We said yes. We got a kick out of the result. The next semester we made doing an artistic project an option for any student who wanted to take it on. And we started getting fabulous work. Students made paintings and sculptures; they wrote plays and made videos; they choreographed Mad dances; they developed websites and blogs; one student designed a dress based on "The Yellow Wallpaper" (Gilman, 1892); another developed three recipes for "Mad food," which I cheerfully ate—the chocolate wontons were especially good. As we saw more and more creativity being displayed by our students, we began to mumble about doing an art exhibit.

And so it was that in April of 2010 the first This Is Madness! exhibit of student art was mounted. The Ryerson Student Union came on board as a partner and the art hung in the student-run Oakham Café for an entire month. The first show featured 14 mixed-media works by 10 student artists. When we mounted the second show—in February of 2011—we had three sponsors, the Ryerson Student Union, the Faculty of

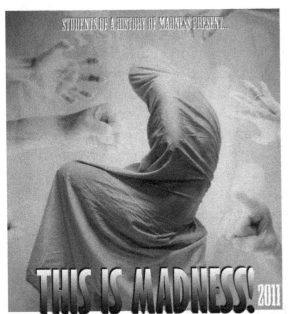

STUDENTS OF A HISTORY OF MADNESS PRESENT...

THIS IS MADNESS! 2011

A STUDENT ART SHOW AT THE OAKHAM CAFE - 63 GOULD ST.
FEBRUARY 1 - 28, 2011

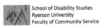 School of Disability Studies
Ryerson University
Faculty of Community Services

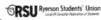 RSU Ryerson Students' Union
Local 24 Canadian Federation of Students

 A-WAY EXPRESS
Toronto's Total Progress Courier
Providing Affordable Same-Day Service Since 1987

FIGURE 12.1: This Is Madness!

The second This Is Madness! exhibition was put on by students in David Reville's History of Madness course in the School of Disability Studies at Ryerson University in February 2011.

Source: Photographed by Claire Critchley and designed by Danielle Landry of the School of Disability Studies, Ryerson University, 2011.

Community Services, and A-WAY Express, a survivor-run business. The second This Is Madness! exhibit profiled the work of 35 student artists and the opening night featured a performance by rap artist Khari "Conspiracy" Stewart. In the fall, we mounted a retrospective of This Is Madness! as part of Ryerson's Social Justice Week.[13]

If You Keep Doing Stuff, Stuff Happens: Talking Back to Psychiatry[14]

So, there I was, teaching Mad People's History to university students, most of whom were not Mad themselves. How could I get more Mad people into the university? I came up with the idea of doing a workshop about the history of the Mad movement. It would be delivered in three 3-hour segments. Off I went to the Chang School with this great idea. "Hmmm," said the Chang School. "We haven't had much success with workshops." I begged and pleaded and finally got the go-ahead. However, if I didn't fill 25 seats at $99 a pop, the workshop would be cancelled. Before the notice of the workshop could appear on the Chang School's website, I had to puzzle out the Chang School bureaucracy. There was the promotions and events co-ordinator in Marketing & Communications; in Program Support, there was the manager and the program co-ordinator; in Digital Education Strategies, there was the web editor; in Academic Program Areas, there was the community service program director. And then—gasp—there was Registration.

We worked out a special registration process. I would get workshop participants to fill out an application and then I would deliver the completed application with a cheque to the program co-ordinator who would then walk the applications and the cheques over to Registration. When I developed the budget for the workshop, I included the cost of a teaching assistant. The Chang School accepted my argument that, when you're reaching out to vulnerable people, you have to do whatever is necessary to make sure they feel able to participate. I wanted to have a TA to watch the body language and intervene when she thought that somebody wanted to say something.

Here's how we dealt with the reality that many psychiatric survivors haven't got $99 for a workshop. Two survivor organizations agreed to send 10 members each; two donors—CMHA Ontario and Accent on Ability, the charitable arm of A-WAY Express, a survivor-run business—agreed to sponsor six participants. Twenty-six psychiatric survivors got to learn about their own history of resistance. I had another objective: I wanted some service providers to sit in the room with psychiatric survivors so that they could see how smart we are when we get a chance to show it. That objective was met when the director of the mental health cluster at George Brown College agreed to send seven teachers. All in all, the workshop attracted 40 people. A convert, the Chang School has scheduled Talking Back to Psychiatry workshops for the winters of 2012 and 2013.

If You Are There, Stuff Happens

Because I am there in the university, students knock on my door and tell me about their own mental health histories. Usually they are enrolled in one of the courses I teach and they have come to me because I use my own Mad story in my teaching. Sometimes, however, students come to me who are not in any of my classes; they've heard about me, perhaps from one of their professors, perhaps from one of their classmates, perhaps from Internet searches. My best mentoring story is about a young woman named Jenna Reid. She was in the first year of the social work program and she wanted to get involved with Mad activism. I made a hot referral to the Mad Students Society. I've been doing this sort of thing for a very long time so I am not surprised if a referral comes to naught. Not this time. Not only did Jenna get involved with the Mad Students Society but, when the time came for her to do her social work placement, she used the connections she made with the Mad Students Society to set herself up with a placement at the Empowerment Council, which is the voice of in-patients at a very large psychiatric hospital. For her master's thesis, she did a study about what it was like to be a Mad student in the School of Social Work at our university. You may imagine my delight when she asked me to give her a reference when she applied to do doctoral studies. I was delighted again when she emailed me that she'd been accepted. Six years after that first knock on my door, I got to sit and beam while Jenna did a guest lecture for A History of Madness. Very smart it was, too. Jenna is one of a number of high-knowledge crazies who will take Mad Studies to the next level. (Update: When Jim Ward retired after the 2012 winter semester, Jenna was hired by the School of Disability Studies to teach a section of DST 500, A History of Madness. The course is now delivered by three mad-identified instructors—a dream come true.)

Bringing the Mad Community into the University

I've been haunted by an irony. The reason I am in the university is because of work I have done in the survivor community. Yet, survivors are barred from the university for all sorts of reasons, the chief of which is that survivors don't have any money. What to do? I have found four ways to get around that problem.

Survivors as Teachers

My courses are built on survivor knowledge, so bringing survivor leaders into the university to teach is an obvious thing to do. Doing a unit on community organizing? You bring in Lucy Costa to talk about the campaign to keep psychiatric patient advocacy independent.[15] You bring Ruth Ruth Stackhouse in to talk about Mad Pride, Becky McFarlane[16] to talk about how survivors can—or cannot—link to other social movements, Pat Capponi to talk about her latest book, and Danielle Landry to talk about the many intersectionalities of Charlotte Perkins Gilman's "The Yellow Wallpaper,"[17] that fabulous turn-of-the-century short story about a housewife who is slowly being driven mad by the rest cure prescribed for her by "wise" men.

Survivors as Learners

I was reading a biography of Daniel Ortega, the Nicaraguan Sandinista leader (Morris, 2010). He was lamenting the fact that Nicaraguans had been prevented from learning their history of resistance to domination by foreign powers and the puppets thereof. Yes, I said to myself, the same is true of psych survivors. What if I could sneak them into the university so that they could learn about the history of their own community's resistance? It turns out that it's easy to sneak survivors in. They can audit courses. Several employees of A-WAY Express have audited courses. Mel Starkman, an early antipsychiatry activist, audited my Mad People's History course, partly because he had been cast in a play Ruth Ruth Stackhouse was developing. Quite a few cast members dropped in for parts of lectures. Another way to get survivors into the university is to convince them to enroll in the Disability Studies program. In October 2011, I got to cry at Ruth Ruth's convocation. I'm looking forward to crying at Becky McFarlane's a few years from now. Diana Capponi[18] has done the introductory disability studies course and I'm hoping to see her online in Mad People's History soon.

Survivor Knowledge as Core Curriculum

This is a subset of survivors as teachers. All my courses are chock-a-block with survivor wisdom. When I wanted to talk about self-labelling and identity, I did video interviews with a dozen Toronto survivor activists. I asked them how they self-identified and why. I have 12 hours of video in the can waiting on the day when time and money allow me to bring that wisdom to students of Mad People's History. I learned how to do this from a master—Kathryn Church. For one summer institute, Kathryn was given the task of teaching DST 613, Strategies for Community Building. It's a core course for disability studies students. She built the whole course around *Working Like Crazy*, a broadcast-quality documentary about survivor business.[19] Out of the experience of working on that film, Kathryn identified seven key elements about community action. When I was assigned to teach DST 613 one summer, I built on Kathryn's approach. And I did the same thing when I was given DST 726 to teach. The course was called Leadership in Human Services. I didn't know enough about leading a human service organization to teach that, so I bent the course through several iterations until it became another course called DST 727, Leadership for Community Action. And, again, I used the survivor movement as my exemplar.

Survivor Authors on the Reading List

I make a point of assigning readings by survivor authors. One of the assignments in Mad People's History is a book review. I have put together a list of 16 books, all of them written by survivor authors. I want to make sure that students read at least one book by a survivor author. The assigned readings for each module include 20 articles and books by survivor authors.

Taking Madness Back Out to the Community

The last thing I want is for Mad people's history to be cloistered in the university. So, whenever I get a chance, I take Mad people's history out to the community. Last year, I gave 14 talks in many different locations; so far this year (2011) I've given 22. One talk was called "Mad Activism Enters Its Fifth Decade" and the audience was the national conference of the Canadian Mental Health Association. Because, in my opinion, CMHA can be very mainstream in its politics, I wanted to speak at its conference so that there would be one speaker who used the word "Mad." Four of the talks were to George Brown College students. These students have at least two things in common: they all have mental health and/or addiction histories; and they are in college programs designed to help students like them get their lives back on track, either through work or continuing education. I gave a talk entitled "Madness and Work" at the annual meeting of A-WAY Express, a survivor-run courier business. Another way to get Mad Studies back out into the community is through the Internet. The Chang School has put my three webdocs on YouTube; as of November 26, 2011, the webdocs have been viewed 7,600 times—that's the equivalent of 190 forty-student classes. You can watch them, too.[20]

We Need to Solve a Problem

Before I conclude, I want to address a problem. I am a part-time instructor; I get paid by the course. The labour involved in developing courses, art shows, and workshops is not paid labour. I did get some money through the Ryerson-RBC Institute for Disability Studies Research and Education, but that money was used up in 2008. My guess is that my financial situation is different from many part-time instructors—I have two pensions plus Old Age Security; in addition, I still do consulting work. Without that income, I would have to teach so many courses a year in order to make a living that I would not be able to do any developmental work. You can't build a new field of inquiry on part-time labour nor can you rely on true believers like me to do it for free. If Mad Studies is going to emerge, there will have to be tenure-track people who will take up the challenge. Or we shall have to raise money from the private sector to fund something like a Mad institute.

Conclusion

Long before now, you've found me out. I haven't really been wondering whether Mad Studies is emerging as a new field of inquiry. Instead I've been telling the story about what we've been doing at Ryerson to make Mad Studies emerge there. If I were to turn this chapter into a quick-and-easy recipe, it would look like this:

1. Find a way into the academy.
2. Once you're in, you have to find your way around.
3. That includes making alliances with like-minded people and making nice with the bureaucrats who make things happen.
4. You have to bring Mad students and teachers in, too.
5. Then you have to find your way back out to the community again.

It's my hope that there are others who will pick up this recipe, adapt it to their local conditions and set about using it. It's time that Mad Studies emerged as a new field of inquiry.

Notes

1   Ontario got its first Mental Health Act in 1968; it was written by Barry Swadron.
2   R.D. Laing's *The Politics of Experience and the Bird of Paradise* was first published in 1967.
3   Often Howie the Harp is credited with starting the mental patients' liberation movement when he formed a group called the Insane Liberation Front in Portland, Oregon, in 1970 (Chamberlin, 1990). I'm hearing rumours that there was a Norwegian group as early as 1968.
4   In 1985, CMHA National published a pamphlet called *Listening to People Who Have Directly Experienced the Mental Health System*. It's an early example of consumer participation or "user involvement" as it is called in the UK (Church and Reville, 1989).
5   This is a rip-off of T.S. Eliot's "The Love Song of J. Alfred Prufrock."
6   Richard is a post-doctoral fellow at the Centre for the Study of Gender, Social Inequities and Mental Health, Simon Fraser University, Harbour Centre campus. His talk at the 2008

conference was called "Mapping 'Mad Studies': The Birth of an In/discipline." For quote, see conference website: http://bccc.syr.edu/DisabilityStudiesConference.htm.

7   In 1985, Kathryn Church, now director of the School of Disability Studies at Ryerson University but then a staff member in the national office of the Canadian Mental Health Association, recruited me as the "consumer" member of the National Mental Health Services Committee. The committee's project was called "The Framework for Support," a conceptual model of how to support people with mental health issues in the community.

8   My public service career spanned 16 years. It included two terms on Toronto City Council, two terms in the Ontario Legislature, four years as Special Advisor to the Premier, and 18 months as chair of the Ontario Advocacy Commission. On March 29, 1996, the Harris government repealed the Advocacy Act and dismantled the commission. That's when I established DRA.

9   For a history of Mad People's History, see Reaume (2006).

10   At Ryerson, a section is 55 students; the demand for DST 500 is so strong that each section gets over-subscribed early. The School of Disability Studies is considering adding two more sections a year.

11   Ruth Ruth Stackhouse is a community theatre director; for years, she was the driving force behind Toronto's Mad Pride celebrations. She has a BA in disability studies from Ryerson.

12   Madness, Citizenship and Social Justice: A Human Rights Conference, Simon Fraser University, June 12–15, 2008.

13   October 17–21, 2011.

14   Part of the subtitle is taken from Morrison, L.J. (2005). *Talking Back to Psychiatry: The Psychiatric Consumer/Survivor/Ex-patient Movement*. New York: Routledge.

15   Lucy Costa is the systemic advocate for the Empowerment Council at the Centre for Addiction and Mental Health in Toronto. In 2005, she founded the Mad Students Society. The Ontario Ministry of Health decided to divest the Psychiatric Patient Advocate Office to the Ontario Division of the Canadian Mental Health Association. Mad activists and mental health lawyers formed a coalition to oppose the transfer.

16   Until recently, Becky McFarlane was the co-director of the Ontario Council of Alternative Businesses (now called Working for Change).

17   A Mad student and activist, Danielle is a research and teaching assistant in the School of Disability Studies at Ryerson. She curated all three This Is Madness! exhibits. You can read "The Yellow Wallpaper" here: http://womenshistory.about.com/library/etext/bl_gilman_yw.htm.

18   Following many years as director of the Ontario Council of Alternative Businesses, Diana became the Employment Works! co-ordinator at the Centre for Addiction and Mental Health.

19   *Working Like Crazy* (1999), National Film Board of Canada.

20   www.youtube.com/watch?v=pxbw7dDMX60; www.youtube.com/watch?v=AKBFYi6A6pA; www.youtube.com/watch?v=9uTbEBPkAAk.

CHAPTER 13

Making Madness Matter in Academic Practice

Kathryn Church

Introduction

> *Practice is understood as something that people do in "real" or everyday life. The doings of everyday life are seen as constituting a foundation for social order and institutions. What people do every day to get their work done, in this view, itself constitutes an explanation of social life, and it enjoys full explanatory status, substituting ... for theories, explanations, norms or ideologies.*
>
> —Miettinen, Samra-Fredericks & Yanow (2009, p. 1312)

For more than two decades, I have worked with psychiatric survivors who are resisting and attempting to change regimes of "treatment" and "help" that are governed by professional knowledge and practices. This political project has continuously unsettled and redirected my own professional practice: as a national organizer for the mental health association (e.g., Trainor & Church, 1984); as a doctoral student doing research on mental health policy-making (e.g., Church, 1993); as an independent researcher studying how psychiatric survivor-run organizations do economic development (e.g., Church, 1997); and as a university professor. My commitment has roots, as well, in personal experiences of "breakdown" and ongoing attention to constituting health. Because I was never formally marked by psychiatry, I do not identify as "Mad." I think of myself as an ally of the "Mad" movement (Bishop, 1994)—not as an achievement but as a process of lifelong learning.[1]

In this chapter, I recall and think through what happened in the School of Disability Studies at Ryerson University to make "madness" an identifiable and substantive part of our program. Over 10 years, the School generated and now regularly runs two courses that assert Mad knowledge.[2] Taught from an insider's standpoint, they are successfully drawing students from our program as well as a range of disciplines across the university. Our experience reveals the strategic importance of curriculum development—of taking curricular risks—and highlights the strength of disability studies as a facilitative context: theoretically, politically, and organizationally. Less obvious is how catalytic these courses have been for other kinds of activities and relationships: for research and publication, for university-wide advocacy, for community organizing and political action, for international education and exchange.

My narrative of "what happened" runs parallel to the account provided by David Reville also in this volume (Chapter 12). It surfaces my dilemmas as a faculty member whose role was not necessarily to do the work but to support the efforts of people who did: people who were "experts by experience" (Anglicare Tasmania, 2009) and unfamiliar with how universities work. A particular quality of this engagement is that, while I have been in the thick of things from the beginning, my labour tends not to be visible. I appear mostly in the background. Yet without a Mad-positive "engaged academic" in the mix (Cresswell & Spandler, 2012), Mad scholarship would not have emerged as it did within the School.

To get at the relational nuances of practice, I focus my attention on two instances of significant collaboration between David and myself. The first traces how he became involved with Disability Studies; the second recounts our struggle to create the online course titled Mad People's History. I take them as "turning moments" of query, negotiation, trust, and experimentation as we put in place structures, relations, and practices that did not already exist. I want to revisit my part in these developments— using my actions *and reactions* as an empirical resource for "reflexive work at the interface of the academic and psycho-political fields" (Cresswell & Spandler, 2012). I view what I do (or cannot do), and how I feel about my "doings"—as fully relevant to a feminist analysis of the broader institutional order (Smith, 2005).

Beginning from "We"?

"Who do you think you are?" she demanded, cool gaze under brim of black hat. "What could you possibly offer to the psychiatric survivor movement? Are you tough enough? Will you go the distance? Or just get what you need and get out? Why should I take a risk on you?" (Church, 2011)

In 2002, I was contracted to develop a research program for an institute run by the School of Disability Studies (DST). At Ryerson, DST is an undergraduate degree-completion program for part-time learners who do much of their coursework online. Sustained by a corporate grant, the institute's primary purpose was to enhance student learning and challenge public perceptions through community-based disability arts and culture. My history with arts-informed research seemed like a good fit for the job (I had just finished touring an exhibit that featured women, domestic sewing, and wedding dresses), and my background in community mental health may have helped. The transition was personally significant. After a post-doctoral decade as an independent researcher, I was finally entering the academy—albeit from outside a tenure-track position.

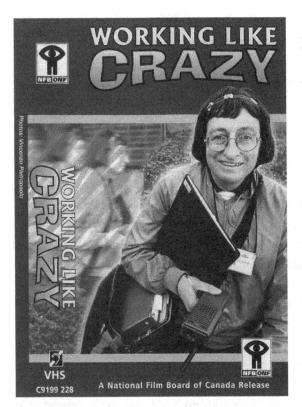

FIGURE 13.1: Working Like Crazy

The 1999 documentary *Working Like Crazy* depicts the community development project that Kathryn Church recounts in this chapter. On its website, the National Film Board observes that the film "takes a unique and compelling look at the daily struggles and victories of psychiatric survivors working in survivor-run businesses."

Source: Sky Works Charitable Foundation and the National Film Board of Canada, 1999.

Soon after, I was asked whether I would also teach in the School. "Everyone at Ryerson teaches," I was told. The course that needed an instructor was called Strategies for Community Building (DST 613). It is one of three required courses that we run each year as a two-week "intensive" in the summer. I took it on, keeping the calendar description intact but orienting the material more towards community organizing than community development: in other words, drawing more from conflict than consensus theories of social change.[3] I organized a new syllabus around seven steps distilled from a particularly strong piece of work by the Ontario Council of Alternative Businesses in Toronto. I hung the whole course on the "skeleton" of a single campaign: the four- to five-year process whereby we created and disseminated the National Film Board of Canada documentary titled *Working Like Crazy* (Church, 2006).

The redesign worked particularly well when I added guests who could animate the course materials from direct experience. David Reville made his first appearance in Disability Studies as one of these guests. The invitation was natural enough given a history of shared projects between the two of us. I realize now that he came as something of a surprise to the students; most are educational assistants or service workers in front-line jobs and settings. By contrast, here was a skilled community organizer and an experienced politician who was "out" with his mental health history. Here was someone who knew how to use his personal story to pursue social change—reinforcing the emphasis on political autobiography ("situate yourself!") that I layered into the course (Church, 1995; Jackson, 1990). Clearly, he had a lot to offer to people in this setting.

In 2004, David and I taught the course as a team. No doubt about it, the classroom was much livelier when we worked it together: his dramatic stories enlivening my more structured lectures; my mappings of the literature balancing his campaign examples. While one of us talked, the other attended to student reactions; pairing up made the classroom a safer space for questions and comments. What was most important, however, was enacting an interpersonal alliance that had strong relevance for community organizing (Bishop, 1994). I am not saying we did this perfectly—only that we took the project seriously. Some of our best class discussions emerged in the mingling of David's expertise and mine: bringing two kinds of knowledge—both engaged, but differently—to the classroom. The hidden syllabus lay in the absolute respect we gave each other as we taught across these differences.

I would not have missed this experiment for anything, or, in subsequent years, our practice of blending and exchanging classes in order to share responsibility for two courses. It was a powerful demonstration of, and learning from, "user involvement" in education (Church with Reville, 2010; McKeown et al., 2010). However, it was not without its dilemmas. One of mine was contending with the gender relations of having a classic "alpha male" co-instructor. Over the course of his life, David has become an accomplished and confident public presence. With his big voice and witty ways, he can dominate the room. By contrast, I still struggle to speak, to say what I think, to become more visible. With David in the classroom, I would allow myself to slip to the side or into the background, to become silent, to ease away from strained or heated moments.

Unlearning that tendency is the reason I value so highly the five years that I taught the course alone. Though it belies the participatory ethos, being solely responsible allowed me to become more self-assured: better prepared, more forward-looking with readings, and more present for students. As an ally, it has been important to relinquish the pedagogical centre. As a woman making my way in an institution that is still surprised we are here—seizing that centre has been essential.

Now You See Me/Now You Don't

I wasn't prepared for those questions, for her refusal to take me as an ally, to trust me, for the disdain in her tone. "How do you feel?" he asked as we walked away. He could introduce me but he could not shield me in this rite of passage. "F... off!" I shot back. But I might have said that I was surprised. Hurt. Annoyed. Angry. Frustrated. Confused. That I was ... unsettled. (Church, 2011)

Something odd happened to me in Disability Studies. As a content area, my expertise is community mental health, specifically the impact that people with mental health histories have on various systems when they attempt to reshape how they operate. But I do not teach in this area; in fact our program has no courses in critical mental health and professional practice. I teach research methodology, and I supervise students as they do the independent study that constitutes their final year in our program. David is our lead on mental health—David and the savvy-sparky doctoral candidates who will inherit the groundwork he has helped to build in the academy. I still puzzle about this situation—and I can be hurt by it. One day David approached me about the impending departure of one of his co-instructors.

"We really need another sociologist," he agitated—into an awkward pause.

"I am a sociologist!" I replied.

When I arrived at Ryerson, Disability Studies was a school in early formation (the electrical cords for my office were still dangling from the ceiling) within a field still attempting to define itself across academic disciplines and sites of practice. I plunged into writing grant proposals and fairly quickly launched more studies than I could handle. ("Don't expect to translate that into a faculty position," I was warned.) As well, I was preoccupied with the need to learn as much as I could, as quickly as I could, about disability communities beyond the mad world where I felt somewhat at home. I acquired new colleagues, renewed my attention to language, picked up new ways of relating and communicating, delved into other bodies of literature, and searched for common ground. Figuring out what to do in these complex worlds—and in the places where they periodically came together—consumed me.

It took a while, then, before I noticed that David was in trouble—not just grumping—but really struggling. He appeared to have secured a strong place for himself as the core instructor for A History of Madness. A popular offering across the university, it was acquiring students and growing sections by leaps and bounds. The glitch appeared in the crossover to Continuing Education (CE) and the translation to an online version of the course—Mad People's History (CDST 504). Somehow, in his accidental ethnography of the university, David had gotten bogged; he had been made befuddled.

How did we decide that I should intervene? I cannot recall. But I went along to several meetings and that meant there were two of us listening to the young course designers. In stark contrast to David's dynamism, they seemed locked into a standard—and standardizing—set of procedures for managing a mass production of courses. By the time I arrived on the scene, they had convinced David that he was doing everything wrong. They were uprooting his autobiography from its roots deep in the oral tradition. They were shifting his polished course materials from inductive to deductive, from stories to conventional lectures. They were extracting the madness from Mad People's History—and smiling politely while they did it.

My presence gave him a witness who was completely on his side, who could say "You aren't crazy! What they are asking for really IS offensive." I weighed in on the side of his voice and creativity. I took up the pedagogical debates and validated the position he knew was right but could not name. I was angry at them and that helped to cut the fear. Then we could strategize about how to resist and reclaim.

Behind the scenes at Continuing Education, Naza Djafarova noticed that things had stalled. No doubt the course designers reported that David was not hitting his "milestones" on schedule. A higher level manager with a mandate for technological innovation, Naza took a risk and jumped "outside the box."[4] Catching the spirit of the material, she free-associated to the website for *Valkyrie*, a film about the failed assassination of Adolf Hitler. The website's graphic timeline of events and pop-up videos suggested a style that she thought would work for the course. Oddly, it was me she called to a meeting; our dialogue went something like this.

Naza: "Would this kind of thing be good?"

Kathryn (peering at the computer screen): "Absolutely—let's do it."

From that point on, the dynamic changed. The initial course designers were replaced with people who had different skills. I connected David with Naza and she connected him to Daniil Novikov, a talented young videographer with a rock band history. That summer, they filmed the scenes and the interviews for three webdocs that have since become iconic in representing Mad People's History to Ryerson and the online world.[5] More at home in these media, David recaptured his vision and energy for the project. Literally wired for sound, he was off and running once more.

"But what about the learning objectives for the course?" I yelled after him.

"You'll take care of that, right?" he threw back and disappeared over the horizon.

In keeping with the university's course management policy, every content expert hired for a CE course must produce a document that lays out its key elements including topic area, teaching methods, and course materials. Because Mad People's History had a fully developed syllabus, we felt we had a jump start on that product. The course has a clear focus on the politics of madness. It asks a question that is raised rarely in academic circles: in their own words, what is the history that Mad people have lived over the centuries and what are the implications of that collective experience for society? Working against the dominant psychiatric paradigm, the course places the perspectives of the "mad, insane, or mentally ill" at the centre of knowledge formation. This fundamental move is embodied by the instructor. Through extensive use of autobiographical voice and personal narrative, David recognizes the lived experience of madness as a fundamental form of expertise that fuels people's resistance to psychiatric definition and oppression.

A provocative offering, to be sure, but before we could proceed we were required to produce "learning objectives and outcomes" for the course as a whole, and for each of its 14 modules. As a resource for the task, I was given a document featuring a "Table of Cognitive Domains" derived from Bloom's Taxonomy[6] (see Table 13.1 on page 187). The table came as something of a shock. Consider, for example, the interruption it causes in the visual field alone.

The guidelines asserted that effective learning objectives are "specific, observable and measureable." Some words are to be avoided because "they cannot be measured or are redundant." Words such as "knows," "learns," "understands," and "comprehends" are prominent examples: thus, the long list of terms in columns one and two that are offered as preferable substitutes for "knowledge" and "comprehension."

TABLE 13.1: Table of Cognitive Domains

Knowledge	Comprehension	Application	Analysis	Synthesis	Evaluation
Choose	Arrange	Adapt	Analyze	Arrange	Appraise
Cite	Associate	Apply	Appraise	Assemble	Approve
Define	Clarify	Catalogue	Audit	Build	Assess
Label	Convert	Chart	Break down	Combine	Choose
List	Describe	Compute	Calculate	Compile	Conclude
Locate	Discuss	Consolidate	Categorize	Compose	Confirm
Match	Draw	Demonstrate	Compare	Conceive	Criticize
Name	Estimate	Employ	Contrast	Construct	Diagnose
Recall	Explain	Extend	Correlate	Create	Evaluate
Recognize	Express	Extrapolate	Criticize	Design	Judge
Record	Identify	Generalize	Deduce	Devise	Justify
Repeat	Locate	Illustrate	Defend	Discover	Prioritize
Select	Outline	Infer	Detect	Draft	Prove
State	Paraphrase	Interpret	Differentiate	Formulate	Rank
Write	Report	Manipulate	Discriminate	Generate	Rate
	Restate	Modify	Distinguish	Integrate	Recommend
	Review	Order	Examine	Manage	Research
	Sort	Predict	Infer	Organize	Resolve
	Summarize	Prepare	Inspect	Plan	Revise
	Transfer	Produce	Investigate	Predict	Rule on
	Translate	Relate	Question	Prepare	Select
		Tabulate	Reason	Propose	Support
		Use	Separate	Reorder	Validate
			Solve	Reorganize	
			Test	Set up	
			Uncover	Structure	
			Verify	Synthesize	

In their recent discussion of academic intellectuals and the psychiatric survivor movement, Mark Cresswell and Helen Spandler argue that the work of a movement intellectual involves

> producing knowledge *for* [the movement] and *within* it, not *about* it and *of* it.... From within such a location, the movement is no sort of "object." Thus, the movement intellectual's *theoretical* work is formulated, not according to the abstract generalizations of the academic intellectual, but upon concrete "case propositions" which analyse pragmatic proposals in practice. (Cresswell & Spandler, 2012)

Further, they suggest that a key question for movement intellectuals is "What is to be done?" in the realm of practical choices.

Being pressed towards evidence-based teaching was just such a moment for me. That mundane little chart, cheerfully provided as a form of assistance, signified a whole battlefield of knowledge and power on which I was already at war, refusing to relinquish the terrain of knowing, learning, and comprehending. But in this situation, with respect to this particular dilemma, what was I to do? I could refuse outright or contest the framework, causing the course to founder in a fresh set of negotiations. I could acquiesce to the framework and weaken my practice. Or I could play strategically within the framework, seeking some kind of momentum for the larger endeavour.

I chose the latter, which is why, for better or worse, for the course as a whole, the learning objectives are:[7]

- To explore the vital importance of language in the course of mad people's history; to examine the role of words in the oppression of mad communities as well as in their resistance;
- To identify the presumptions about madness held by societies past and present within the context of their broader socio-economic circumstances;
- To link therapeutic interventions with modernist notions of scientific progress; to situate the theories and practice of psychiatry with respect to gender, race, class, and sexual orientation;
- To recognize the lived experience of madness as a fundamental form of human knowledge; to take a mad people's standpoint on social history;
- To situate first-person narratives as expressions of knowing that have been suppressed and subordinated over time, and collective story-making/telling as vital work in building a social movement;
- To introduce the central phases of the psychiatric survivor/consumer movement from the 1960s to the present; to identify the major debates and activities, leaders and allies who have characterized that movement throughout.

The student will:

- Add new words to his/her repertoire as substitutes for terms in medical and popular use; be able to explain to a friend why those words have become important;
- Critique portraits of "mental illness" in contemporary mainstream movies and books from the standpoint of the mad community;
- Query the view of "madness" embedded in other university courses and various academic disciplines;
- Think twice before saying "That's just anecdotal" in response to hearing a personal story from someone who identifies as "mad";
- Recognize the names of psychiatric survivor leaders when they appear in the media (old and new), and read further to find out how the work of the movement is portrayed.

Thus, the template got filled, the document was accepted, and we moved on.

Some months later, the Canadian Association for University Continuing Education presented David Reville and the Chang School of Continuing Education with the award for best continuing education course in Canada. He and I attended the awards luncheon together, savouring his rare moment of academic recognition. There were surprised faces around the table when I walked in; a couple of people had to skooch over to make room. At one point, one of the CE managers leaned over to fill me in on the origins of Mad People's History.

"We have quite a tight team on this project," she reassured.

"Is that so?" I replied.

Conclusion

I continue to experience myself as a sort of hybrid creature: neither in nor out, betwixt and between the survivor community and the academy; familiar with but uncomfortable in both. My location is shifting again but I am still engaged with the problematic of being a mad-positive scholar. As always, I believe that engagement itself will produce the next step forward. (Church, 2011)

I conclude with just two comments on the relatively simple stories I have told in this chapter. Most obvious in my account are the structural inequities that separate my career trajectory from David's within the academy. As we have worked together, with David in the lead, my circumstances have steadily improved while his have remained the same—or become worse. I got a limited-term faculty contract, a tenure-track position and, finally, tenure. I was promoted from assistant to associate professor, and am now director of the School of Disability Studies. My salary has reached the point where it is a matter of public record.[8] David is adjunct professor—I made that happen in my first weeks as director—but he is still paid as a sessional instructor, still experiencing the restrictions of that role, and working hard to draw boundaries around the amount of unpaid labour he does for the School. In a university context, he and I are compelled to live out our collegiality in ways that are not of our own choosing. We work that difficulty through with constant discussion. We also pay a price for it.

But even this outrage is far from simple. Embedded in the faculty/sessional divide are complicated subjectivities that give rise to other kinds of divides. Here I have been particularly fascinated by situations in which I "disappear": sometimes stepping back voluntarily, sometimes pressed back by various rules or relations; sometimes content with it, and sometimes disturbed. As I work at living out my particular heritage of privilege and disadvantage, I think about how "disappearing" is also a political act, not always comfortable, yet integral to the practice of an engaged academic. Knowing when to be present or absent, verbal or silent, is a skill. Performing that skill is highly gendered emotional labour that is undervalued in both academic and activist contexts. I react to the tension of it every time. I remain as curious about the emotional patterns that cause me to feel stuck as I am about the institutions that more tangibly bind me (Smith, 2003). In my practice, I have found it necessary to create strategies for dealing with both.[9]

Notes

1   I am taking the terms "Madness," and "Mad positive," and "Mad Studies" as terms-in-use in my work context. It is not my purpose in this chapter to define them, or analyze them in comparison to other terms that are also in use.

2   As director of Disability Studies, Melanie Panitch played an important role in opening the doors to Mad curriculum at Ryerson.

3   For an excellent theoretical delineation, I recommend the chapter titled "Exploring Models, Theory and Learning from History," written by Eric Shragge for his 2003 book on activism and social change.

4   Naza Djafarova has since become director of Digital Education at the Chang School of Continuing Education, Ryerson University.

5   "Introducing Mad People's History": www.youtube.com/watch?v=AKBFYi6A6pA&feature=relmfu; "Presenting the consumer/survivor/ex-patient movement": www.youtube.com/watch?v=9uTbEBPkAAk; "Self-labelling and identity": www.youtube.com/watch?v=pxbw7dDMX60&feature=relmfu

6   "Writing Effective Learning Objectives," handout, G. Raymond Chang School of Continuing Education—Distance Education Unit, no date.

7   As I mentioned, each of the 14 modules has learning objectives. If you are interested in what they are, contact David Reville at dreville@ryerson.ca, or me at k3church@ryerson.ca.

8   In Ontario, anyone making more than $100,000 as an employee of a public institution is part of a public registry of salaries.

9   My thanks to David Reville, Jijian Voronka, Lucy Costa, and Helen Spandler for honest and helpful comments on the first draft of this chapter, and to the editors for their skillful editorial interventions.

PART IV Law, Public Policy, and Media Madness

The five contributions to Part IV converge around the politics of resistance in the public sphere. Each chapter, in its own way, considers how critical activism against biopsychiatric powers and practices can express itself variously through legal jurisprudence, the realm of public policy, and both conventional and alternative forms of media. By turn, the chapters address: (1) the contradictory role of law as a forum for Mad struggle, (2) the poverty of official justifications for abrogating human rights, (3) the spatial regulation of psychiatrized people through residential zoning, (4) the discriminatory implications of mental health literacy campaigns, and (5) the strategic potential of news media as a resource for anti-sanist practice.

Chapter 14, "Mad Patients as Legal Intervenors in Court," is authored by Toronto rights activist Lucy Costa, who has worked at the CAMH Empowerment Council for nearly a decade. In her historical overview of milestones in consumer/survivor/ex-patient (c/s/x) activism in Ontario from the 1970s to the present, Costa recounts how early initiatives in Mad movement and citizen participation in "mental health" policy laid a foundation for more recent ventures in legal activism by and in alliance with psychiatrized people. In this post-Charter era of judicial activism and direct litigant involvement in rights challenges, rich possibilities have opened up for engaging in legal "rights talk," and for shaping the content and course of jurisprudence. Moreover, Mad patients and their allies have seized these initiatives with energy and ingenuity, securing important victories in the realms of both civil and criminal law. In exploring law's capacity to combat discrimination against members of Mad communities, Costa takes up the often-overlooked 1999 Supreme Court of Canada holding in *Winko*—a case where the appellant, with the support of intervenors including the Queen Street Patients Council, argued that the procedures under Part XX.1 of the federal Criminal Code violated the section 7 and 15 Charter rights (to life, liberty, and security of the person, and to equality) of persons found "not criminally responsible" (NCR). While the majority of Justices ultimately ruled against this Charter-based challenge, the Supreme Court did find that the Part XX.1 provisions had been breached in *Winko* in several important respects; and in laying down a number of new procedural protections the Justices "effectively 'reread' the law, reminding Review Boards to follow the provisions." As Costa observes, whether the partial "win" in *Winko* had any enduring impact on the liberty and equality rights of psychiatrized people in conflict with the criminal law remains an open question. As countless feminists, racialized people, queer activists, and other rights-seekers have learned through the years, the law can prove to be a fickle instrument of social change, and the courts sometimes a decidedly unfriendly terrain for human rights activists. Still, there may be good reason for Canadian Mad intervenors to sustain and even expand, however warily, their recent agenda of legal activism. "The challenges ahead for c/s/x engagement with advocacy and legal mobilization as a means of empowerment," concludes Costa, "require … [an] approach … that takes into account psychiatry, law, and other intersecting governmental arms in order to understand not only how to deal with emergent issues of representation, identity, class, and poverty, but also to learn how best to represent these matters in court (if at all)."

Gordon Warme's commentary in Chapter 15 offers a practising psychiatrist's take on the "terrifying" moral calculus involved in depriving Mad people of their basic human rights. Author of *Daggers of the Mind* (2006) and other writings on the politics of madness, Warme turns his attention in this chapter to the unyielding attitudes that fuel his profession's enduring addiction to systems of diagnosis and biomedical accounts of human (dis)order—and its seemingly unquenchable thirst for pharmaceutical "solutions" to mental difference and distress. Psychiatry's capacity to dominate public culture and organizational practice, cautions Warme, is inexhaustible. "Nothing," he writes, "can shift our intoxication with the doctor archetype, dislodge her from being embraced as the primary helper, healer, and counsellor." So it is, too, with the institutions that the profession has erected in its name. "Like soaring Gothic cathedrals, our hospitals now have soaring atriums. Science, especially medical science, is horning in on religion—it *is* a religion; our faith in medical progress is boundless." This entire edifice, he continues, is built on a bedrock of false premises, if not outright falsehoods—among others, that "mental illness" exists as a scientific and experiential entity; that clinicians are capable of detecting and curing it; that "disordered" people are dangerous, biochemically different beings; and that the Mad frequently require involuntary constraint, in our/their own best interests, until medicine can restore us/them to a state of normalcy. Aside from the professional hubris and false sense of certainty that such belief systems foster, the equation of mental experiences (however traumatic they may be) with physical illness allows psychiatry to effect a number of self-empowering "manoeuvres"—to present itself to the world as a benevolent healing profession; to colonize judicial spaces and dictate the content of "mental health" laws; to insist on autonomy within its own ever-growing professional sphere; and to efface the moral and political roots—and often devastating consequences—of its interventions into people's lives. Unless and until clinical practitioners can divest themselves of this bifold "delusion"—to the effect that they are practising scientists, and their patients are biochemically damaged, non-agentic beings—the prospects of refashioning psychiatry into a genuinely humanistic, self-critical, just, and progressive discipline seem remote.

Using a psychiatric survivor analysis that incorporates a nuanced understanding of the multiple manifestations of sanism and "examines socio-legal circumstances in the context of deeply embedded power relations," Lilith "Chava" Finkler (Chapter 16) provides a scholarly assessment of the impact of land use law and social planning upon psychiatric survivor housing. She argues convincingly that "a psychiatric survivor analysis [serves] as a perspectival antidote to the ways in which planning practices, such as zoning, ignore psychiatric survivor realities" and reinforces systemic discrimination in blatant and exceedingly painful ways. These include issues such as the way in which spatial restrictions are imposed based on minimum separation distance zoning bylaws, which are enacted based on the discourse of "social mix," as well as the parallel arguments made within a land use law context between psychiatric survivor housing and waste manage facilities, such as garbage dumps. For example, Finkler reveals that "concentrations of psychiatric survivors, like concentrations of 'garbage,' breed rejection and resistance. Prospective neighbours, municipalities, and sometimes adjudicators link psychiatric survivor housing to undesirable developments such as garbage dumps and toxic waste sites. The distance between the loony 'bin' and the garbage 'bin' evidently remains close." The detailed analysis Finkler provides in relation to systemic sanism in the restriction and prevention of housing for psychiatric survivors, and the social, linguistic, legal, political, emotional, spatial, and practical ramifications for psychiatric survivors, is unique in both the fields of social planning and Mad Studies.

In Chapter 17, Kimberley White and Ryan Pike deliver a searing analysis of recent Canadian policy initiatives in "mental health" and their representations in mainstream media. White and Pike are centrally concerned with the power relations and belief systems fuelling the 21st-century campaign for mental health literacy (MHL). As elsewhere, MHL initiatives in Canada have proven themselves to be inherently exclusionary, to the extent that they advance a narrow and objectifying disease model of "mental illness" that privileges official-professional knowledge claims and marginalizes antipsychiatry and survivor-centred perspectives on madness. As the authors insightfully observe, the current "national mental health strategy," as institutionalized in the Mental Health Commission of Canada (MHCC), is grounded in an ironic appropriation of anti-stigma and recovery models, which—when processed through the machinery of neoliberal marketing strategies and biogenetic disease discourse—"calls forth the very histories and representations of madness they claim to dispel." Similarly, in their analysis of commentaries by journalists André Picard and Joseph Brean, White and Pike show how any gesture by the MHCC or others towards denaturalizing "mental illness," decentring brain science, promoting strategies of empowerment and peer support, and embracing a "language of rights" inevitably incurs the wrath of "mental health" policy-makers and opinion leaders alike. In a political and cultural environment dominated by medicine and the marketplace, not only is the anti-stigma focus of MHL unproductive, but it has the effect of further marginalizing those who are considered or cast beyond the reach of government-sanctioned programs. "[R]ather than identifying social stigma as the primary barrier to the empowerment of the mentally ill," conclude White and Pike, "a more significant barrier to achieving meaningful social justice may in fact be the state failure to recognize its own participation in past injustices and the lack of the courage it would take to initiate a radical change."

Chapter 18, by Victoria-based writer, journalist, and educator Rob Wipond, is a primer of sorts for "pitching" human rights issues in ways that might resonate with the gatekeepers of mainstream media and fit the frame of expectations for what is newsworthy. Making inroads with news producers, and through them the public, requires challenging the governing paradigm of professional expertise, biochemical mental illness, and pharmaceutical cure that dominates media discourse. It hinges on unravelling what Wipond terms the "knot of wires"—the power-sustaining tangle of prejudicial cultural beliefs about the supposed "irrelevance" of human rights concerns, the "scientific" status of psychiatry, the "benign" influence of corporations, the "independence" of stakeholder organizations, the "pernicious" effects of social welfare, the inherent "dangerousness" and "difference" of the Mad (and their "unreliability" as news sources), and the "terrible and irreversible" human condition that is madness itself. Singling out the media as a key battlefield of this war over hearts and minds, Wipond canvasses a number of strategies for working with, through, and beyond mainstream news producers to contest this dominant paradigm, and to commence reframing madness as a matter of human rights, not medical science. Further, he advocates forging strategic alliances between activists and sympathetic mental health workers, lawyers, and critical academics who might harness their cachet with news producers to bring psychiatric survivor perspectives—and even more basically, the very notion that varied perspectives on "mental health" exist—to public light. In the end, Wipond (in contrast to some: see, for example, Warme, Chapter 15) remains upbeat about the prospects for successfully contesting psychiatric power and celebrating the experience of human and neuro-diversity: "Biological psychiatry cannot lay claim to the definitive explanations of what it means to be wholly, healthfully human," concludes Wipond. "Still today, vast territories of our psyche remain unconquered and uncharted in all their vital, beautiful multifariousness. That's a message the world needs to hear."

CHAPTER 14

Mad Patients as Legal Intervenors in Court

Lucy Costa

O ver the past three decades there has been an increase in "rights talk"[1] within the consumer, psychiatric survivor, and ex-psychiatric patient (c/s/x) movement.[2] The adoption of the Canadian Charter of Rights and Freedoms in 1982 played an important role in advancing rights for the c/s/x community and, as a result, section 7 (the right to life, liberty, and security of the person) and section 15 (equality before and under law and equal protection and benefit of law) of the Charter have allowed the c/s/x community more than one channel through which to address issues of equality and discrimination.

In this chapter I discuss some of the general themes raised in social movement organizing for the c/s/x community both in policy and in law. I follow with a discussion of the Supreme Court of Canada case *Winko v. British Columbia* (1999)—a case that included evidence from the Queen Street Patients Council, an organization that was made up of psychiatric survivors and ex-psychiatric patients. I conclude by analyzing *Winko*'s designation as a "win" for the c/s/x community and discuss considerations for future psychiatric and legal reforms and organizing.

Setting the Stage for Legal Intervention

The evolution towards more political opportunity, policy reform, and resource mobilization for the psychiatric survivor legal intervention from 1999 onward occurred because of the grassroots work in earlier movement building. As with all movements, the c/s/x movement encompasses a diversity of views on psychiatry; but there are nevertheless several core values and objectives that have endured over time. These values include the ability to have choice in psychiatric treatment, access to information about treatments, protection of legal rights, and promotion of self-determination (Chamberlin, 1978; Morrison, 2005).

By briefly touching on the historical context of the 1970s and 1980s I highlight why legal interventions were possible in later years. Canada's publicly funded health care system came into being in 1957 (Freeman, 1994). In the 1960s, a number of professional lobbying efforts began to educate and organize for funding for services in mental health. In many ways, the 1960s delivered the first major public education campaigns, not only about the need for universal health care but also for specific health care dollars aimed at "mental illness." The Royal Commission on Health Services of 1961 complained of the "small, closed nature of the mental health policy community" (Hartford, Schrecker, Wiktorowicz, Hoch & Sharp, 2003, p. 66). In 1963 the Canadian Mental Health Association's *More for the Mind* promoted the idea that "mental health be dealt within the same organizational, administrative and professional framework as physical illness" (Griffin, 1963, p. 38).

By the mid-1970s, Ontario began to feel the effects of waning health care dollars from cuts to federal transfer payments (Boyce, 2001; Lightman & Aviram, 2000). After a decade of deinstitutionalization, institutional and psychiatric professionals' efforts continued to raise awareness about the urgency in mental health care. However, internal politics within the Ministry of Health were tumultuous, with administrative and financing issues becoming intertwined with service delivery and professional territorialism. In 1972, a task force entitled the Committee on Government Productivity tried to incorporate recommendations from earlier meetings and protests that favoured using more democratic processes as a cure for the "deficiencies of big bureaucracy" that had preceded (Simmons, 1990, pp. 147–150). In this context and in response to pressure from service users and other stakeholders, new terms such as "citizen involvement" and "citizen participation" became more common in policy development (Simmons, 1990, p. 148).

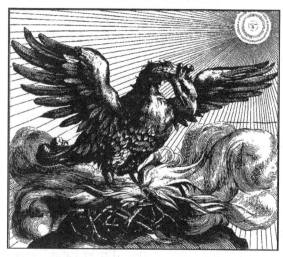

FIGURE 14.1: Phoenix Rising

The phoenix rising, a symbol of resilience and renewal, has been adopted by the Mad movement to represent its vision of overcoming and survival. This image was associated with the iconic psychiatric survivor journal of the same name, which was published in Toronto between 1980 and 1990. Back issues of *Phoenix Rising* are available in their entirety on the Psychiatric Survivor Archives of Toronto website.

Source: Psychiatric Survivor Archives of Toronto

As these insular discussions amongst policy and medical professionals unravelled, in Toronto the first ex-psychiatric patients' group, the Ontario Mental Patients Association (OMPA), was formed in 1977.[3] At the time, no other groups run by ex-psychiatric patients existed and members of OMPA described their vision for autonomy as a "crazy dream" and something that had to be "fought to be made real" (Phoenix Rising, 1980, p. 3). With no funding, support from allies became invaluable. For example, some of the founding members of the group wrote:

Armed with idealistic convictions, we approached an understanding *Toronto Star* reporter, Bob Pennington, in early August of 1977. He listened as we told him a little bit about ourselves and why we wanted to start a group totally controlled by ex-psychiatric inmates. He agreed to write a story for us; it was that story which was largely responsible for bringing almost 150 people to our founding meeting on August 9th in All Saints Church—our first home thanks to the Reverend Norman Ellis. (On Our Own, 1980, p. 3)

Other evidence in Ontario of psychiatric survivors' attempts to advance this growing movement's goals can be found in the Toronto-based magazine *Phoenix Rising*,[4] which ran for a decade, playing a pivotal role in documenting rights issues and the testimony of the current and ex-patient community. The magazine's information was disseminated both to people in psychiatric hospitals and to agencies that provided mental health services. This distribution of *Phoenix Rising* helped forge the beginnings of an accessible and very public critique of psychiatric practices. In the late 1970s psychiatric survivor Pat Capponi had led Minister of Health Larry Grossman on a tour of the Parkdale neighbourhood, where people were living in deplorable conditions. Grossman, in partnership with other advocates, helped form the Psychiatric Patient Advocate Office (PPAO) in 1983 (PPAO Report, 1994, p. 5). In 1985, psychiatric patients were finally granted the ability to vote inside psychiatric facilities. Significant strides were being made in advancing patient rights.

When the Liberals replaced the Progressive Conservatives in the provincial election of 1985, their health strategy included the development of a clearer policy vision for mental health and they did this by commissioning the Graham Report in 1988. During consultations, Robert Graham, the report's lead author, heard from both professionals and c/s/x groups; this was a first in having patients participate in policy discussion. One of the recommendations of the Graham Report stated that "greater efforts should be made to solicit views and opinions of consumers" (Graham, 1988, p. 61). In the same year, a new anthology, *Shrink Resistant*, published and funded by the Canada Council, further documented examples of resistance with its collection of stories about "dehumanization through psychiatric abuse" (Burstow & Weitz, 1988, p. 19).

Following the election of the New Democratic Party (NDP) in 1990, new enthusiasm was ignited for rights reform with their Ontario Advocacy Act (Advocacy Act, 1992; Boyce, 2001; Hartford et al., 2003; Lightman & Aviram, 2000). New groups such as the Ontario Psychiatric Survivors' Alliance (OPSA), created in 1990, also responded to rights violations affecting people in the psychiatric system. For instance, in one of their newsletters, OPSA wrote about 37 allegations against staff in the maximum security psychiatric facility Oak Ridge Branch of Penetanguishene Mental Health Centre, describing scenarios of abuse and violence such as staff "using a fire hose on some patients in lieu of a shower, aiming for the face and genitals, refusing to flush patients' toilets, and denying drinking water (forcing patients to drink out of a dirty toilet)" (OPSA, 1992). Media reports in the 1980s had also publicized hospital deaths due to medications and overcrowding (Burstow, Gower & Weitz, 1988), but the Ontario Advocacy Act, "intended to provide a generic system of social advocacy to vulnerable adults not paralleled in non legal areas" (Lightman & Aviram, 2000, p. 26), was the hope for ameliorative remedy.

In 1992 the Ministry of Health and Long-Term Care committed itself to support hospitals in allocating some of their budgets to patient councils, which would be run by patients or ex-patients of the institution. The Kingston Psychiatric Hospital was the first pilot to be funded by the Ministry, followed by the Queen Street Mental Health Centre in Toronto (Claxton, 2008, p. 83). This role enabled patient councils to lobby the government to be more proactive in responding to increasing stories of abuse inside psychiatric facilities. Unfortunately, when the Progressive Conservatives were re-elected in 1995, the Ontario Advocacy Act was repealed, and in its place amendments were enacted under an Advocacy Consent and Substitute Decisions Statute Law and Amendment Act (Lightman & Aviram, 2000).

In the late 1990s new challenges for patient rights arose with the proposition of Bill 68, a private member's bill later passed in December 2001 amending the Mental Health Act and launching Community Treatment Orders (CTOs), a mechanism for mandatory psychiatric treatment and monitoring in the community (Dreezer, Bay & Hoff, 2005). In response, psychiatric survivors in 1999 formed the No Force Coalition (NFC), which came together to address institutional violence and stereotypes. In its short existence, the NFC created a number of information pamphlets: *Electroshock Fact-sheet*, *The Miracle Drug Myth*, *The Violent Mental Patient Myth*, and *Bill 68— Ontario New Psychiatric Law*.

On Our Own, Phoenix Rising, OPSA, NFC, and many other emerging organizations were initiatives that shared a commitment to addressing inequalities, neglect, and violence that arose not from madness but from the very institutions aimed at helping. The Women's Legal and Education Fund (LEAF) and the Council for Canadians with Disabilities had also been advocating for clear definitions of equality, and in 1985 successfully pressured the government to establish a Court Challenges funding program for equality seekers (Peters, 2004). As with other groups, entering into the legal arena was an inevitable progression for the c/s/x movement.

Mad Patients Dispute Mad Laws

From the 1980s onward a number of key legal challenges went before the courts, culminating in a groundswell that led to the possibility of c/s/x involvement in legal cases addressing rights for individuals deemed "incapable" or "not guilty by reason of mental disorder" under the provincial Mental Health Act or the federal Criminal Code.

The Ontario Mental Health Act of 1968 contained some minimal rights provisions. For example, under the new legislation, "capacity" was assessed and if a patient was assessed as "financially incapable," the Public Guardian and Trustee would take over the management of property until the patient was made "capable" once again (Bartlett, 2001, p. 28). Diagnostic descriptors such as "epileptic," "alcoholic," and "retarded" were replaced with "mental disorder" (Pollock, 1974, p. 318). In the mid-1970s, the Canadian Civil Liberties Association argued that 70 percent of psychiatric patients were not a risk but were being detained illegally (Bay, 2003, p. 15). In September 1979, lawyer and psychiatric survivor Carla McKague gave a talk entitled "Myths of Mental Illness" at CMHA in Kingston stating, "What we need first of all is friendship, understanding, people that do not shy away from us because they don't quite understand us and we're a little bit different from the rest" (McKague, 1979, p. 8).

In 1983, several electroconvulsive shock survivors mobilized to start the Ontario Coalition to Stop Electroshock, holding public forums in Toronto's City Hall. In December 1983, this same coalition supported legal efforts to address the case of "Mrs. T," which went before the Supreme Court of Ontario (On Our Own, 1984, p. 26; Weitz, 2008). Mrs. T had been declared a "competent" patient but her doctor insisted on ECT treatments (Savage & McKague, 1987, p. 96). She refused treatment and her psychiatrist then attempted to obtain consent from Mrs. T's husband and brother, who both opposed the doctor's opinion. Her doctor then proceeded to get second opinions from two other psychiatrists. The case gained much attention, raising concern about psychiatrists' ability to override both the patient's and family's wishes. Mrs. T won her case; ECT was not administered and Mrs. T was transferred to another facility (pp. 95–99). In 1987 Carla McKague with colleague Harvey Savage published *Mental Health Law in Canada*, calling for legal reform and a patient bill of rights. The book was the first to speak directly about how mental health law was impacting patients. That same year, a psychiatric patient and appellant named Mr. Reid brought a similar case challenge, claiming that the Psychiatric Review Board[5] ignored his and his substitute decision-maker's role in executing his prior capable wishes (not to be treated with neuroleptic medications), and thus contravened the doctor's power to act in the patient's "best interest." In *Fleming v. Reid* (1991), the Court of Appeal agreed that bypassing a patient's prior capable wishes "rendered the Mental Health Act meaningless and unconstitutional" (p. 13).

The 1990s also had changes in store for the "criminally insane." In 1992 Parliament rewrote a new section of the Criminal Code of Canada. Part XX.1 established legislation that would deal with "mental disorder." The rewritten Criminal Code would establish forensic Review Boards and their role in each province (Carver & Langlois-Klassen, 2006). A year earlier, *R. v. Swain* (1991) became the first case challenging the constitutionality of restriction of liberty under the Charter. Mr. Owen Swain had been charged with aggravated spousal assault but was found not guilty by reason of insanity (NGRI). His case questioned the state's authority to detain psychiatric inmates at the "pleasure of the lieutenant governor" where no due process existed to review when or if a sentence could be terminated. Through its challenge of "indefinite sentencing" for persons labelled NGRI, the *Swain* decision obliged the federal government to amend the legislation via Bill C-30, which modernized the Criminal Code and helped set the stage for the arguments in *Winko v. British Columbia* (1999).

Though "mental disorder" and "disability" have had separate historical trajectories from the nineties onward, the Charter began to conflate these two disparate categories and created a subtle shift in "mental disorder" discourse towards one of "psychiatric disability." *Swain* helps interject a new "positioning" for the "criminally insane" towards individuals in need of rehabilitation and equal rights by virtue of "psychiatric disability." This shift was also aided by cases such as *Battlefords v. Gibbs* (1996), where the court upheld a decision supporting a discrimination charge by Betty-Lu Clara Gibbs on the grounds of "mental disability" and "historical disadvantage." In *Swain*, Justice Lamer had also provided analysis on "historical disadvantage" experienced by persons with "mental disabilities"[6] (*R. v. Swain*, 1991; see Carver & Langlois-Klassen, 2006).

Mad Patients as Intervenors

"Intervenors" can include groups, organizations, or individuals who have a special interest in an issue before the court and are generally seen (by law) as being able to bring a unique perspective or expertise that is different from other parties' evidence.[7] *Winko* was the first legal case where a c/s/x organization applied for standing to intervene. This signified the beginnings of a new role for the c/s/x community to further articulate and mobilize the goals of self-determination, access to treatment choice, and protection of rights via litigation.

The Queen Street Patients Council (QSPC) was born in 1992 to provide systemic advocacy for the patients of what was then called the Queen Street Mental Health Centre.[8] By the 1990s the QSPC was not only acting on behalf of patients within the hospital, but had also begun to participate in advocacy outside of the hospital, for instance into the inquest of Edmond Yu who was shot by police in 1997 (QSPC & Urban Alliance on Race Relations, 2002). In 1999, the QSPC had attempted to join forces with the Toronto Rape Crisis Centre, Multicultural Women Against Rape, and two patients from within the forensic system (Cinderella Allalouf Ad-Hoc Litigation Committee) to seek standing into the inquest of Cinderella Allalouf. The coroner rejected involvement of the QSPC; he felt that they did not have a direct interest and that the PPAO should instead address the advocacy issues (*Cinderella Allalouf Ad-Hoc Litigation Committee v. Lucas*, 1999). The involvement of the QSPC in *Winko* signalled new opportunity

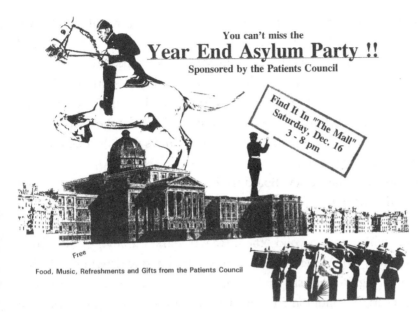

You can't miss the
Year End Asylum Party !!
Sponsored by the Patients Council

Find It In "The Mall"
Saturday, Dec. 16
3 - 8 pm

Free

Food, Music, Refreshments and Gifts from the Patients Council

FIGURE 14.2: Year-End Asylum Party

This poster announces a year-end patients' celebration at the site of the former Queen Street Mental Health Centre in Toronto (now the Centre for Addiction and Mental Health, or CAMH). As recounted here and by Erick Fabris in Chapter 9, the Queen Street Patients Council was an early example of a peer support organization, funded by the Ontario Ministry of Health and run by survivors, patients, and consumers of the Queen Street site.

Source: Psychiatric Survivor Archives of Toronto

for c/s/x perspective in litigation where none had existed previously in Canada. This access to more direct participation with the law signified a shift in c/s/x involvement and over the years has led to other opportunities for intervention in lower and higher courts, inquests, and, more recently, in processes of court diversion.[9] As intervenors, the Queen Street Patients Council applied for standing in order to reposition questions of "dangerousness" and "risk" as a responsibility of the court and not of an accused found "not criminally responsible" (NCR). Like *Swain*, *Winko* challenged historical prejudices and stereotypes embedded within medico-legal psychiatric processes. It is also considered a leading precedent on the application of section 672.54 to an accused deemed NCR (other mental health legal cases influenced by the Charter post-*Swain*, and of particular significance for the inclusion of c/s/x organizations as intervenors, include *Starson v. Swayze* (2003), *Pinet v. St. Thomas Psychiatric Hospital* (2004), *Mazzei v. British Columbia* (2006), and *R. v. Conway* (2010)).[10]

"Facts of the Case"[11]

Mr. Joseph Ronald Winko was charged with aggravated assault and possession of a weapon. He had previous contact with the psychiatric system and was deemed by the court "not criminally responsible" when he was arrested in 1983 for attacking two pedestrians on the street. In 1995, the British Columbia Psychiatric Review Board granted Mr. Winko a "conditional discharge" and Mr. Winko appealed this decision to the Court of Appeal and also challenged the constitutionality of section 672.54 of the Criminal Code, arguing that it violated sections 7 and 15 of his Charter rights as it placed on him a "burden of proof." The BC Court of Appeal upheld the Review Board's decision and did not grant an absolute discharge, and so Mr. Winko took his case to the Supreme Court of Canada.

Section 672.54 confers on the Review Board the responsibility of balancing the need to protect the public with the rights of the accused deemed to be suffering from a "mental disorder." The Criminal Code defines "threat to public" as "significant threat to the safety of the public," which goes beyond "the merely trivial or annoying" (*Winko v. British Columbia*, 1999, p. 44). As such, it was the role of the court to determine whether Mr. Winko would be a "significant risk" and, if so, if he would continue to be detained or be discharged with certain conditions. The BC Court of Appeal ruling noted that the Review Board has the responsibility to be reminded that, "A past offence committed while the NCR accused suffered from a mental illness is not, by itself, evidence that the NCR accused continues to pose a significant risk to the safety of the public" (p. 5).

Winko emerged out of British Columbia and was co-joined with the similar case of Mr. Gordon Bese and Mr. Denis LePage in Ontario. The Queen Street Patients Council became involved because they had made arguments in lower courts for Mr. LePage, who was detained in the Oak Ridge Branch of Penetanguishene Mental Health Centre. All the cases represented similar fundamental concerns about the treatment of psychiatric patients detained under forensic Review Boards.[12] Mr. LePage had entered the forensic system in 1978 for the possession of a number of weapons.[13] Like Mr. Winko he was charged and found NCR. After being detained for 17 years he brought a challenge before the Court of Appeal on the constitutionality of his detention. The QSPC argued that, as it stood, the provisions in Part XX.1 of the Criminal Code were dependent on an unreliable exercise of prediction of dangerousness (Factum of the Intervenor, QSPC, n.d.).

Queen Street Patients Council Evidence

As intervenors, the Queen Street Patients Council's lawyers[14] argued that Part XX.1 of the Criminal Code violated section 7 and section 15 of the Charter because it restricted the liberty of persons deemed NCR irrespective of the nature of the index offence, and it did not give NCR individuals the benefit of procedural protection against the possibility of error.

Legal arguments on behalf of the QSPC echoed critiques raised in the eighties by Savage and McKague (1987) on Review Board procedural fairness (pp. 81–86).

However, other well-known section 15 (equality) cases such as *R. v. Swain* (1991), *Vriend v. Alberta* (1998), *Andrews v. Law Society of British Columbia* (1989), and *R. v. Turpin* (1989) provided the judicial frame whereby arguments could be made and simultaneously legitimated (in the law's eyes) for what was and continues today to be a historic fight to protect against discrimination and bias towards persons with psychiatric disabilities. The intervenors used the *Andrews* case as legal precedent and applied a two-step approach adopted in *Andrews* to convince the court of differential treatment under section 15 (Factum of the Intervenor, QSPC, n.d., p. 2).[15] A portion of this argument relied on a comparison between an NCR accused and an individual convicted in the regular criminal justice stream. With the latter, there exists a clear designation of length of sentencing, whereas an NCR accused is often in the position of unclear and sometimes "indefinite sentencing." The QSPC argued discrimination on the basis of "mental disability." Putting NCR appellants in the position of being detained for an indefinite period, they submitted, violated the rights not only of the individual but also of all members of that group on the basis of "preconceived perceptions and characteristics of the group; namely, that all persons who have been incapacitated by the effects of mental illness and have committed some act proscribed by the Criminal Code are a significant threat to society" (Factum of the Intervenor, QSPC, n.d., p. 7).

The QSPC quoted *Swain* (1991) and *Battlefords v. Gibbs* (1996) as Supreme Court cases that supported the argument that, "the mentally ill have suffered 'historical disadvantage,' have been negatively stereotyped, and are generally subject to social prejudice" (Factum of the Intervenor, QSPC, n.d., p. 6). They also claimed that the court's role in imposing indefinite state supervision following a finding of NCR perpetuated a correspondence between violence and mental disorder. In an effort to remedy the burden of proof placed on an NCR accused, the QSPC suggested three revisions to section 672.54 of the Criminal Code so that ultimately the courts are put in the position of having to justify any restriction of liberty on an NCR individual. In doing this, the intervenors claimed that the "twin guiding principles"[16] would be honoured by both the legislature and the court.

Mad Patients and Future Legal Reform

The Queen Street Patients Council deemed the ruling a success, although there was no finding of sections 7 and 15 violations. Having found that the Review Board had not properly followed the law, the Supreme Court effectively "reread" the law, reminding Review Boards to follow the provisions. Like other case law *Winko* has become a baseline by which to evaluate the ability of the psychiatric system and Review Boards to apply the law's intent. As the application of constitutional rights is contingent on the ability of the court to implement change vis-à-vis its relationship to the state, future c/s/x mobilizing must carefully evaluate how it can best utilize law as a tool for social change.

The Justices presiding in *Winko*[17] ruled 7 to 2, and Justice McLachlin wrote for the majority, concluding that section 672.54 of the Criminal Code did not infringe on Mr. Winko's Charter rights. The Supreme Court made a number of findings. First, it held that "properly read, the section does not impose a burden of proving lack of dangerousness on the NCR accused" (p. 36). In other words, there is no presumption of dangerousness in the law. Second, according to Criminal Code section 672.54, "dangerousness" has a specific restricted meaning of "a significant threat to the safety of the public," and a two-step interpretation of section 672.54 should differentiate between "dangerousness" and a finding that an NCR accused is "not a significant threat to the safety of the public." Therefore, the court established that there must be evidence to support a real risk (pp. 38–41). Subsequently, if the Review Board fails to provide positive evidence that the NCR accused will pose a significant threat to the safety of the public, it must grant an absolute discharge. The court reiterated Parliament's stipulation that the "least onerous and least restrictive disposition" must be enacted to an accused (pp. 47–48). Finally, the court instructed that Review Boards have the responsibility of assisting an NCR accused to their fullest potential by meeting needs and assisting them to "cascade" through the system.

Measures of "success" via litigation should raise questions about whether legal victories have any impact on the lives of the psychiatric patients they purport to help. Although an increase in absolute discharges occurred after *Winko*, it is difficult to gauge whether this trend was necessarily due to the *Winko* ruling or rather to hospital bed shortage or more people appearing before the Review Board (Balachandra, Swaminath & Litman, 2004). Statistics collected by the Ontario Review Board in fiscal year 2008–2009 reported an increasing number of new accused entering the forensic system with no corresponding increase in discharge rates (see Appendix 14.1). The responsibility to assist an NCR accused to their fullest potential is affirmed in declarations such as the following:

> In its purpose and effect, it reflects the view that NCR accused are entitled to sensitive care, rehabilitation and meaningful attempts to foster their participation in the community to the maximum extent compatible with the individual's actual situation. (*Winko v. British Columbia*, 1999, p. 57)

It appears on the surface that the law aims to be delicate and fair; however, ensuring in practice that "sensitive care" and rehabilitation occur is another matter. Alongside the challenges of limited resources, staff and patients within the system are barely aware of case law such as *Winko*. In order for law to be effective, legal knowledge must be diffused within and across an organization (Barnes, 2007). Only a small number of lawyers are versed in mental health law, and on how to apply *Winko* to counter the evidence presented by hospital counsel or the Crown. Further, the problems of "translation" from both the client to his/her counsel and vice versa are often fraught with a number of challenges besides the accessibility of legal processes, and leave limited room for NCR accused to become anything other than medico-legal classifications (Dhand, 2009; Menzies, 1989). Thus, future intervenors must explore how the law may potentially legitimate itself by the inclusion of c/s/x knowledge. Activists such as Jijian Voronka are beginning to theorize how the "mad informant" is used in bridging the unknown experiences of Mad people with that of mainstream mental health, and establishing what are the conditions and consequences of such participation (Voronka, 2010).

In order to "fit" the legal framework, the QSPC had to translate opinions, experiences, and observations into legalese that could be argued before the court.[18] Though Winko, Bese, and LePage were claiming unequal treatment, none of the judges agreed. Razack has suggested that participation offers marginalized groups only the opportunity to "reveal" to the courts what they need to know and how to build a fair and impartial legal system. While participation may bring feeling back into the court, real change and transformation are not readily evaluated or even available (Razack, 1998, p. 38). For instance, the intention of legislation to have forensic clients "cascade" runs in contradiction with Ontario Review Board figures (see Appendix 14.1) and media reports that claim "mentally ill offenders [are] swamping prisons," as one *Globe and Mail* article mentions (Makin, 2010).

The points in *Winko* that create hope for constitutional remedy (the "win") lie in the interpretation by Justices Gonthier and L'Heureux-Dubé. These two minority judges agreed to some extent with the arguments put forward by McLachlin, affirming that Charter rights had not been violated. However, a discrepancy lay between Justice Gonthier's and Justice McLachlin's interpretation in the section, "Rules of Responsibilities of the Review Board." Justice Gonthier pointed out that the court had a duty to clearly define "significant threat to the safety of the public" and to provide evidence of this threat. To clarify, on the second point (in "Duties of the Review Board"), Justice Gonthier rewrote and added the following new point to the original paragraph:

> Relevant factors include the nature of the harm that may be expected; the degree of risk that the particular behaviour will occur; the period of time over which the behaviour may be expected to manifest itself and the number of people who may be at risk. (*Winko v. British Columbia*, 1999, p. 37)

A number of other significant points were rewritten by Justice Gonthier, including the need to release the accused absolutely if no evidence is found of dangerousness. If the Review Board "harbours doubts as to whether the NCR accused poses a significant threat to the safety of the public," it must unconditionally discharge (p. 37) as there is no constitutional basis for confinement (p. 38). The Review Board must also make all disposition that is the least restrictive possible of the NCR accused's liberty (p. 48). Finally, the Review Board has a responsibility in any regard "to consider the accused's personal needs" (p. 57).

In practice, the effort to meet the personal needs of NCR individuals continues to be challenging as patient numbers increase and other demands arise within the operations of the institution (increasing demands of electronic health documentation, compliance with hospital policies aimed at liability reduction, etc.). Debates continue to unfold in the Canadian courts regarding what authority Review Boards bear when it comes to meeting the rehabilitation needs of an accused (*Mazzei v. British Columbia*, 2006; *R. v. Conway*, 2010). The challenges ahead for c/s/x engagement with advocacy and legal mobilization as a means of empowerment require a more complex and nuanced approach—one that takes into account psychiatry, law, and other intersecting governmental arms in order to understand not only how to deal with emergent issues of representation, identity, class, and poverty, but also to learn how best to represent these matters in court (if at all).

Understanding the impact of c/s/x intervention in the courts requires more empirical research that describes the degree to which intervenors can influence the way judges vote. In an essay published in 2010, Alarie and Green report having discovered some evidence that intervenors do matter—although the motivations behind how judges vote, or what ends are met by allowing certain interests to influence the "acceptability" of certain court decisions, remain unknown. While legal forums remain fraught with power imbalances and other problems, perhaps these findings lend psychiatric survivors and their allies hope for the future. The law allows two sides to come together, to engage in a conversation. Perhaps acting as a witness to these structured interactions, in the hope of altering them for something less harmful, is a step forward.

Conclusion

The consumer, psychiatric survivor, and ex-patient movement has changed over the years from a silent and invisible community to one that speaks out, and acts as a voice of resistance against dominant medico-legal discourse. The nineties led to increasing "rights talk" and engagement with human rights systems, including the Supreme Court of Canada. *Winko*'s place in the history of organizing for rights protection is not widely known. In part, making *Winko* and other legal decisions more accessible for discussion and debate has been the purpose of this chapter. A number of future considerations worth scrutinizing might include more robust discussions about how to evaluate legal success, and whether working with legal processes helps or hinders goals of self-determination for the c/s/x community. While there have been symbolic "successes" through judicial victories, the c/s/x community is still struggling to ensure that those rights are protected.

Notes

1   By "rights talk" I mean the accumulation of text and subsequent discourse (policy, legislation, legal rulings, and activist political writings) that inform current understandings and assumptions about people's experience of the psychiatric-legal system (see Barnes, 2004; McCubbin & Cohen, 1998).

2   Over the last three decades, identity politics within the "Mad" community have grown and changed beyond "patient," "psychiatric survivor," and "consumer." Individuals use numerous terms to reflect political and non-political relationships or identities to the psychiatric system(s). For this chapter, I predominantly use the generic acronym "c/s/x" or the term "psychiatric survivor," as these are the terms that were widely used in reference to activism and advocacy in the 1980s and 1990s.

3   In Canada, the first psychiatric patients' group, the Mental Patients Association, was started in Vancouver in 1971 (Reaume, 2002, p. 416).

4   *Phoenix Rising* issues can be viewed online by visiting the Psychiatric Survivor Archives website at www.psychiatricsurvivorarchives.com.

5   Review Boards have jurisdiction over individuals who have been found by a court to be either "unfit to stand trial" or "not criminally responsible" due to "mental disorder." For more information on the mandate of Mental Disorder Review Boards, please see the Criminal Code of Canada, section 672.38(1).

6   "Mental disability" is used in *Swain* as opposed to "psychiatric disability."

7   The rules for intervenor status are different at every proceeding and every level of court. For more information on the rules for the Supreme Court of Canada, please see "Guidelines for Preparing Documents to be Filed," Rule 42.

8   The QSPC existed from 1992 until 2002. At the time a merger of all four hospital sites (the Clarke Institute of Psychiatry, the Addiction Research Foundation, the Queen Street Provincial Psychiatric Hospital, and the Donwoods) forced the QSPC to reconstitute itself into the Empowerment Council (EC). The EC continues to provide systemic advocacy, which now includes advocacy for addiction clients.

9   Psychiatric survivor/consumer organizations, the Queen Street Patients Council, the Empowerment Council, and the Mental Health Legal Advocacy Coalition have all intervened in lower/higher court cases and/or inquests and at tribunals. In 2007, the Dream Team (Toronto consumers/survivors advocating for affordable, safe, supportive housing) filed a complaint with the Ontario Human Rights Commission against Liberal provincial Member of Parliament, Tony Ruprecht. Sound Times, a consumer/survivor initiative, began assisting with release-from-custody plans in mental court diversion in approximately 2004 (personal correspondence with Sound Times staff Laura Horsman, September 2011).

10   The Supreme Court in *Winko* ruled that the court could not detain a "not criminally responsible" accused without proving they would be "a significant threat to the safety of the public." *Starson* became a precedent-setting Supreme Court case that ruled in favour of the appellant, Scott Starson, and his "capacity" to understand the "reasonable and foreseeable consequences of refusing" drug treatment. *Pinet* helped to ensure that dispositions are "the least onerous and least restrictive to the accused." In *Mazzei*, the court decided that the Ontario Review Board is responsible for supervising and managing treatment care plans. The case stemmed from the request of Vernon Mazzei (an Aboriginal inmate) for treatment that was culturally appropriate to his needs. At issue in *Conway* was whether the Ontario Review Board has the

authority under section 24(1) of the Charter to provide remedies. A two-step "Conway Test" was established to address the aforementioned question.

11   Legal cases will often include a section entitled "Facts of the Case," which on the surface is meant to reproduce a summary of relevant main points of the case. However, the construction of such legal narratives as "factual" can be misleading. For more on the construction of case files, please see Robert Menzies' *Survival of the Sanest* (1989) and Sherene Razack's *Canadian Feminism and the Law* (1991).

12   Often cases will be combined at the Supreme Court level when related questions are before the lower courts.

13   These weapons included a 12-gauge shotgun, a .357 snub-nose Magnum, and a box of 12-gauge Magnum shells and handcuffs. He also had a number of other previous charges in his criminal record.

14   Dan Brodsky served as counsel for Mr. LePage, and Paul Burstein acted on behalf of the intervenor Queen Street Patients Council.

15   The *Andrews* "two-step" approach is a legal test that determines whether an individual's rights have been violated based on personal characteristic within the section 15 criteria.

16   The twin guiding principles would ensure that both individual rights and public safety are protected.

17   The Supreme Court judges for this case included Justices McLachlin, Lamer, Cory, Iacobucci, Major, Bastarache, Binnie, L'Heureux-Dubé, and Gonthier.

18   For example, among the medical records used in the case, the QSPC included evidence of Mr. LePage's psychiatric treatment, which subjected him to experimental therapies by the now infamous Dr. Elliot Barker. Barker's "therapy" involved the use of LSD-induced psychosis, humiliation, deprivation, and restraint to "break down" "psychotic ego."

Appendix 14.1: Ontario Review Board Statistics

Year	New Accused (NCR & Unfit to Stand)	Absolute Discharges	Total # under Board Jurisdiction
2008/09	255	90	1,419
2007/08	318	88	1,330
2006/07	311	76	1,241
2005/06	269	131	1,044
2004/05	193	129	995
2003/04	148	135	983
2002/03	208	102	991
2001/02	179	96	1,086
2000/01	219	134	1,055
1999/00	200	111	913
1998/99	252	42	824
1997/98	196	40	754
1996/97	239	38	656
1995/96	222	39	662
1994/95	219	24	550
1993/94	210	31	465
1992/93	198	46	426
1991/92	80	36	391
1990/91	72	36	390
1989/90	82	25	409
1988/89	94	21	416
1987/88	73	20	386

Source: Ontario Review Board, www.orb.on.ca/scripts/en/resources.asp.

CHAPTER 15

Removing Civil Rights: How Dare We?

Gordon Warme

The inability to take an unfamiliar life seriously, creates monsters.

—Heinrich Mann

Although I complain about how my psychiatric colleagues practise, my complaints are careful. I don't insult and denounce; I explain that psychiatric problems are enigmatic and complex. I'll therefore go after the civil rights problem warily, making sure that it's clear why psychiatrists practise as they do, and why denunciations and harsh criticisms won't change their practices. Getting them to change their *attitudes*—as opposed to their practices—will be *very* tricky. Suppressing their improper behaviours—forbidding electroshock, banning certain drugs, cancelling their power to commit patients involuntarily—would simply mimic what *they* do: suppress psychiatrists' practices because they suppress their patients' practices. Although the law has always been designed to make it hard for psychiatrists to remove patients' civil rights, in practice, a psychiatrist's claim that her patient has a psychiatric "disease" or that her patient is "a danger to himself or others" has usually been accepted by the authorities without question. This is still true, but in recent years psychiatrists, knowing that Review Boards no longer automatically uphold psychiatric recommendations that patients be kept in hospital, are less willing to commit patients against their will. What is obvious is that these changes haven't reformed the *thinking* of the medical profession; psychiatrists still believe they ought to have the power to hospitalize patients—and to "treat" them—even against their will.

Today's psychiatrists have chosen drugs as their favourite medical tool, a treatment method that, after being given some of these drugs, transforms despairing, peculiar, and silly people into subdued, compliant *zombies*. Antipsychotic drugs (they are not really antipsychotics; the proper term is neuroleptics) definitely suppress patients, but there's no evidence that this is a treatment, that they cure or correct psychosis; like lithium and benzodiazepines, antipsychotics are powerful sedatives. These antipsychotic drugs have grave neurological side effects—which all psychiatrists know about. Every year, 1 percent of the neurons in the frontal lobes of patients who take them are destroyed (Andreasen, 2008). Even though they may not have been destroyed, many more cells are functionally impaired, perhaps permanently damaged. In addition, there are other neurological effects, peculiar tics and abnormal movements, effects that are common and disfiguring.

Also worrisome are the hematological and general metabolic consequences of taking antipsychotics (Cohn et al., 2006). The blood effects are occasional, but when they occur, they are a serious death hazard. General metabolic changes are commoner—pretty well universal—but apart from the immediate and obvious obesity, are slowly cumulative, in the long term lethal. Some observers report that, because of these drug effects, "people with depression, bipolar disorder, and schizophrenia are losing twelve to twenty years of life expectancy compared to people not in the mental health system" (Whitaker, 2010, p. 176). Although the obesity problem is common knowledge, the more insidious effects—diabetes mellitus and heart disease—get little attention. Yet the shortened life expectancy of Mad people is almost certainly due these drug-induced effects.

Doctors are used to drug side effects and, when powerful drugs are necessary in the treatment of serious disease, we expect them. Were it indisputably necessary to give antipsychotics to Mad people, this risk would be part of good medical practice, nothing more than one of the burdens of being a doctor. Balancing the risks of a dangerous disease against the risks of taking certain drugs is part of every doctor's day-to-day work.

This is not simple information, a hazard attendant on practising psychiatry. It's about a routine practice that is risky, yet nowadays taken for granted. The routine is to automatically give these powerful drugs to Mad people, a protocol rarely called into question. Were a doctor not to do so, he'd at least raise eyebrows, and might get into trouble with his professional college. The drugs are also given wholesale to people who live in total institutions: jails, nursing homes, and chronic care facilities. In such places, anything disruptive is quickly medicalized. Ordinary behaviours—getting up in the middle of the night, noisiness, pacing, complaining, horsing around—are treated as evidence of psychopathology. In institutions, these behaviours are recorded by guards, nurses, and attendants, translated then into symptoms of mental dysfunction, and "managed" with drugs, most commonly neuroleptics, the drugs that destroy brain cells, interfere with normal metabolic functions, and render patients lethargic and emotionless.

I've just watched a horror show, a DVD documentary (Citizen's Commission on Human Rights, 2006) that exposes these evils, the ones that, in the name of medical help, psychiatrists have visited on the odd, the crazy, and the marginal. It's all there: the shackles, cages, electric shocks, insulin comas, ice picks tearing into brain tissue (lobotomy), and drugs that make patients fat (with all the social prejudices and medical complications that go with it). If seen on this DVD, it's obviously a scandal; in an actual hospital, prison, nursing home, or chronic care facility, the scandal is insidious. It is easy to be fooled, tricked by a system that, if you actually see what goes on, looks calm and careful, and which is insistently defined as helpful. The DVD misrepresents modern psychiatry: overt brutalities are nowhere to be seen.

The atmosphere in a psychiatric hospital looks benign. The staff are careful and thoughtful, and patients are spoken of with compassion. This very medical atmosphere renders what's happening more dangerous than it would be if abuses were blatant; the sensationalism of the DVD misleads us. My guess is this: were they to see this DVD, antipsychiatry activists would cheer that the sensational images are revealing the truth; most other people would react by saying, "Wow, isn't it awful how psychiatry used to be practised."[1] The apparently civil and careful practices on real psychiatric wards aren't at all like what's on the DVD. It takes restraint and thoughtfulness to figure out that the practices on real psychiatric wards are wrong, ignorant, and wicked.

Many are convinced that the solution is to abolish psychiatry, transfer the care of Mad and unhappy people to kinder citizens, perhaps social workers and volunteers, wiser helpers who would minister humanely, work in the community, and help overburdened and despairing families. However, they forget this: from time immemorial, in every culture, certain citizens have been designated as special helpers. It's no surprise that, in our scientifically enthusiastic culture, this respect and authority is given to doctors: without an aura of authority and power, how could a technologically ambitious doctor inspect our nakedness, insert instruments into our bodies, surgically remove abnormal tissues?

In many other parts of the world, the designated practitioners have been priests, shamans, and medicine men. But even in the latter places, in Africa, Dawson City, and rural China, for example, doctors are taking over. Partly this is due to a global health strategy, but to a surprising degree, there is an indigenous urgency to take on Western—read: "American"—ways. The Shanghai students I supervise on Skype are desperate to adopt American/Canadian psychiatric practices, and are bewildered at my skepticism and my unwillingness to persuade them to adopt those ways. Misled about the benefits of psychiatry, practitioners all over the world, keen to take on Western ways and Western thinking, are shifting the care of madness and social unhappiness to doctors, including the enlistment and training of psychiatrists.

Nothing—I repeat, nothing—can shift our intoxication with the doctor archetype, dislodge her from being embraced as the primary helper, healer, and counsellor. Furthermore, the prevailing psychiatric superstition—the widespread belief in the magic powers of science—further immunizes my profession against criticism, largely because scientists—*medical* scientists—are no more doubted than were doctors who in past centuries practised humeral medicine. Like soaring Gothic cathedrals, our hospitals now have soaring atriums. Science, especially medical science, is horning in on religion—it *is* a religion; our faith in medical progress is boundless. On the walls of hospital atriums are commemorative plaques that celebrate donors, not unlike the commemorative plaques on the walls of Gothic cathedrals that celebrate bishops, kings, and electors. When built, and in anticipation of our superstitions, the priests in charge of these cathedrals were doing the reverse, horning in on medical science. They *were* science—superstitious version of "science": temples of healing through suggestion, prayer, absolution, penance, and offerings, a legitimate route to getting cured. Superstition infects all societies, and ours is no different; we hold precious a host of believed-in health manoeuvres, usually impervious to contrary evidence when they don't work, convictions that reveal our credulity, dead ringers for the delusions of insane people. Lots of current enthusiasms capitalize on the word "science": Christian Science, household science, social science, Scientology. Science is a holy word, sanctified not by the Pope, but by analytic philosophy, the bastard child of British logical empiricism and Viennese positivism.

My ideal psychiatrist abhors diagnosis, but she's like everyone else: she has automatic reactions to the strangeness of psychiatric patients, the depersonalizing reactions that cloud our thinking. For example, if her patient is despondent or terror-stricken she'll instinctively think of him as being "afflicted" with something, that he is tragic and helpless. By reacting in this human way, feeling badly and worrying, the psychiatrist risks underestimating her patient and losing her most important therapeutic leverage: hope. Tragic or not, as long as a patient's suffering is an expression of ordinary humanity—is, as I repeatedly insist, a social practice—the psychiatrist will carefully reflect on her own automatic reactions of alarm and distaste. It's essential that she be flexible, adopt other points of view, work hard at being curious and intelligent, lest defeatism and surrender come into play. Rather than coming to diagnostic conclusions, then following a pre-scripted plan, the psychiatrist's job is crueller. She must tolerate contradictory emotions, live with unsteadiness and uncertainty. But being unsure has a payoff: it keeps her thinking, coming up with new and imaginative responses to human suffering.

Had her patient a real disease, my drug concerns wouldn't matter. Faced with an indisputable pathological fact, treating her patient as someone helpless in the face of an affliction makes sense—especially if there is an effective treatment. But since there are no psychiatric diseases, there are no treatments. The psychiatrist has to forget about the imaginary diseases that exist only in the theories of ideologues, stick to her guns about this, and insist that the patient has within himself the potential for change. Like every medical treatment, this therapeutic attitude has risky side effects, perfectly analogous to the side effects caused by drugs or surgery: deprived of the notion that her patient has a disease, the psychiatrist or the patient's family and friends could conclude that the patient is a faker, someone wilfully acting peculiarly, perhaps cowardly or manipulative. Through discretion and courtesy, an experienced psychiatrist should be able to minimize this hazard, but it can easily happen that a patient will be insulted.

Neither wilful action nor being the victim of an affliction adequately explains why a patient acts as he does. This is why the psychiatrist must keep a close eye on her own reactions, especially on her oscillation between theoretical models, thinking of the problem as something the patient is possessed by at one moment, as real-but-peculiar purposes in action the next. In practice, she'll lean towards the idea that her patient is the creator of his own life—not on theoretical grounds, but because this attitude gives both her and her patient hope, the idea that, if he has a hand in how he lives his life, he can change it. Like the fussy grammar check on my computer's word processor, I'm discouraging (but not forbidding) the psychiatrist from using the passive voice. As with any patient, this attitude not only gives the psychiatrist hope for a person who acts blatantly insane; it immunizes her, just a bit, against treating him as an alien, someone with no legitimate place in our culture. It's the psychiatrist's duty to push herself beyond tolerance, to go so far as to think of her patient as skilled: only someone who knows the category of madness well can be convincingly mad; only someone who lives according to pattern "B" in a culture that heartily accepts only pattern "A" can successfully occupy the role of insanity. What's easier—almost automatic—is to think crazy people aren't up to snuff, aren't capable of occupying a proper role.

Such a courtesy—treating her patients as fully human—isn't the only payoff: it's a wedge that undermines our culture's unfortunate way of reacting to psychiatric patients, and would influence psychiatric practices. Were "treating our patients as fully human" deeply realized, committing and treating people against their will would be impossible. These problems are acute with the patients that concern us most: those who, because they are distressingly bizarre, are hard to talk to, and because we fear what they might do. Each of these patients is so different that, although we try our best to invent rules about how to intervene, in practice no rules could possibly work as well as we'd like. Therefore, when called on to write out involuntary commitment and compulsory treatment orders, psychiatrists realize—I hope they realize—that the guidelines for how to fill out the required forms never quite fit the situation.

It's no surprise that the rituals through which we confine a person are sometimes applied too quickly, in other cases too delayed; by nature rituals are imprecise, and how one psychiatrist commits an individual (a priest serves the mass, a mullah calls believers to prayer, an employer deals with harassment in the workplace) differs from case to case and from context to context. Although the patient in question hasn't usually broken the law, the situation he presents us with is pressing and urgent. For years, I told myself that these procedures are tolerable because they keep the community safe and comfortable: the system gets society through awkward predicaments. But I was wrong.

Every case is unique, so the officials involved—usually a psychiatrist, but sometimes the police, judges, or other social agent—need wide discretionary powers. But whenever arbitrary powers are given, there must be officials who oversee and monitor—carefully monitor—what is going on. This bears repeating: if we agree to bend the law in the service of a social value, and if we recognize that social values are arbitrary and personal, and if we know that every tyranny is tyrannical precisely because it promotes what it thinks is an obvious social value, then we'll make sure our monitoring system is powerful and alert.

In Ontario, the jurisdiction in which I work, there is a system, a set of rituals, that works pretty well. It gives the psychiatrist discretionary power *and* is carefully monitored; a person can be confined to a hospital quickly and efficiently. When the psychiatrist fills out the required form, she gives her *opinion*, a privilege granted to her by the law, just as expert witnesses in courtrooms are permitted to give an opinion. In her opinion, the person to be committed must be seriously at risk of harming himself or others, and must suffer from a mental disease. Once committed, the patient can appeal—this may take several days—and appear before a Consent and Capacity Board, a panel of officials, citizens, and doctors. In the presence of lawyers for both sides, these boards make decisions, this time on the basis of *evidence* rather than *opinion*: the original commitment is reappraised, thereby monitoring the psychiatrist's earlier decision. I've reviewed a series of such hearings—they are published on the Internet by the Province of Ontario—and found that, first, once such appeals are heard, many patients are released;[2] and, second, when the boards rule that a patient must continue to be confined, the ones I studied were distressing to read about, and I could well imagine that someone might guess—note "guess"—that they were a danger to themselves or to others.

This power is granted to a psychiatrist on the basis of her opinion. Yet we all know that it's best to be skeptical of mortal opinion: I doubt my neighbour's opinion that I should go to Lourdes for my rheumatism. This makes the commitment process tricky; despite what we think, a psychiatrist cannot predict better than anyone else that a person will do harm to himself or others, nor can she certify that a psychiatric patient has a disease—yet that's what she is obliged to say. But saying so lets the emergency ritual work. To say the psychiatrist is wrong or lying is to miss the point. Rather than submitting scientific information, such a doctor is using language to soothe distressed people, moving a bad situation into a more comfortable place. That her euphemisms can be misused is obvious; in an imperfect world, what else can we expect?

However there are problems. First, many patients don't understand that they can appeal, or if they do, are too passive to make such an appeal. Furthermore, the antipsychotic drugs these patients are encouraged to take subdue them, further reducing their will to act on their own behalf. Second, the efficient management of a crisis is a relief for those upset by a patient's behaviour, but not for the person who is confined: his civil rights have been removed. That the loss of civil rights is temporary doesn't mean we are off the hook; that because there are safeguards, the way things are is okay. Third, once certified as mentally diseased, the person is forever stigmatized, discriminated against when applying for jobs or insurance, and when seeking political office or romance (I'm not making a joke; romance is a vital part of life).

I've described the situation as neutrally as I can. But if I stretch my mind, force myself to face facts, my neutrality fades away. What if a racialized youth is hospitalized against his will because his upper-middle-class parents—especially if they are influential—have persuaded a psychiatrist that there is something seriously, perhaps "dangerously," wrong? They are distressed and frightened by his clothes (crotch of pants near the knees, baseball hat backwards, t-shirt several sizes too big), are appalled that he speaks a language adopted from his peers ("chill," "hood," "peace out"), doesn't work, and is rebellious and provocative? Couldn't happen, you say? Consider this. Forty years ago, abortion was allowed in Canada only if a doctor certified that there was a compelling medical reason why a pregnancy was dangerous to the mother or foetus. The law was easy to override: I saw women in my office, married and unmarried, teenagers and women, and wrote letters on their behalf. Although I didn't lie, I nudged and winked. The magic word, the key word, was "worried." That word, plus the fact that the letterhead made clear that I was a psychiatrist, implied that the patient might be suicidal and, lest they might someday be held responsible for a death, no authority or hospital board would override that implication. No one could criticize me for this; all I'd said was that I was worried about an unhappy person who'd come to my office. The analogous thing happens when a crazy person is *committed*: reports are written in such a way that it is *implied* that something serious may happen. This coerces and terrifies the powers that be.

Because of this possibility, lots of people can be committed. The current logic applied to the mentally odd and different is based on three arguments: they are dangerous; they are biologically flawed; there are reliable experts available to testify to this (the expert's only tool is opinion). Here are a few opinions that nowadays seem preposterous, but not long ago were commonplace. Note carefully that these practices are supported by the same kinds of arguments now used to confine Mad people:

- Some Jews ought to be committed because they are dangerous (dangerously shrewd/shady businessmen, too tribally loyal, hence having undue influence in business and banking, a dangerous advantage over those of us who never, ever, ever give favours to kith and kin). It's biological, of course; because they have Jewish genes, they can't help it. Hitler and his Nazis went too far, but if you think about it …

- Under certain circumstances, women, especially certain immoral women, must be restrained without due process—committed, in other words. We all know that women are dangerously provocative, *sexually* provocative (psychiatrists recognize this when we say that many women are "borderline" or "hysterical"; rapists recognize this when they tell us that women are "bitches who have it coming to them."). All you have to do is look at how they dress. In his book *Sex and Character* (admired by James Joyce, Karl Kraus, Robert Musil, Arnold Schoenberg, Gertrude Stein, William Carlos Williams, and Ludwig Wittgenstein), Otto Weininger (1903) had it right. Because they have two X chromosomes, they are biologically disadvantaged.

- Can anyone doubt that homosexuals are radically different from the rest of us? That their biology is different from ours? Haven't you seen them in the Gay Pride Parade, publicly cavorting in the nude? This lack of restraint must not be tolerated, even if there are no explicit laws that have been broken. Society is at risk, don't you know? They are dangerous.

In 2013 we live in what we call a democracy, yet, because I'm a doctor, I'm an officer of the state. I can therefore deny someone his personhood with a stroke of my pen. At my whim, without due process, and if you set foot in my jurisdiction, I can remove your personhood, too; the committal forms are in my desk. It's a power I shouldn't have. When I've use such forms, I was always haunted by three fears:

- I'm a coward. I'm filling out this form because I'm afraid that if I don't, I'll get in trouble with my professional college. It's the way North American doctors practise in today's risk-obsessed society: hyper-cautious, perfectionistic, concerned about lawsuits.
- If I don't commit this patient, the patient's family, who so badly want their relative hospitalized, will hate me, and make things difficult and awkward.
- I'm taking the easiest way out of a tough spot. I'm passing on to the hospital a problem that causes me anguish, a practice recognized in the profession by calling it a "dump."

Like madness, liberty and self-invention are not concrete things, iron facts, or holy truths to be upheld forever. They are practical, ways of thinking about how people live their lives, important in our culture and worth fighting for—a lot of the time. However, we are not well served by extolling liberty when faced with delirious, bewildered babblers on street corners. At this point mental flexibility comes to our rescue: we can change our minds, re-describe what's going on, decide that—for the moment—it's best to say someone is sick, unwell, "unable" to care for himself. Yet such a decision shouldn't be easy, for sure not formalized or official.

In *On Liberty*, John Stuart Mill advises that, "Neither one person, nor any number of persons is warranted in saying to another human creature of ripe years, that he shall not do with his life for his own benefit what he chooses to do with it" (1986, p. 133). He also cautions against paternalism, that a person's own good, either physical or moral, is not sufficient reason to restrain him. Mad people aren't usually harmful, nowhere near as dangerous as drivers who drink or drive fast, so when people are committed ("for the physical or moral good of the mad," as some might say), Mill's directive against paternalism has been breached.

However if someone is institutionalized, the psychiatrist has been assigned a task—why else would someone be in a hospital? The psychiatrist is expected to *treat* the patient, but since there is no disease to treat, this is a euphemism for what she really does and is expected to do: pacify or subdue the patient, usually with drugs. There are a few medical circumstances when the patient doesn't decide for himself that he should receive treatment, and this is one of them. The others are: unconsciousness; children whose health isn't being attended to by their parents; unusual and risky-to-others disorders (HIV, typhoid fever, tuberculosis) that the victim—the carrier—is unaware of or ignores. In all these cases, *objective evidence must be demonstrated.*

But not in the case of a psychiatric patient who is committed.

The "treatment" that follows upon committal is not a treatment: certain behaviours are, plain and simple, suppressed. I'm unpopular if I insist that these are moral, not medical, decisions—but they are. It's vital to remember that the psychiatrist's job is, or should be, to *not* act as a moralist, to *not* suppress odd behaviour, even if families and friends complain, even if they put strong pressure on us to do something. On the other hand, whether committed by the crazy or the sane, antisocial behaviour *must* be suppressed by someone—for trivial things, a reminder or a good scolding; for serious things, real sanctions and restraint. But this ought not to be done by a psychiatrist *qua* psychiatrist; this is a matter for the law and its proper instruments: the police and the courts. When we call this "treatment," we are either lying or stupid. Society has no choice but to censure, contain, or suppress those who: have sex on the subway; pee on their neighbour's front door; obey God's command that City Hall be burned down. But these are not psychiatric problems. Although drunk drivers, rapists, and gangsters need more than censure—obviously, their actions demand containment, restraint, and suppression—their civil rights are removed only if they are suspected of a major crime; this is rarely the case when people stigmatized as mentally diseased have their rights removed.

Legislators won't change the laws until psychiatrists have changed their attitudes about madness; doctors are the ones called upon by legislators for expert opinion, and that opinion is that psychiatric patients are biologically abnormal. Because most psychiatrists believe this, they are convinced that civil rights have pushed society's liberalism too far, that license and social mayhem are in the air. Because the psychiatrist believes this, she's liable to gum up the system and give legislators bad advice. She'll hint at suicide and dangerousness, or make ominous pronouncements about nonexistent diseases that "need" to be treated—thereby luring legislators into letting her continue to violate her patients' civil rights. And because medical doctors are held to be experts, her pressure on legislators to *not* repeal commitment laws will often succeed.

Obviously, if Mad people commit legal offences, something has to be done. Ordinarily, the law has its own ways of dealing with offenders, methods they are uncomfortable using with Mad people. But of course madness makes all of us uncomfortable. The justification for giving drugs to odd or bizarre offenders is that, if they have a disease, penalties don't make sense—except that, inconveniently, they don't have diseases. So should they be sent to trial, or should they be subdued with drugs? Unusually, I'm of the opinion that they should be subject to legal charges and their consequences.

The most poignant madness story is about the suffering of families and friends. Their anguish and worry can't be exaggerated, nor can the intensity of their wish that the loved family member or friend be induced to quit acting so oddly, settle down, and once again be the person he once was: it's a problem for families and friends, not for the designated psychiatric patient. I can't "treat" someone who, first, doesn't have a disease, and, second, doesn't want to be treated. And they hardly ever want it.

It's a mess.

Doctors want to do the right thing, so it's important to keep in mind that we commit people to hospitals for social, rather than medical reasons. Calling on social utility—we've got to *do something* about insane people—is to walk a slippery slope. Every show trial, every tyranny, every wink and nudge between judge and witness is rationalized on the grounds of social utility. So if, earlier in this piece, I sounded as though I might argue on behalf of an open falsehood—that sometimes commitment is okay—in the final analysis, I must eat my own words. Since social utility always seems justified to the person invoking it—I don't have to look beyond my own opinions to know this—we must be very, very careful. Or must we be more than careful? Must we be absolutist and inflexible about justice? *Fiat iustitia, pereat mundus* [Justice be done though the world perish]. I don't know the answer to this terrifying ("terrifying" is the only satisfactory word) dilemma, but I do know that "social value" has a weaker claim on our actions than does the law.

And what would be the fate of manic, phobic, and crazy kleptomaniacs if, when they commit a crime, they were charged with a crime? The answer is easy: pedophiles, CEOs, children, and drug dealers are charged with crimes and the courts accommodate. Besides, if an offender, Mad or sane, is convicted, prison isn't the only option. Should the following categories of people be obliged to undertake psychotherapy, take drugs, be confined?

- Madmen?
- Derelicts?
- Atheists?
- Christians who claim to eat the body and blood of Christ on Sundays?
- Psychiatrists who believe schizophrenia exists/is a disease of the brain?
- Psychiatrists who don't believe schizophrenia exists/is a disease of the brain?
- The 3,000 self-identified witches in Quebec?

The only solution is pressure—more and more pressure. But not on legislators: they want re-election and therefore go with public and expert opinion, the opinions that incorrectly emphasize dangerousness, and agree with the psychiatrists who tell them that psychiatric diseases exist. There are three kinds of pressure:

1. Defend doctors who, because they practise properly, are vulnerable to being disciplined by their professional regulatory bodies or by the courts. Psychiatrists who understand that their patients have no diseases can lose their licenses if they practise in accord with what they know.

2. Defend patients who have committed no crimes, but are legally confined against their will (I don't know where the money will come from).

3. Write critical articles that point out that psychiatrists, when they write about their patients, rarely follow the elementary rules of science: replication, prediction, objective evidence. I'm suggesting that we be scientific nags; that slowly but surely, our nagging will have an effect.

Notes

1 Note: "used to." The public relations campaigns of psychiatric hospitals and drug companies work only too well.

2 Some colleagues involved in commitment hearings tell me that my observation is unique to the day I read the reports on the Internet, that fewer are released than I think; others tell me that the situation is dire, that to their chagrin, it's nowadays impossible to keep people in the hospital.

CHAPTER 16

"They should not be allowed to do this to the homeless and mentally ill":
Minimum Separation Distance Bylaws Reconsidered[1]

Lilith "Chava" Finkler

> *How would anybody in this room like it if somebody came up to you and said "We do not want you living in our neighbourhood"? It does not matter why they say it to you; it is wrong. People are not allowed to prevent Blacks, gays or Jews from living in their neighbourhood because it is considered a hate crime and they should not be allowed to do this to the homeless and mentally ill either.*
> —Philip Dufresne, cited in Standing Senate Committee on Social Affairs, Science & Technology (2006, p. 12)

Introduction: Towards a Psychiatric Survivor Analysis of Land Use Law

A significant housing literature examines psychiatric survivor experiences (Capponi, 1992; Corring & Cook, 2007; Forchuk, Nelson & Hall, 2006a,b,c), preferences (Johnson, 2001; Walker & Seasons, 2002), and quality of life (Depla, De Graaf & Heeren, 2006; Nelson, Sylvestre, Aubry, George & Trainor, 2007). Scholarly planning articles discuss implications of the "not in my back yard" (NIMBY) phenomenon, citing neighbourhood opposition as a factor in decreased housing availability (Dear, 1992; Schively, 2007; Takahashi & Dear, 1997). However, there has been little comment on the impact of land use law upon psychiatric survivor housing (Dear & Laws, 1986). I write this chapter to fill the gap and examine land use law within the parameters of a psychiatric survivor analysis.

A psychiatric survivor analysis considers the impact of social and legal processes upon psychiatric survivors as central, rather than peripheral, to scholarly understanding. Such an analysis reframes social or legal practices by posing questions that challenge commonly accepted beliefs. Although many survivors offer a psychiatric survivor analysis (Beresford, 2005; Chamberlin, 1978), one need not be a survivor to present such an analysis (Kaiser, 2001; Perlin, 2008). I suggest a psychiatric survivor analysis as a perspectival antidote to the ways in which planning practices, such as zoning, ignore psychiatric survivor realities. While mental health policy-makers acknowledge that survivor perspectives must be included in decisions regarding service provision (Government of Ontario, 2011), they rarely apply a psychiatric survivor analysis to land use planning and law.

A psychiatric survivor analysis incorporates an understanding of sanism, a form of systemic discrimination similar to sexism or racism, which targets psychiatric survivors. As Perlin (1991) notes, "The concentrated efforts to 'zone out' group homes and congregate residences for the mentally disabled offers a paradigm of sanist behaviour" (p. 92). Sanism, however, is not limited to spatial aspects of exclusion. Psychiatric survivors have often been denied access to mental health care (Abraham, 2008; Ontario Psychiatric Association, 2008) and physical health care (Kisely et al., 2007), have endured exploitation of their labour in sheltered workshops or hospitals (Reaume, 2004), have been forcibly sterilized (Cairney, 1996; Woodson, 1994), have disproportionately lost custody of their children (Mosoff, 1997), and have been vulnerable subjects of research (Collins, 1988). Clearly, sanism is evident in multiple manifestations.

Scholars such as Zippay (2007), Takahashi and Dear (1997), and Dear and Taylor (1982) discuss prospective neighbours' rejection of psychiatric survivor housing in an attitudes research framework that individualizes systemic sanism. Attitudes research examines non-survivor perceptions of psychiatric survivors; sources of community opposition are construed as individual feelings and thoughts. The proposed solution to the rejection of psychiatric survivors is to eliminate the "stigma of mental illness" (Ontario Psychiatric Association, 2008). The displacement of ex-psychiatric patients from their homes in some neighbourhoods may well be spurred on by individual negative feelings of neighbours (Slater, 2004). However, gentrification processes also provide economic gain to real estate developers and investors (Slovenko, 2009; Wong, 2007). A psychiatric survivor analysis, then, does not simply seek psychiatric survivor perspectives or preferences, but rather, examines socio-legal circumstances in the context of deeply embedded power relations. Of course, these power relations are mediated not only by psychiatric survivor status but also by gender, race, class, ability, etc. An examination of the intricate, and often invisible, connections between social and political locations can inform and enhance a psychiatric survivor analysis.

In the land use law context, a psychiatric survivor analysis distinguishes between the interests of landlords and those of their tenants. Care providers in land use disputes typically articulate tenants' needs.[2] Sometimes, the interests of housing providers may conflict with those of their tenants. For example, landlords may seek permission to increase density. However, municipal approval might translate into shared bedrooms for tenants. Alternatively, landlords may wish to assure neighbours there is little risk of fire and prohibit tenants from smoking inside the building. However, smoking is a significant part of psychiatric survivor culture (Wilton, 2004) and cigarettes often serve as an alternate form of currency exchange in hospital settings (Lawn, 2005).

Because cigarettes are so central to psychiatric survivor lives, tenants may resent not being able to smoke in their own home.

Unfortunately, even housing advocacy publications lack a critical psychiatric survivor analysis. The Wellesley Institute report, *We Are Neighbours*, offers evidence that the presence of psychiatric survivor housing does not decrease property values (De Wolff, 2008), a traditional housing provider response to neighbourhood opposition (Galster, Tatian, Santiago, Pettit & Smith, 2003). A psychiatric survivor analysis might challenge the preliminary assertion by asking, "Why are property values so important?" If an assessment proved subsequently that the presence of survivors does lower property values, ought survivors to be removed from residential areas?

Sanism in a Housing Context

Sanism manifests not only in restrictive zoning bylaws but also in the language used in the land use law context. For example, disturbing parallels are often made between housing for psychiatric survivors and waste or waste management facilities such as garbage dumps. During deinstitutionalization, residents' associations sometimes described psychiatric survivors being "dumped" into the community. One writer connected use of such terms to NIMBY sentiment:

> Stories about the "dumping" of mental patients into local communities are a perfect example.... Just the very word "dumping" has a derogatory connotation—garbage dump, dumping garbage. That the state or the media may view mental patients as garbage may not be too far off the mark ... the public is left with many misconceptions about mental patients, increasing the reluctance of communities to accept them in their midst. (Linter, 1979, pp. 415–416)

Even some psychiatric survivors internalized this comparison:

> I perceived myself as having a serious mental illness ... as having been relegated to what I called the "social garbage heap" ... I would do things such as standing away from others at bus stops and hiding ... in the far corners of subway cars. Thinking of myself as garbage, I would even leave the sidewalk in what I thought of as exhibiting proper deference to those above me in social class. The latter group of course included all other human beings. (Gallo, cited in Corrigan & Watson, 2002, p. 35)

One could argue that associations between psychiatric survivors and garbage are an unfortunate historical phenomenon. However, one published report (De Wolff, 2008) described incidents in which psychiatric survivor tenants living in non-profit housing dealt with garbage dumped onto their site: "[O]ne neighbour was dumping his garbage in our back yard. I guess he thought this was public property and that because we were crazy people, we would not notice" (p. 21).

A newspaper report illustrates this same association. Neighbours in Georgina, Ontario, complained about the behaviour of psychiatric survivor tenants in a local boarding home. When asked by a reporter to comment on opposition to tenants wandering about town, one councillor replied: "We all produce garbage, but we have no mega dumps. We enjoy super highways but we have no super highway in Georgina.... Sometimes we're more average, sometimes we're less.... We don't want to look like hypocrites or NIMBYs" (Kibble, 2009).

This link between psychiatric survivors and waste has also been noted by researchers investigating the NIMBY literature. Ross (2007) notes:

> What is disconcerting is that the understanding derived from waste-related research is often considered transferable to NIMBY directed at social service land uses. In some cases, research on NIMBY still addresses the two types of uses—hazardous waste and human service facilities—in the same discussion.... This methodological approach is problematic as it inherently legitimizes a demeaning attitude towards persons with mental illness, who are indirectly labelled as "hazards" in such research. (p. 3)

As indicated by psychiatric survivors, researchers, and social commentators, concentrations of psychiatric survivors, like concentrations of "garbage," breed rejection and resistance. Prospective neighbours, municipalities, and sometimes adjudicators link psychiatric survivor housing to undesirable developments such as garbage dumps and toxic waste sites. The distance between the loony "bin" and the garbage "bin" evidently remains close.

Land Use Law Processes

Planning is governed by provincial law in Canada. Municipalities are created by provincial legislatures and are granted specific powers such as the ability to enact zoning bylaws within their own borders. In recent years, appeal court decisions have strengthened municipalities' powers to enact bylaws. A "broad and purposive" (*Croplife Canada v. Toronto (City)*, 2005) reading of such powers has emboldened municipalities to assert their authority on multiple fronts, including rebuffing human rights complaints initiated by disabled persons. Despite case law and statutes, which militate against use of exclusionary zoning, municipal munificence has not been extended to psychiatric survivors challenging discriminatory bylaws (*Dream Team v. Toronto (City)*, 2011).

A Supreme Court of Canada decision prohibits enactment of zoning bylaws based on the user rather than the use (*R. v. Bell*, 1979). Section 35(2) of the Ontario Planning Act states that the municipal authority to zone does not include the authority to differentiate between persons who are related or unrelated with regard to their occupancy of a building. Section 2(1) of the Ontario Human Rights Code prohibits discrimination based on disability. Despite court decisions (*Aurora (Town) v. Anglican Houses*, 1990; *Children's Aid Society of the Region of Peel v. Brampton (City)*, 2003) and statutes, municipalities in Ontario enact bylaws that can discriminate against psychiatric survivors (Finkler & Grant, 2011).

One such bylaw, which establishes minimum separation distance (MSD), can restrict or prevent the establishment of psychiatric survivor housing. MSD bylaws stipulate that particular forms of housing must be a specific distance away from another of the same type. MSD bylaws typically apply to group homes, boarding homes, lodging houses and/or homes for special care, all of which are forms of potential psychiatric survivor housing. I focus here exclusively on group homes, a form of congregate housing in which many psychiatric survivors live. The group home is clearly defined in provincial law.[3] Cases litigated in Ontario and Manitoba determined that group homes are permitted in residential areas (*Aurora (Town) v. Anglican Houses*, 1990) and that MSD applied to housing specifically for disabled persons constitutes a Charter violation (*Alcoholism Foundation of Manitoba v. Winnipeg (City)*, 1990).

Despite these court decisions, Ontario municipalities continue to enact zoning bylaws that effectively restrict housing for psychiatric survivors. Of course, Ontario is not the only jurisdiction in which zoning bylaws are used to such effect. Zoning is a common planning instrument used to reinforce social control. As Margo Huxley (2002) notes,

> [d]evelopment controls and the classification and distribution of uses of land in space use normalizing techniques to produce and reinforce taken-for-granted forms of environments, uses and users and their inter-relations. The most obvious of such social controls could be found in the socially exclusionary zoning … which at times has regulated the size of families and the rights of unrelated people to share housing. (p. 145)

Locational restrictions, such as MSD, impose an unfair burden on housing providers seeking a development site, and upon future tenants. If developers wish to establish a group home close to a similar residence, providers must apply for a minor variance to a municipal Committee of Adjustment. If the application is denied, the developer may appeal to the Ontario Municipal Board (OMB), an administrative tribunal adjudicating land use disputes. This legal process extends timelines and increases costs. It is easier for housing providers to consult and compromise with the opposition, rather than proceed legally. As a result, developers may cream (Goetz, 2003) applicants and admit the tenants that are least likely to offend opponents

(Knowles, 2000). By creaming, service providers ensure that the success rate for the program is high and will receive continued funding. Providers may offer tenant profiles to neighbours, seeking advance approval (Bordone, 2003). They may remove structural elements to reduce or eliminate overlook and limit visibility through installation of window coverings (Finkler, 2006).

My focus on MSD as it pertains to group homes does not reflect uncritical support for congregate forms of housing. Survivor tenants have indicated a strong preference for increased privacy (Fakhoury, Murray, Shepherd & Priebe, 2002), control of their own space (Dorvil, Morin, Beaulieu & Dominique, 2005; Nelson et al., 2007), and the power to determine when and from whom they receive services (Nelson et al., 2007; Stanhope, Marcus & Solomon, 2009). Scholars have noted that most survivors prefer their own apartments (Kyle & Dunn, 2008; Sylvestre et al., 2007) rather than congregate settings. Fakhoury et al. (2002) observed that, "Privacy, independence, personal choice, convenient location and proximity to mental health services have all been reported to be significantly more important to residents in community housing than to their case managers" (p. 310). Clearly, tenant priorities vary considerably from those of their landlords and reflect tensions inherent between those invested with institutional power and those without.

Nonetheless, supportive housing has helped reduce homelessness and hospitalization rates and can enhance survivors' basic coping skills (Kyle & Dunn, 2008; Nelson & Saegert, 2009). Group homes and other communal living arrangements offer possibilities for peer support and the creation of a psychiatric survivor community (Habitat Services & OCAB, 2010). Compared to shelters, prisons, or hospitals, supportive housing is less costly for government (Culhane, Metraux & Hadley, 2002).

Historical Context

In the 1960s, the Ontario government instigated deinstitutionalization of psychiatric survivors and required alternate economical housing (Marshall, 1982; Simmons, 1990). In contrast to asylum architecture in which high walls barred escape, group homes were considered liberating locations. Nonetheless, tenants were restricted to specific spaces within the community. Restrictive zoning replaced physical obstacles.

In the 1970s, the Ontario government explicitly supported group homes. The province encouraged municipalities to regulate group home location and structure (Dear & Laws, 1986). Provincial leaders hoped, given this power, that city councillors would not oppose group home establishment. Margaret Birch, former member of provincial Parliament, stated in her speech to the Provincial/Municipal Liaison Committee in 1978, "You may wish to introduce distance separation requirements as between group homes or requirements as to the type of dwelling unit, which is best suited for use as a group home in your community."[4]

When group homes were first established, most municipalities required site-specific zoning bylaw amendments (Secretariat for Social Development, 1983). Group home developers applied for amendments on a case-by-case basis. Public meetings required under the Planning Act permitted neighbours to voice opposition. By 1986, some municipalities were permitting group homes in residential areas, subject to MSD (Burbridge, 1986). Group homes became routine; a zoning bylaw amendment was not required. This change eliminated the statutory requirement for public meetings and increased the pace of psychiatric survivor housing development. MSD was perceived as a balance: a preventive measure to ensure no single neighbourhood contained disproportionate numbers of group homes. Both the provincial government and housing developers perceived these municipal changes positively.

Since 1986, group homes and related communal residences have proliferated. Today, most Ontario municipalities have enacted group home bylaws, usually coupled with MSD requirements (Finkler & Grant, 2011).

Case Study

This chapter is based upon mixed methods research conducted between 2005 and 2008. I read approximately 200 OMB decisions, used grounded theory (Glaser & Strauss, 1968) to analyze two case files in detail, conducted 26 semi-structured interviews (including adjudicators, housing providers, planners, and lawyers), and compiled municipal MSD bylaws across Ontario. Here, I examine OMB Case 1 and OMB Case 2 in light of municipal use of MSD and efforts exerted by a developer to challenge their implementation. OMB Cases 1 and 2 both dealt with disputes in a town I call "Placeville" and were ultimately decided by the OMB. In OMB Case 1, the developer requested municipal rezoning to permit a group home on his property. The building had previously housed 16 extended family members; the developer wished to house 16 tenants, psychiatric survivors who had lived together elsewhere. There were no changes to the physical structure. Placeville had no group home bylaw. The municipality viewed group homes as residential uses; however, due to the number of homes for disabled persons near the business district, Placeville council refused the rezoning application. The developer appealed the municipal refusal to the OMB and subsequently won the case. In OMB Case 2, the same developer appealed enactment of an MSD bylaw pertaining to group homes. The developer lost the second case and Placeville's MSD bylaw was formally adopted. Both cases addressed multiple issues; however, the MSD bylaw and discussion of tenants' psychiatric history dominated municipal meetings and OMB hearings.

During interviews, both Placeville's lawyer and town planner justified use of MSD by insisting that bylaws facilitated the community integration of psychiatric survivors. The town lawyer stated:

In order to ensure ... successful integration within the community ... the minimum separation distances were established. It is not in the interest of the residents of group homes to be ... ghettoized—by finding themselves living ... in the same block on a particular street in the town. The idea is integration into community, not isolation within a part of the community, and by forcing them all to be in an environment where they're all ... lumped together ... in order to achieve this objective of integration and belonging in a community, some distance separation was considered appropriate.

Similarly, Placeville's town planner stated:

The Official Plan said that [Placeville] would "provide appropriate special needs housing." We did not think [XYZ Street] was an "appropriate" location for a group home. "Appropriate" means integration, not over-concentration. We were trying to help group home residents integrate into society. We don't think that would happen if they were concentrated in one area.

A second planner concurred with this view:

Separation distances are estimations of what a reasonable amount of separation is to ensure that they do not form a concentration or an agglomeration. We have separation distances for group homes.... We have separation distances for adult entertainment facilities so they don't form a conglomeration.

In comparing group homes to adult entertainment facilities, the second planner ignored the nature of uses. Group homes are homes where tenants may live for years. Adult entertainment facilities are commercial venues that may cater to transient populations. The one thing both land uses have in common is the opposition they attract from neighbours.

Adjudicator #1 (who addressed MSD in another OMB case) noted that:

Minimum separation distances are useful [if] they are ... trying to enhance the quality ... of services provided.... If the concentration of a certain social service in a neighbourhood means ... people are not being well served because auxiliary services are overwhelmed, then ... [MSD] serve a purpose.

On one hand, municipal employees cited MSD benefits of community integration. In that situation, MSD was good for psychiatric survivors. An OMB adjudicator, on the other hand, noted MSD might prevent care providers from becoming "overwhelmed." In that case, MSD was good for social workers.

In OMB Case 1, the adjudicator decided that since Placeville had not enacted an MSD bylaw at the time of the group home application, town employees could not apply one retroactively. The adjudicator stated, "The physical location of this home is critical to integration within the community whose residents have opportunities for access and choice." While Placeville staff used community integration as a justification for implementation of MSD, the adjudicator rendering the decision used the same philosophical approach to reject the town's position.

Subsequently, Placeville enacted a group home MSD bylaw. The group home operator in OMB Case 1 appealed enactment of the bylaw, leading to OMB Case 2. At the second hearing, the operator argued that the bylaw was "discriminatory" but presented no arguments to support the assertion. Placeville staff insisted the bylaw's purpose was ameliorative and garnered the support of local service providers. Ultimately, a second adjudicator approved Placeville's MSD bylaw.[5]

The evidence strongly suggests that MSD was justified by the concept of community integration and its parallel in the planning arena, an idea known as "social mix." In the current context, community integration refers to the extent to which psychiatric survivors are physically, psychologically, and socially connected to others in their neighbourhood (Wong & Solomon, 2002). Social mix, in contrast, is a municipal government policy response that attempts to address social problems associated with concentrations of poor tenants in public housing. Social mix involves dispersing or integrating tenants on social assistance into areas with a large number of homeowners and private renters. The redevelopment of Regent Park (Kipfer & Petrunia, 2009) and Lawrence Heights (Sunshine, 2011) in Toronto are contemporary examples of social mix.

Planners depicted MSD as preventing an over-concentration of group homes. The term "over-concentration" describes a high density of social services in particular vicinities. MSD bylaws, a municipal response to perceived clustering, are used to decentralize and enforce distribution of social services as well as their recipients.

Although proponents of deinstitutionalization spoke in favour of community integration in the 1970s and 1980s, evidence indicates that supportive housing facilitates only limited social integration (Abdallah, Cohen, Sanchez-Almira, Reyes & Ramirez, 2009; Aubry & Myner, 1996; Zippay, 2007). Supportive housing, especially group homes, may facilitate peer support (i.e., tenants offering support to one another) (Corring & Cook, 2007; Wong & Stanhope, 2009).

Community integration, however, has been construed solely as spatial proximity between psychiatric survivors and non-survivors. Emotional proximity between psychiatric survivors is not considered integration. Sometimes, psychiatric survivor relationships are actively discouraged. As one example, in-patients at psychiatric hospitals are often, as a matter of policy, refused permission to visit friends on a ward once discharged (Neugeboren, 1997).

In OMB Case 1, tenants had pre-existing relationships with one another and wanted to continue to live together. As Town Councillor #1 attested:

> Some men had been together in a group home for close to fifteen years ... they were definitely a family and had not caused any issues within the community ... he [tenant who testified] touched my soul ... he did not want to be split up from his family which was the only environment that was safe and loving that he'd really known.

In their haste to integrate psychiatric survivors, town planners in OMB Case 1 may have inadvertently disregarded the social supports tenants offer one another.

The over-concentration argument assumes that psychiatric survivors have few connections with each other. However, persons previously institutionalized may continue their relationships for years after deinstitutionalization (Jones, 1992; Sinson, 1993). In the past, bonds between psychiatric in-patients were forged on hospital wards (Reaume, 2000). Today, friendships flourish in boarding homes (Capponi, 1992; Habitat and OCAB, 2010), shared accommodation (Boydell, Gladstone & Crawford, 2002; Dorvil et al., 2005), or at psychiatric survivor community events (Finkler, 1997). The perception that large numbers of psychiatric survivors in the same neighbourhood constitute an over-concentration negates the possibility that a critical mass of psychiatric survivors is necessary to create and sustain community.

The proliferation of peer support groups also offers an eloquent rebuttal to planners' dispersal recommendations. Peer support provides a foundation for community organizing (Chamberlin, 1978) and often lowers rates of re-hospitalization (Solomon, 2004). The literature suggests that some elements of self-imposed segregation offer significant health and social benefits. Academic and activist accounts of self-help illustrate ways in which psychiatric survivor-centred analyses can inform both theory and practice (Clay, 2005).

Finally, the concept of community integration incorporates the idea of the normal, the "madman" and the "man of reason" (Foucault, 1962, p. 240)—that is, psychiatric survivors integrating with non-survivors, reinforcing socially accepted notions of human behaviour. However, as Goffman states, "the normal and the stigmatized are not persons but rather perspectives" (Goffman, 1963, p. 138). The suggestion that community integration of psychiatric survivors with non-survivors will lead to social betterment for the former group belies a lack of acceptance of the contributions that psychiatric survivors can make to "men of reason" and to members of their own community. To presume otherwise is to reinforce yet another manifestation of sanist attitudes.

Sanism is certainly not silent in the municipal milieu. Instead, psychiatric survivor actions are analyzed and interpreted through a medical lens that pathologizes human behaviour. Actions considered acceptable when performed by non-survivors become problematic in those labelled by the psychiatric system. In the current context, many non-survivor friends or extended family members rent a home and live together. When survivors choose to share space, it can constitute a bylaw violation.

Dynamics of Invisibility

Restrictive bylaws can pressure developers to compromise with opponents. Developers then foist results of negotiations upon tenants in an effort to circumvent bylaw constraints. As one non-profit developer elaborated:

> The windows were deliberately replaced to eliminate or decrease sightlines.... Windows were bricked to accommodate neighbours.... In two apartments, lighting ... could be better but tenants have lots of [other] amenity space.

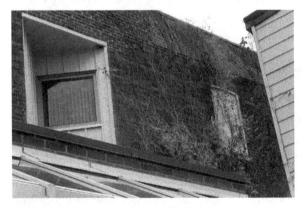

FIGURE 16.1: Inverted Windows

This window was inverted so prospective psychiatric survivor tenants would not be able to look down at their non-disabled neighbours.

Source: Lilith Finkler

These negotiations regarding structural overlook reflected neighbours' concern that they not see or be seen by psychiatric survivor tenants. The housing provider's willingness to accede to neighbours' demands and the subsequent structural alterations demonstrate ways in which architecture spatially reproduces social hierarchy.

The all-knowing, medical/visual interrogation, described by Foucault (2007) as the clinical gaze, manifests in tensions between psychiatric survivor tenants and their neighbours. While the clinical gaze exercises its authority by examining the less powerful, those in control can also implement its reverse. Because of such tensions, tenants can become conscious of their precarious presence in the neighbourhood and attempt to avoid notice. Tenants internalize the constant scrutiny of staff (Drinkwater, 2005) and neighbours. Boydell, Gladstone, Crawford, and Trainor (1999) noted in their study of psychiatric survivor tenants that

> in order to ... integrate into their neighbourhoods, they adopted passing strategies ... that included blending in, being invisible and minding one's own business. Several people talked about staying out of trouble and not drawing any undue attention to themselves. (p. 14)

In some situations, developers may insist upon a low profile when moving into a neighbourhood. MSD bylaws, or fear of their application by hostile neighbours, result in pressure to escape notice (Gash, 2011). This pressure, felt by developers, is subsequently exerted onto tenants. Aubry, Tefft, and Currie (1995) note:

> This strategy entails moving facilities into neighbourhoods without informing or consulting neighbourhood residents. In many cases, it has proven successful in minimizing obstacles to facility placement. However, the adoption of a low profile in neighbourhoods may also impact negatively the neighbourhood integration of tenants by encouraging them to remain all but hidden from their neighbours. (p. 50)

MSD bylaws and other forms of restrictive zoning not only limit psychiatric survivor housing, they simultaneously "discipline" (Foucault, 1979) survivor tenants by insisting upon their own invisibility.

The Implications of Integration versus Segregation

There are well-publicized problems with urban concentrations of poverty (Goetz, 2003; Jones & Newman, 1998). Planners have written in the context of race, arguing that segregation can be positive or negative, depending on circumstances. Scholars such as Qadeer (2005) and Peach (1996) have distinguished between forced residential segregation and voluntary association.

Tenants may live in congregate housing not by "choice" but due to economic necessity. Certainly, moving from one area to another is contingent on income or assets, something survivors may have in limited supply. However, they simultaneously may seek neighbourhoods in which other psychiatric survivors reside. One historical account of rooming houses noted:

> Low-income singles may feel more comfortable in a neighbourhood where there are other low-income singles, just as most affluent middle-class families want to live surrounded by other affluent middle-class families. This is not the same thing as "ghettoization," which implies a lack of choice, it is more like solidarity and sociability. For example, one boarding house in the High Park area [in Toronto] had great difficulty attracting and retaining residents, since it was too far away from the familiar Parkdale setting that the ex-psychiatric patients preferred. (Campsie, 1994)

The insistence that a concentration of psychiatric survivors always constitutes segregation and must be dispersed also ignores the possibility that psychiatric survivors may be

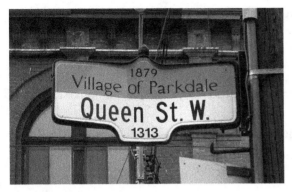

FIGURE 16.2: Parkdale

In contrast to other municipal street signs that indicate culturally specific composition in the Toronto municipal region (e.g., Little Italy, Little Portugal), the street signs for the Parkdale community do not mention the large psychiatric survivor population.

Source: Parkdale Village Business Improvement Area

poorly treated in integrated environments. Milner and Kelly (2009) note:

> The less palatable reality for many people with disabilities is that they often take significant psychological and sometimes physical risk being in many mainstream contexts because ... their spatial and economic inclusion also includes the "normality" of discrimination, abuse, intolerance and more subtle forms of personal exclusion. (p. 53)

Community Integration and Social Mix

The idea of community integration as articulated by housing advocates and academics (Yanos, Stefanic & Tsemberis, 2011) has, as its distant parallel, the idea of social mix among planners. In both intellectual frameworks, the solution to concentrated poverty is to disperse poor persons among the middle class. Prevailing assumptions dictate that living among those with privilege and power offers social and political advantage to marginalized persons.

Ontario planners have espoused the philosophy of social mix, touting the benefits of mixed income communities in local print media, in particular with regard to redevelopment of public housing (Barmak, 2008). It is an unfounded presumption that a social mix of housing tenures (i.e., public housing, private rental housing, and home ownership) is a positive form of social planning (Arthurson, 2012; August, 2008). Research described in planning literatures indicates that social mix has not eliminated urban concentrations of poverty; it has merely moved them from the centre to the periphery (Crump, 2002). Evidence suggests that benefits of social mix are sparse. Many scholars emphasize the dangers associated with uprooting or dispersing poor tenants (Bartz, Joseph & Chaskin, 2011).

The literature suggests that the development of upscale private market housing in traditionally low-income neighbourhoods does not necessarily result in friendly interaction between low-income tenants and new middle-class homeowners (August, 2008; Mazer & Rankin, 2011). Poor people may become more aware of class disparities and their own economic marginalization (Arthurson, 2002). Nor are employment opportunities necessarily enhanced. Research examining the development of social networks of dispersed tenants living in subsidized housing indicates that poorer residents are less likely to discuss job opportunities with neighbours than when they lived in public housing in segregated settings (Atkinson, 2005). Enhanced shopping opportunities fail to cement common bonds. Limited transit service often means people living on low incomes shop locally while those earning more shop farther afield (Ruming, Mee & McGuirk, 2004).

Damaris Rose, a researcher conducting an analysis of social mix in Montreal, Quebec, observes that interviewees, all of whom had recently purchased modestly priced condominiums,

> acknowledged ... that the appreciation of socio-economic diversity is a luxury granted to those who can choose to experience it as part of their personal trajectory of upward social mobility. (Rose, 2004, p. 293)

Clearly, the notion of social mix is inherently problematic in its conception of socio-economic diversity. There is little consideration of social mix as it pertains to psychiatric survivors (Mazer & Rankin, 2011). It is instructive to examine the South Parkdale neighbourhood in Toronto, an area famous for its large concentration of psychiatric survivors. Middle-class inhabitants have long sought to gentrify the area by moving psychiatric survivors out. Rooming house bylaw 67–78, for example, specifies that

> no person shall erect or use a building for the purpose of a rooming house in the area known as South Parkdale except where the residential building was legally used as a rooming house on January 30, 1978.[6]

The bylaw, designed to limit the number of boarding homes in the area, reflects municipal efforts to facilitate gentrification (Slater, 2004; Whitzman & Slater, 2006). Boarding homes are the primary form of housing used by psychiatric survivors in the area. Certainly, concerted attempts at gentrification have been successful. According to one article, condominiums in Parkdale increased in value by 18 percent during the fiscal year 2010–2011 (Farley, 2011).

As housing prices rose, property taxes and, consequently, rents in Parkdale also rose. This development may displace psychiatric survivor tenants, as they are often social assistance recipients. Middle-class homeowners, new to the area, are not kindly disposed towards old timers, referring to them as "real low life, pathetic creatures" and "people who checked out of the mental hospital too early" (Slater, 2004). Such attitudes do not encourage integration or contribute to enhanced employment opportunities. Rather, they reinforce established patterns of spatial segregation.

In one exchange documented by an academic living in Parkdale, the very existence of psychiatric survivors in the area was erased by changing the neighbourhood's name. Carolyn Whitzman recounted her conversation as follows:

> Whitzman: I just finished reading a book about Parkdale. It's called, "Landscapes of Despair."[7]
>
> Real estate agent (quickly): You can see why we prefer the term "Roncesvalles Village." (Whitzman, 2009, p. 151)

Roncesvalles Avenue, Parkdale's western boundary, offers an array of bustling gourmet food outlets and expensive cafes, catering to local upwardly mobile inhabitants. In sharp contrast, storefronts on Queen Street West feature social services, discount stores, and donut shops. Whitzman's (2009) exchange with the real estate agent illustrates the latter's efforts to make invisible not only psychiatric survivor tenants but also, by association, the poverty in which they live.

Cheryl Teelucksingh (2002), in a study that analyzed aspects of spatial justice, noted that in the context of opposition to psychiatric survivor housing in Parkdale, newly arrived homeowners justified NIMBY sentiment by pointing out that "improving the look of the community serves everyone's interests, not just their own, by bringing pride to the community, especially for marginalized residents" (p. 34). Teelucksingh (2002) pointed out that homeowner interests were reconstituted as collective interests. Marginalized tenants had limited power and privilege to challenge this assertion or to influence formal proceedings.

Mazer & Rankin (2011) note increased pressure upon psychiatric survivors by police:

> From the perspective of rooming house tenants … worsening police harassment plays a crucial role in the diminishment of safe social spaces. Police—along with drug related crimes—were cited among several dangers faced by local psychiatric consumer/survivors and low income residents. (p. 830)

In Parkdale, the influx of non-psychiatric survivor homeowners has not enhanced psychiatric survivors' lives but has led instead to increased efforts to displace them. An increase in variety of housing tenures has not benefited psychiatric survivors, although municipalities have used social mix philosophy to justify the gentrification process.

Challenging Discriminatory Zoning

There have been advocacy efforts exerted to end discriminatory zoning and establish human rights entitlements in a land use law context. In January 2012, the Dream Team, a psychiatric survivor housing advocacy group, received permission to proceed with their application at the Human Rights Tribunal of Ontario (2012 HRTO 25). Unfortunately, positive decisions such as the case heard before the Manitoba Court of Appeal in 1990 (*Alcoholism Foundation of Manitoba v. Winnipeg (City)* [1990] 69 D.L.R. (4th) 697), which established that the use of minimum separation distances infringed upon the equality provisions of the Charter and discriminated against disabled persons, has had little real impact. The City of Winnipeg still uses separation distances to separate homes for disabled persons from one another more than 20 years after the decision was rendered. Lack of enforcement of court decisions means that separation distances are still enacted and supported. In attempting to understand why discriminatory zoning exists despite legislation and case law to the contrary, we can draw upon the insights of Michel Foucault. Foucault has asserted that power functions not only in its consolidated sense, as within the state, but also in its dispersed form.

> One impoverishes the issue of power if one poses it solely in terms of legislation and constitution, in terms solely of the state and state apparatus. Power is quite different from and more complicated, dense and pervasive than a set of laws or a state apparatus. (1980, p. 158)

In an interview conducted with the collective of *Quel Corps*, Foucault elaborated upon his analysis:

> I don't claim that the State apparatus is unimportant, but, it seems to me that among all the conditions for avoiding a repetition of the Soviet experience and preventing the revolutionary process from running into the ground, one of the first things that has to be understood is that power isn't localized in the State apparatus and that nothing in society will change if the mechanisms of power that function outside, below and alongside the State apparatuses, on a much more minute and everyday level, are not also changed. (1980, p. 60)

Psychiatric survivors experience multiple intrusions daily, whether at home, work, or in public spaces. Leaving the asylum does not translate into freedom from oppression. One-dimensional interpretations of sanism focused solely on critiques of state power do not incorporate understandings of such intrusions. The comparison of psychiatric survivors to garbage, described at length earlier, illustrates the social/linguistic impact of sanism.

Historian Lesley Topp (2007) comments:

> Despite these lingering remnants of what was seen as the crude prison/asylum of the past, what the "free treatment" of the insane in the villa asylum depended on most of all was the invisible order imposed by the house rules,

legitimated by the medical authority of the director and enforced by his assistant psychiatrists and the nursing staff. Michel Foucault's analysis of asylums focused precisely on this point—it was when physical restraints were gradually dispensed within the name of humane treatment and the confining walls, chains and locks were beginning to dissolve, that doctors developed systems of order and internalized discipline that were that much more interesting for Foucault because they were transferable, and independent of the particularities of a specific contained place. (p. 245)

It is precisely this awareness of the invisibility of power stretching its tentacles beyond asylum walls that is so pertinent to analysis of discrimination in land use law. Zoning bylaws fall within traditional realms of law. Municipalities maintain discriminatory zoning bylaws and simultaneously circumvent results of unfavourable court decisions. Because municipal authority is, by its very nature, dispersed, local governments can force opponents to fight discrimination in each municipality individually. Foucault's (1980) analysis of dispersed power then, links the state and its use of zoning to control of psychiatric survivor presence in the "community."

My assessment of MSD bylaws and their intellectual and pragmatic relationship to social mix provides evidence that while community integration serves as an ideological justification, there are inherent contradictions that alienate, rather than incorporate, psychiatric survivors. First, community integration may not be necessary or even desirable for psychiatric survivors. Second, zoning restrictions limit availability and affordability of housing. Third, minimum separation distances specifically are related to the notion of "social mix"—a concept hailed as "progressive" by municipalities but widely criticized by planning academics. Finally, separation distances extend asylum function into residential neighbourhoods by restricting psychiatric survivor presence and enhancing the powers associated with the clinical/supervising gaze. If psychiatric survivors are to be welcomed in city spaces, urban designers, planners, and activists must remove exclusionary zoning, enhance accessibility of residential areas, and celebrate psychiatric survivors' presence in specific neighbourhoods such as Parkdale.

Notes

1   Thanks to Jill Grant whose feedback helped clarify my arguments and strengthen my writing, and to Howard Epstein whose incisive knowledge of land use law provided ongoing guidance. Thanks also to SSHRC and the Trudeau Foundation who funded the research on which this chapter is based. Finally, I wish to acknowledge members of the psychiatric survivor community for our conversations without which I would not have developed or advanced my conceptions of a psychiatric survivor analysis.

2   *Simcoe Community Services v. Township of Springwater*, [2007] OMBD No. 2227; *Stanley Grandison v. Toronto (City)*, [2007] OMBD No. 885. 87388; *Ontario Limited (c.o.b. Dowling*

Rest Home) v. Toronto (City) Committee of Adjustment, [2005] OMBD No. 695; *Centre for Addiction and Mental Health v. Toronto (City)*, [2004] OMBD No. 201.

3 Ontario Municipal Act, s. 163(3): "'group home' means a residence licensed or funded under a federal or provincial statute for the accommodation of three to 10 persons, exclusive of staff, living under supervision in a single housekeeping unit and who, by reason of their emotional, mental, social or physical condition or legal status, require a group living arrangement for their well-being." Despite this legal definition, municipalities may include boarding homes and homes for special care in the group home category. For example, in the case study discussed here, the home in dispute, which offered shelter to 16 psychiatric survivors, was considered a "group home" by all hearing participants, including the Ontario Municipal Board, despite the Municipal Act definition. Law and practice can diverge considerably.

4 File Number RG 54-3, Archives of Ontario.

5 Due to confidentiality requirements, case citations for this section are not mentioned.

6 The definition of "rooming house" is fluid. The City of Toronto has applied the term to boarding homes specifically geared to psychiatric survivors. See *87388 Ontario Limited (c.o.b. Dowling Rest Home) v. Toronto (City) Committee of Adjustment*, [2005] OMBD No. 695. The Rupert Coalition is preparing an appeal to the Ontario Human Rights Commission. It seeks a ruling that the city's zoning bylaw is discriminatory (Rooming House Working Group, 2011).

7 *Landscapes of Despair* (Dear & Wolch, 1987) describes psychiatric survivor housing issues in Parkdale, among other places.

CHAPTER 17

The Making and Marketing of Mental Health Literacy in Canada

Kimberley White and Ryan Pike

Introduction

We are witnessing a pervasive movement in Canada, and in the West more generally, to concretize and promote a unified body of knowledge on mental health and mental illness, now generally referred to as *mental health literacy* (MHL). The explicit political aim of MHL programs is to ensure all Canadian citizens know how to recognize, prevent, and seek "proper" (usually meaning professional) help for mental disorders.[1] However, in examining the broader social and political *function* of MHL work as a regulatory practice, we suggest that both large- and small-scale efforts to homogenize opposing ideologies and culturally diverse ways of understanding, living with, and responding to madness[2] around a central dogma, or set of hegemonic principles, are fundamentally exclusionary and non-democratic. In this chapter we raise two primary concerns regarding the mass making and marketing of MHL.

Our first concern has to do with the instilled processes and administrative structures through which only certain kinds of mental health knowledge become *official* knowledge. In the context of MHL we predominantly find closed interpretations of madness, where madness is reduced to mental illness, and mental illness is further reduced to a disease. In this way, madness has been subjected to and defined through the self-referential and exclusionary business practices that currently drive the production of most any form of official/professional/expert knowledge. Our intention in this short chapter is not to expose a concerted state conspiracy to silence and oppress Mad peoples in Canada (that would be a different chapter), but rather simply to show how the systemic corporatization of state institutions, operating in accordance with efficiency models and social marketing strategies, in effect limit the possibility of establishing meaningful ideological diversity in MHL.

As social actors, it is important that we pay attention to the socio-political and economic processes through which our common sensibilities around mental health and illness are informed, structured, and maintained. In examining *how* mental health/illness is made sense of, we may also learn who is entitled to participate in the production of mental health knowledge, who has the ability, or inability, to control what becomes "common" knowledge, and moreover, who is permitted, or not, to be seen and heard in the making of MHL (Rancière, 1994, pp. 12–13).

Our second concern focuses on a particular motif in contemporary MHL that steadily promotes mental *illness*, both as a medical condition and social identity, as a *disease*, like diabetes or heart disease. We presume it is fair to say without further qualification that madness/mental illness does not occupy the same cultural, political, or even medical space as diabetes. But in directing the public—through a variety of organizations, media outlets, and policy reports—to align mental illness with cultural concepts of disease, we should then anticipate a similar response to mental illness as we have to other diseases; we typically defer to professional/expert authority over diagnoses and treatments, and we accept certain forms of segregation and state intervention—medical, social, or institutional—as both legitimate and necessary. Borrowing powerful symbolic and linguistic representations of illness and disease also suggests that mental health can be restored and the *ill* recovered, but only if the illness is effectively reigned in, decoded, and worked upon by professionals. In translating madness, a vastly diverse and arguably unquantifiable human condition, into the more definitive vernacular of illness and disease, we simultaneously erase the subjects of mental illness, namely, the mentally ill, from society, from culture, and from humanity.

It is not any one particular group of state or professional actors we address in this analysis, nor are we insisting in any way that mental illness does not exist as a social and experiential reality. Rather, we suggest that the making and marketing of MHL programs ought to be scrutinized. To work towards a unified, or worse, a *universal* language around mental health and illness may make things appear simpler, more governable, pragmatic, and transferable, but when examined as a state-authorized regulatory practice, MHL also has the implied legitimacy to perform the social role of hegemonic training.

Making Mental Health Literacy

Considering for a moment the use of the term *literacy* in the context of mental health literacy sheds some light on both the representational and political significance of establishing a national, international, or even global initiative around mental health literacy. The United Nations Educational, Scientific and Cultural Organization (UNESCO) conceptualizes literacy in a culturally grounded way to specifically recognize that "there are many different practices of literacy embedded in different cultural processes, personal circumstances and collective structures."[3] The definition of "health literacy" is more specific and not directly grounded in culture or experience. Health literacy refers only to the assessment of an individual's "ability to read, understand and act upon health care information," to make decisions and follow instructions for treatment (Kickbusch, 2001, p. 292).

Mental health literacy is also defined as a form of knowledge that is not necessarily tethered to culture and experience. A report entitled *Mental Health Literacy in*

Canada, compiled by the Canadian Alliance on Mental Illness and Mental Health (2007), offers the following definition:

> Health literacy is defined as the degree to which people can obtain, process and understand basic health information and services they need to make acceptable health decisions. Mental health literacy may be understood similarly as knowledge, beliefs and abilities that enable the recognition, management or prevention of mental health problems. Enhanced mental health literacy is thought to confer a range of benefits: prevention, early recognition and intervention, and reduction of stigma associated with mental illness. (Bourget & Chenier, 2007, p. 6)[4]

This definition reflects the agenda of most social and public policy research on MHL, which is designed primarily to document *what* the public knows and believes about mental health and mental illness: Can they identify common signs of mental disorder? What do they believe about the causes of mental illness? Do they know what treatment options are available? Do they think some treatment options are more effective than others, and why? What factors do they believe are important for mental health? In compiling such information, the aim is to determine what educational, interventional, or corrective measures would most efficiently improve MHL within particular targeted groups. In this context we do not often see questions that ask *how*—how have we come to recognize or acquire knowledge about the signs, causes, and treatments for mental illness in the first place?

Nineteenth-century notions of madness and insanity in British North America centred on home care and treating the Mad as a family and community responsibility (Moran, 2000, p. 4). With emergent fears of the mentally ill as immoral and dangerous, so developed the idea that the mentally ill were not capable of self-care or self-control. This belief coincided with the industrialization era, which saw a restructuring of the family unit and an increased reliance on medical science (Moran, 2000, pp. 8, 115). In this climate, asylums were established for custodial care—institutions characterized by restraining and subduing patients, which remained in place for much of the 20th century (Frankenburg, 1982, p. 172). The asylum prevailed as the primary form of care until the rise of the rights movement and the (partial) deinstitutionalization movement over the 1960s and 1970s (Anthony, 1993, p. 11). During this time provincial mental health policy development remained stoically focused on matters of administration, management, and institutionalization, and has since changed very little.

Alberta provides an example that is archetypal, though not exceptional. In 1964, Alberta passed a new Mental Health Act (AMHA) with the explicit goal of protecting the rights and dignity of patients. The act replaced the Mental Diseases Act, 1924, and the Mental Defectives Act, 1919 (Angus, 1966, p. 423), the former of which granted physicians greater power to admit patients, while the latter was an instrument of the eugenics movement. The AMHA, lauded as a vanguard in mental health policy, aimed to replace the two outmoded acts (Angus, 1966, p. 423). Any patients who had been detained under the previous acts were to be admitted and detained in a hospital under the new AMHA. The AMHA was also guided by the Child Welfare Act, the Public Inquiries Act, the Alberta Hospitals Act, the Criminal Code of Canada, and a number of other provincial mental health policies, some sections of which were reproduced verbatim.[5] The most notable changes introduced by the new act concerned voluntary and involuntary admission, detention, and release, all of which claimed to put at the centre the rights and well-being of the patient (Angus, 1966, p. 423). Each step in the incarceration process required at least one physician to confirm whether a patient was experiencing a "mental disorder," defined in the AMHA as the state of "suffering from mental illness, mental retardation or any other disorder or disability of the mind" (Alberta Mental Health Act, 1964, p. 195). Despite the act's patient-centred "innovations," and in some cases as a *result* of them, many patients in Alberta were still housed in Calgary prisons,[6] and many still underwent sexual sterilization.[7] The 1964 act was replaced in 1990 under an only slightly modified name, Alberta's Mental Health Act, which remains the authority today.

Alberta's Mental Health Act, 1990, does not show substantial change from its predecessor, either in format or content. The act refers to 20 different federal and provincial policies of which the most cited is the Alberta Hospitals Act, 1989.[8] The structure of the 1990 Mental Health Act differs only marginally from the 1964 version. For example, while organized in much the same format, the AMHA, 1990, introduces a new section, "Mental Health Patient Advocate." Here, a patient advocate is defined as an individual appointed by the Lieutenant Governor in Council to investigate complaints from patients or subjects of Community Treatment Orders (Alberta Mental Health Act, 1990). In the AMHA, 1964, a section entitled "Investigation of Complaints" stipulates that an appointed review panel consisting of three people within each hospital should review patient grievances (Alberta Mental Health Act, 1964, pp. 200–201). The "Administration" section (Alberta Mental Health Act, 1990) introduces the only original procedure to be found in the new act, detailing the responsibility of mental health care professionals to properly inform patients of their rights during admittance, detention, and release (Alberta Mental Health Act, 1990).

Across regions and over time,[9] mental health policies in Canada are consistently found to be self-referential and reveal an exclusive deference to previously adopted policies, acts, and other legislation. Often with the clear goal of creating continuity and stability across the country,[10] policy-makers have historically assumed as an official starting point that mental health knowledge produced under the authority of the state is the most legitimate knowledge, the authority and legitimacy of which seems to rest in the virtue of its very existence. When provincial inquiries or commissions were established to survey and report on mental health policy concerns, the official reports reflected little more than the consolidation of several prior policies and procedures deemed outdated—policies that had also been constituted through the amalgamation of knowledge that had informed pre-existing policy, legislation, and procedure.

As another example, consider the current Mental Health Act of Ontario (OMHA), written in 1990 and most recently amended in 2010.[11] The OMHA references five other acts[12] and the Criminal Code of Canada to define both terminology and procedure. The most cited authority in the OMHA is Ontario's Health Care Consent Act of 1996, which itself makes reference to 19 different acts[13] including, most often, the 1990 Ontario Mental Health Act. In this self-referential process, the Health Care Consent Act adopts the official definition of "mental disorder" to be "any disease or disability of the mind" in accordance with the OMHA. However, the definition of mental disorder that is relied upon in the OMHA is both unexplained, and un-referenced (Ontario Mental Health Act, 1990). Aside from the definition adopted in Ontario, nearly all other provinces and territories define the term "mental disorder"—with little or no variation—as "a substantial disorder of thought, mood, perception, orientation or memory that grossly impairs judgment, behaviour, capacity to recognize reality, or ability to meet the ordinary demands of life" (Alberta Mental Health Act, 2000).[14] In fact, of Canada's 12 provincial and territorial mental health acts, none make reference to *outside* sources, or suggest there might be more than one way of defining or explaining experiences of "mental disorder."

Over the past decade, there has been increased movement towards the creation of a national mental health system that is cost-efficient and accessible to every person living in Canada. At the same time there has been an across-the-board adoption of the corporate business model in the administration of state institutions and organizations.[15] The effects are clearly seen in the manifestation of contemporary MHL, particularly in the exclusionary practices through which mental health knowledge is made. In 2003, the Government of Canada organized the Standing Senate Committee on Social Affairs, Science and Technology to study mental health, mental illness, and addictions in Canada. The committee released a report of its findings in 2006, entitled *Out of the Shadows at Last: Transforming Mental Health, Mental Illness and Addiction Services in Canada*, also referred to as the Kirby Report. The general mandate of the committee was to capture the full value of Canada's mental health system and recommend actions for better delivery of services. However, a business model is not structured to allow for variations in the interpretation of "value" and does not allow space for the possibility of different, yet equally meaningful, ideological frameworks to operate simultaneously. Using a business model, the standing committee's broad goals and recommendations are necessarily transcribed into a series of units packaged neatly as measurables, outcomes, and deliverables.

Among the 118 recommendations in the Kirby Report was a call for a national mental health strategy, which precipitated the establishment of the Mental Health

Commission of Canada (MHCC) in 2007. Along with the development of a national mental health strategy, the MHCC was also mandated to design and deliver a 10-year national anti-stigma campaign, and to establish an evidence-based knowledge exchange centre to ensure that *proper* information about mental health and mental illness is made available to all Canadians and across the mental health sector. The MHCC released a report in 2009 in which it recommended improved access to treatments, services, and supports; early recognition, diagnosis, and intervention, especially among children and youth; programs to target people and communities at risk for mental health problems and illnesses; and the wide promotion of mental health literacy (MHCC, 2009b, p. 16). However, when filtered through the exclusive vernacular of MHL, which is transformed into a desired form of mental health knowledge, certain concepts may lose meaning for some people, and subsequently some people may further lose power over their own self-determination. For instance, in the MHCC strategy for mental health and well-being, the very premise of *recovery*—originally conceived by psychiatric survivor/consumer/ex-patient communities as a resistance model to traditional psychiatric treatment approaches—has been appropriated and reconfigured to fit within the domains of various mental health care systems, policy initiatives, and psychiatric treatment models. The political significance of recovery as a form of empowerment or resistance is changed.

In examining *how* official mental health/illness knowledge has been produced in Canada, we are able to explain, at least in part, why institutional practices tend to enforce closed interpretations (Rancière, 1994) of "mental disorder" and "mental illness." We can also observe here the profound power of official knowledge. As MHL is routinely organized, legitimized, and disseminated through reductive, homogenizing evidence-based research, we lose (whether by choice or by chance) the ability to more broadly define Mad experiences, cultural expressions of madness, and Mad identities that exist beyond the allowable terms of reference. In the next section, we focus on the recurring motifs of illness and disease in the production and public dissemination of mental health knowledge in Canada to explore some of the implications of formalizing a universal vision of what mental health literacy should look like.

Marketing Mental Health

The universalizing habit by which a system of thought is believed to account for everything too quickly slides into a quasi-religious synthesis.... In fact, inter-pretation and its demands add up to a rough game, once we allow ourselves to step out of the shelter offered by specialized fields and by fancy all-embracing mythologies. The trouble with visions, reductive answers and systems is that they homogenize evidence very easily. Criticism as such is crowded out and disallowed from the start, hence impossible.... Far from taking in a great deal,

the universal system as a universal type of explanation either screens out everything it cannot directly absorb or it repetitively churns out the same sort of
thing all the time. (Saïd, 1983, p. 143)

Overwhelmingly, the determinants of mental illness, and thus by association the
determinants of mental health, have been proffered by medical experts and social
reformers of a particular ilk. Indeed, the official recognition of *mental health*, as a
matter of national importance and civic responsibility, has been a preoccupation of
Canadian governments since the early 20th century (Dowbiggin, 2011) and remains
deeply inculcated in contemporary clinical ideologies of psychosocial well-being and
professional models of recovery.

Early in the establishment of the Mental Health Commission of Canada[16] there
emerged a general consensus (reached not without disagreement) from the Board
of Directors to employ the language of "disease" in order to promote the idea that
individuals and families are not to blame for mental illness—that mental illness is a
disease just like any other.[17] The expressed hope in naming mental illness a disease,
like diabetes or heart disease, was that it would help lift associated feelings of shame
and reassure Canadians that the experience of mental illness (directly or indirectly)
is relatively common, that we are all the same. Except, we are not all the same.
The repeated attempt to *naturalize* mental illness rested somewhat uncomfortably
alongside the commission's other major public relations initiative, which has been to
bring national attention to Canada's looming mental health "crisis."[18]

In June 2008, in the midst of the economic downturn, the *Globe and Mail*, one
of Canada's national newspapers, published the first in a series of special reports
titled, "Breakdown: Canada's Mental Health Crisis."[19] The introduction to the series
assuredly outlined the parameters and severity of Canada's mental health problem:

FACE IT. FUND IT. FIX IT. At least 1 in 5 Canadians will experience some
form of mental illness in their lifetimes. "There's nobody in our country,"
renowned psychiatrist David Goldbloom says, "who can stand up and say,
'Not my family—not my aunts or uncles or cousins or grandparents, children, siblings, spouse or self.'" Yet unlike any other group of diseases, mental illness today remains surrounded by shame and silence, concealing the
almost unequalled devastation it wreaks on Canadian families, workplaces
and health-care and justice systems. Through the next week, The Globe and
Mail will tell those stories and seek solutions.[20] (*Globe and Mail*, 2008)

The official mandate of the MHCC anti-stigma initiative Opening Minds is, like every
other mental illness anti-stigma campaign, to dispel popular myths about the nature
and danger of mental illness and to educate the public on what mental illness *really*

is. While the MHCC denounces more politically charged terms such as "madness" as derogatory and loaded with negative connotations, in employing social marketing strategies to pique public concern and gain political and corporate buy-in for various anti-stigma projects, the commission's official message on mental illness, as a *disease*, calls forth the very histories and representations of madness it claims to dispel.[21] More disconcerting is the fact that there appears to be a complete lack of awareness or appreciation of this irony.

MHCC officials claim that while mental illness *is* a disease, at the core we are all the same and thus should not think in terms of "us" and "them" (MHCC, 2009b, p. 13). On that premise, the central theme of the Opening Minds campaign is to bring "mental illness out of the shadows," and to encourage those living with mental illness to come "into the light" in order to make themselves seen and heard in every aspect of social life.[22] Echoing the message in the "Breakdown" series, the public is again informed of the many ways in which stigma prevents those "suffering" with mental illness from seeking the appropriate professional treatment they need in order to recover into fully functioning, productive citizens. However, as Gilman points out, "the banality of real mental illness comes into conflict with our need to have the mad be identifiable, different from ourselves," and thus "madness must express itself in a way that is inherently different" (Gilman, 1988, pp. 13–14). It is therefore significant that the call is expressly for those living with "mental illness" to come out of the shadows, and not the "Mad." Those who do not on the surface reflect the desired, enlightened vision of mental illness and health are likely to remain in the shadows where they will retain their status as mad and dangerous.[23]

For instance, we know that historically the mad often occupied the same physical and ideological spaces as criminals and that these proximities have over time produced and maintained strong associations between crime, madness, disease, and danger (Foucault, 1962; Menzies, 1989). Today still, it is typically these individuals—the mad *and* criminal—who are represented as the most disordered, dangerous, and unrecoverable, and who thus make unsuitable candidates for anti-stigma programs.[24] These stories of madness and mental illness are not simply the fodder of popular fiction or sensational media misrepresentation. Such representations of mental illness and those deemed "mentally ill" are also routinely maintained and disseminated through the production of institutional knowledge.

Consider a different news report in the *Globe and Mail* titled "To Heal and Protect." This article, published in January 2011, was intended to expose the inability of the Correctional Service of Canada to manage and treat the "staggering" number of "mentally damaged" individuals currently "flooding" the criminal justice system and "clogging" jail cells (Makin, 2011, pp. F6–F7). However, the three-page special feature also exposed the ease with which we are able to recall and deploy historically informed alignments between mental illness, disease, and danger. In outlining the inevitable social costs that come with failing to properly manage the "sick and demented" through appropriate risk assessment and medication, the report describes the situation in Canadian prisons as a "revolving door to disaster." The article is punctuated with fearful messages about a decaying system out of control, and about the inability of mental health experts to effectively detect dangerous individuals before "disaster" strikes. Concern regarding the effects of stigma seems not so prominent in this context where mentally ill inmates are likened to animals on a "range" wandering around "like a herd of deer, they appear docile, yet leery; most are heavily medicated." In this context, the "primary concern" is simply "getting medication and the right treatment" (Makin, 2011, pp. F6–F7).

This institutional story is familiar to us, capturing a vision of mental health knowledge in which the mentally ill are seen as hopeless, nameless, faceless, and feared. The images assembled in "To Heal and Protect" appear at first to contradict the positive, hopeful messages conveyed about mental illness by the MHCC. However, it is precisely these *other* institutional stories that help define and give meaning to anti-stigma campaigns and other mental health literacy initiatives. We must be able to recall cultural images of *madness* in order to characterize and control the image of *wellness*. The Opening Minds anti-stigma campaign is designed to ensure that all people living with mental illness are treated as full citizens with equal opportunities to participate in society and in everyday life. Those who will remain locked away and out of sight, or who are otherwise victims of social death—the herds of damaged, deranged, and disorderly—will never have such an opportunity.

Despite the unprecedented resources that have been poured into the Opening Minds campaign, the MHCC has encountered some challenges in making its messages heard. The work, and even existence, of the MHCC is not well known among the general Canadian public, even among those whom the work of the MHCC is supposedly intended to help. Chair Michael Kirby recently commented on the fact that over the past three years there has been little reporting in Alberta (where the MHCC is based) about the commission in general and little progress on the anti-stigma front in particular. According to Kirby, "[i]f people get the *right* help, there is hope. But you can't even get started if people aren't willing to talk about it. Once we take away the stigma, we can begin the work" (Fortney, 2010). The insistence that the necessary starting point is getting the mentally ill to talk about mental illness immediately screens out those who are unable or unwilling to talk, as well as denies the historical processes of social, political, and economic exclusion that systemically silenced Mad people in the first place.

In May 2010, the *National Post,* another of Canada's national newspapers, published an article entitled "Mad Pride: Movement to Depose Psychiatry Emerges from the Shadows." Here readers are warned of the counter-hegemonic Mad Pride movement's plan to "overthrow" psychiatry. In the report, the Mad Pride movement, an international grassroots organization, is sharply dismissed by well-known Canadian medical historian Edward Shorter as a group inspired by the "hidden hand of Scientology," a cult-like "hobby" that also "opposes medical psychiatry even as it believes in aliens," suggesting that to reject psychiatry is a sure sign of madness itself (Brean, 2010a).

The article refers to delegates (academic and non-academic) of an international conference titled PsychOUT, held at the University of Toronto in the spring of 2010, as "fringe advocates," "self-absorbed crackpots," and "ideological zealots" who deserve no place, or voice, in a respected university. The risk of such movements, the *National Post* reporter explains, is that they will "discourage people from seeking mental health care, and increase stigma and suicide." The message is that there is only one rational response or course of treatment for mental illness, and that resistance to the institution of psychiatry is not only *crazy*, but also subversive and dangerous to society. The article triggered a number of heated responses and again revealed the challenges in reconciling, or making space for, different systems of thought.

The public dispute regarding mental illness also lays bare the strict policing of hegemonic order, a process that keeps at the periphery those perspectives and practices interpreted as social transgressions, or simply "at odds with the mainstream" (Brean, 2010b). Understanding the principles of social marketing and the need for some recognizable form of consensus, the MHCC must work continuously to maintain its legitimacy by appearing focused, decided, and strategic, not open and flexible. The public is warned in the *National Post* article that for an institutional forum (such as the MHCC) to be seen as too accepting of divergent and diverse views on mental illness is "ignorant and dangerous" (Brean, 2010b). This skepticism resounded again in the media in August of 2011, following the leak of a "confidential" draft of the MHCC's mental health strategy report. In an article published by the *Globe and Mail* entitled "Mental Health Strategy Draft Doesn't Go Far Enough," the reporter pointed out some "subtle, yet important differences between the tone and content of Out of the Shadows at Last and the draft strategy" (Picard, 2011).[25] The language in the draft strategy is described as "wishy-washy" and "circumspect" with "far too much emphasis on the 'recovery model'—the notion that everyone will get better with support—and not enough emphasis on brain science." While the recovery model may be considered a "legitimate approach" for those with minor mental health problems, the reporter was concerned that it was not appropriate for those with "severe conditions." The author also expressed further concerns:

> There are distinct—and sometimes clashing—views in the mental health field. But the strategy gives far too much credence to social science and not enough to neuroscience. It also pays far too much attention to the views of "psychiatric survivors" who hide their vehemently anti-treatment views in the promotion of

"peer support" and the language of "rights." But hope—and false hope—cannot be allowed to take the place of care. Where in the strategy, for example, is the call for investment into brain research, psychiatric beds and more addiction treatment facilities? The draft also gives short shrift to the sickest of the sick ... who populate our streets and prisons. They don't need the right to refuse treatment, they need the right to be well. (Picard, 2011)

Subsequently, in October 2011, the *National Post* published an article entitled "Mental Health Commission Struggles to Find Balance in Developing Strategy," in which it is reported that the MHCC "has been squirming under accusations of dysfunction, antipsychiatry bias and neglect of the most serious illnesses" (Brean, 2011b). According to this report, the MHCC is looking for a way to balance, at least in theory, two conflicting ideologies of mental illness: "empowerment, based in social science, in which recovery is seen as a personal growth experience; and psychiatry, based in neuroscience, in which recovery sometimes must be imposed against a delusional will" (Brean, 2011b). There is a notable discomfort in this report with the recasting of patients as "survivors," "consumers," or "experts with experience," and the call to end the seclusion and restraint of psychiatric inmates. The reporter points out that the word "recovery" is mentioned 67 times in the 30-page document, and "support" is mentioned 125 times, with "no reference to psychiatry. Or schizophrenia or bipolar." The sentiment expressed by this news article, and by other critics of the leaked report, is that it is not a strategy about mental illness at all, but rather one about *mental health*. While the MHCC claims to stand by the fundamental principles of the draft report, the organization's chief executive announced a promise in a "letter to Canadians" to "correct" the strategy before its official release in 2012, concurring that "the draft does not sufficiently reflect the essential role neuroscience, treatment and psychiatry have to play" (Brean, 2011b). Media responses to the draft national strategy by the MHCC demonstrate two things quite clearly: our inability to have two or more legitimate and equal interpretations of mental health/illness and recovery operating at the same time, and a deep reluctance to accept "new" knowledge, even knowledge produced and funded under the authority of the Canadian government, that appears at odds with current mainstream thinking.

The official function of the MHCC, following the direction of previous government organizations, inquiries, and working groups on mental illness/health, is to generate a set of strategic frameworks as reassurance that cost-efficient and effective solutions for change are *possible*. We argue that in effect it is precisely this kind of moral policing of mental health knowledge that undermines the possibility of meaningful change. Thus, rather than identifying social stigma as the primary barrier to the empowerment of the mentally ill, we argue instead that a more significant barrier to achieving meaningful social justice may in fact be the state failure to recognize its own participation in past injustices and the lack of the courage it would take to initiate a radical change.

Conclusion

From the closed interpretation of mental illness as a disease there follows an imperative remedy, or conclusion. The premise of illness or disease acquires its *truth* in part through the remedy of professional diagnosis and treatment. At the same time, the implied truth in the premise of illness or disease renders the imperative conclusions (diagnosis, treatment, state intervention) *true*. Such imperatives legitimize the exclusion and subjugation of those so declared as ill, as well as those who might resist dominant models or identities of mental illness.

Even a cursory analysis of Western mental health literacy initiatives reveals the insistence on a linear logic that presumes that mental health literacy improves as one's thinking comes more in line with professional research-based knowledge; that the popularization of professional knowledge will lead to a reduction in social stigma; and that a reduction in social stigma will increase the likelihood that individuals with mental health problems will seek out *appropriate* professional treatment. Again the assumption typically is that if the social barriers of stigma are removed, the *natural* inclination for those we consider to be suffering from mental health issues will be to seek professional treatment.

A moderate Mad/consumer/survivor/ex-patient perspective might challenge this narrow interpretation and call, at the least, for a more comprehensive reading of mental health literacy in which educational and intervention programs are designed to also include the development of social skills that support mental health promotion and the ability to assess and act upon one's individual determinants of mental health and mental illness. A more radical perspective would oppose outright the formalization of mental health knowledge and the mandates of state-authorized mental health literacy programs. It is from this more radical perspective that we question the making and marketing of a single, official vision of mental health/illness that constitutes contemporary mental health literacy. We are not confident that MHL programs as implemented in Canada necessarily represent a progressive act of social justice that will correct historically informed power imbalances. Mental health literacy training might also be seen as a manifestation of a collection of ongoing cultural practices through which the "mentally ill" are socially and institutionally identified and managed.

Notes

1   In exploring its possessive nature, Nicholas Fox refers to professional care as "the Proper." According to Fox, "caring becomes a relation of dominance and disempowerment for those who are cared for" (Fox, 1994, p. 93).

2   We use *madness* to reflect a more inclusive and culturally grounded human phenomenon that encompasses various historically and contextually specific terms such as insanity, feeble-minded, mental disorder, and mental illness.

3   UNESCO does not advocate a single "model" of literacy. The understanding of who is literate and who is illiterate has evolved considerably over the years, giving rise to new implications for both policies and programs (UNESCO, n.d.).

4   The Canadian Alliance on Mental Illness and Mental Health (CAMIMH) is an alliance of mental health organizations composed of health care providers, as well as "the mentally ill" and their families. CAMIMH's mandate is to ensure that mental health is placed on the national agenda so that persons with a lived experience of mental illness and their families receive appropriate access to care and support (CAMIMH, 2011). See also the World Health Organization (WHO) Mental Health Atlas, 2011, retrieved November 13, 2011 from www. who.int/mediacentre/multimedia/podcasts/2011/mental_health_17102011/en/.

5   The AMHA, 1964, copied portions of Saskatchewan's policy on establishing panels (rather than judicial committees) to review appeals. This "new venture" was itself based on British Columbia's decision to do the same in 1940 (Angus, 1966, p. 427).

6   In 1965, an official opposition member confronted the Minister of Health in the Alberta Legislature concerning the fact that mental patients were being held in Calgary jail cells—an apparent result of a lack of communication between physicians and law enforcement (Angus, 1966, p. 1).

7   Sterilization was implemented under the Sexual Sterilization Act of Alberta until the Eugenics Board was disbanded and the act was repealed in 1972 (Grekul, Krahn & Odynak, 2004, p. 366).

8   This includes the Alberta Hospitals Act, Personal Directives Act, Regional Health Authorities Act, Child, Youth and Family Enhancement Act, Adult Guardianship and Trusteeship Act, Government Organizations Act, Youth Criminal Justice Act, Recording of Evidence Act, Health Information Act, Occupational Health And Safety Act, Canada Health Act, Medical Professions Act, Nursing Profession Act, Health Professions Act, Health Disciplines Act, Public Trustee Act, Public Inquiries Act, Public Service Act, Mental Health Amendment Act, and Young Offenders Act (which was repealed in 2003).

9   Canada does not have a national mental health policy.

10 Though we do not have space to provide a comprehensive history of mental health policy, a comparative analysis of provincial mental health policy reveals that, in general, policies within and across provinces show little variation over time.

11 However, most revisions in the act were made between 1990 and 2000.

12 This includes the Health Care Consent Act, Health Protection and Promotion Act, Personal Health Information Act, Substitute Decisions Act, and the Regulated Health Professions Act.

13 This includes the Ontario Mental Health Act, Substitute Decisions Act, Long Term Care Homes Act, Regulated Health Professions Act, Drugless Practitioners Act, Private Hospitals Act, Public Hospitals Act, Family Law Act, Personal Health Information Protection Act, Public Services of Ontario Act, Law Society Act, Mandatory Blood Testing Act, Statutory Powers Procedure Act, Home Care and Community Services Act, Child and Family Services Act, Legal Aid Services Act, Solicitors Act, Consent to Treatment Act, and the Consent and Capacity Statute Law Amendment Act.

14 This excludes British Columbia and New Brunswick, which both use the term "mental disorder," but leave it undefined.

15 This can be seen in the operating models of schools, hospitals, political offices, committees, etc.

16 A permanent Mental Health Commission of Canada (MHCC) was first proposed in November 2005, and officially mandated and incorporated in March 2007. The official MHCC website is under a steady state of reconstruction and much of the information on the original terms of reference and early initiatives has been "updated" or edited out.

17 The diseases the MHCC most often juxtaposes with mental illness are diabetes and heart disease, not other historically stigmatized diseases such as leprosy, cancer, or AIDS. Occasionally breast cancer is mentioned as a comparator, but it is the success of the Pink Ribbon campaign to bring awareness to breast cancer that is aligned with the Opening Minds campaign, not breast cancer the disease.

18 The use of the term "crisis" is particularly significant here if we consider that a crisis in health typically marks a turning point of a disease when an important change takes place, indicating either recovery or death.

19 While the "Breakdown" series was not explicitly presented to *Globe and Mail* readers—demographically identified as upper-middle class, educated, and right-leaning—as an advertisement for the MHCC, neither can it be said to be an independent news report. The idea for the special report was originally conceived by the commission's then director of communications as a strategic initiative to shine a spotlight on pre-selected issues to be addressed by the MHCC. An open forum, including an official Facebook group, for the ongoing *Globe and Mail* special report can be accessed through the MHCC website under "resources" or at http://v1.theglobeandmail.com/breakdown/.

20 Dr. David Goldbloom is also a member of the MHCC Board of Directors and a senior administrator at the Centre for Addiction and Mental Health in Toronto. These affiliations are not mentioned in the *Globe and Mail*'s news coverage.

21 For further analysis on how the corporate organization of the MHCC has forced a particular set of administrative structures that in every way has directed the production of knowledge within that organization, see Kimberley White, "Out of the Shadows and into the Spotlight: The Politics of (In)visibility and the Implementation of the Mental Health Commission of Canada" (White, 2009).

22 The metaphors of shadow and light play an important role in MHCC messages. For example, the banner on the MHCC website home page reads "out of the shadows forever," which is taken from a Senate report in 2006 titled "Out of the Shadows at Last: Transforming Mental Health, Mental Illness and Addiction Services in Canada." Also, in 2009, the MHCC organized a national conference titled Into the Light: Transforming Mental Health in Canada as a forum to discuss the "framework" for the national mental health strategy (MHCC, 2009a).

23 The seven-day "Breakdown" series included full-page articles on a range of mental health issues including: a history of madness, as experienced by Alice G., at the Queen Street asylum in Toronto; the cost of mental illness to the workforce and corporate revenue; practical strategies to "solve" the crisis; the virtues of "deep brain stimulation" (electric shock therapy); and the pressures that the mentally ill put on Canada's bulging criminal justice system. The series wrapped up with an essay written by Michael Kirby, chair of the MHCC, titled "Fighting the Stigma" (*Globe and Mail*, 2008).

24 One rare, and brief, reference to historical processes—the only we have seen in official MHCC publications—states that: "For far too long, people who have been given a diagnosis of mental illness have been seen as fundamentally different. There was a time—not that long ago, even in Canada—when they were sent away and locked up, never to be seen again" (MHCC, 2009b, p. 13). This quote seems quite out of touch with institutional reality in Canada, where we still lock people up, some never to be seen again.

25 In this piece, Picard echoes an earlier article by Susan Inman, "Suppressing Schizophrenia" (2011b), in the *Tyee*, August 29, accessible at http://thetyee.ca/Opinion/2011/08/29/Review-Mental-Health-Strategy/.

CHAPTER 18

Pitching Mad:
News Media and the Psychiatric Survivor Perspective

Rob Wipond

Major North American news media rarely cover mental health, civil rights, and psychiatric survivor issues accurately, critically, or fairly, if at all. Here's why—and how it can be changed.

On a random day while working on this chapter, I searched for the word "schizophrenic" on a global Internet news aggregator. This is what appeared at the top of the results:

- *Paranoid Schizophrenic Cut Woman's Arm with Screwdriver* (Reoch, 2011)
- *Son Who Stabbed Father to Death was Schizophrenic, Court Hears* (Brown, 2011)
- *Police Search for Missing Schizophrenic Patients* (Staff Report, 2011)

When I combined "schizophrenic" with "civil rights," only one widely reproduced story appeared. The Associated Press reported that police officers searching for a car burglar in a poor area of Fullerton, California, confronted a "schizophrenic" man, Kelly Thomas, and asked to search his bag. Thomas ran in fear. According to witnesses and videos from the scene, police officers then chased Thomas down, shocked him repeatedly with a stun gun, and beat him to death. The article concluded: "The Police Department has … placed on paid administrative leave six officers involved in the beating. The FBI also opened a probe into whether the officers violated Thomas' civil rights" (Flaccus, 2011).

These are apt examples of how mental health issues tend to be covered in major, mainstream English-language news media—an observation demonstrated in detail in a report prepared for the Canadian Mental Health Association, *Mass Media and Mental Illness: A Literature Review* (Roth Edney, 2004). Running down the top six ways that most people gather information about mental illness, the report identified TV newsmagazine shows, newspapers, TV news, newsmagazines, and radio news. At number five, TV talk shows are the only information source to break that iron grip by news media, and farther back in influence are other commercial magazines, the Internet, and books. We can presume the Internet has been climbing those rankings— yet much of that climb would be coming courtesy of online news.

Most studies show that news stories are replete with inaccurate information and biased perspectives, recounts report author Dara Roth Edney, yet can be so powerful that they often "override people's own personal experiences in relation to how they view mental illness" (ibid). Two-thirds of these stories link mental illnesses to crime and violence, Roth Edney notes, even though people diagnosed with mental illnesses are statistically less likely than the general population to be violent while some 90 percent of news stories are not about crime. Roth Edney adds that first-person accounts and interviews of people who have been labelled mentally ill occur in a mere 1–7 percent of stories about mental illness.

Another study published in *Psychiatric Services* in 2005 noted previous studies had found "as many as 75 percent of stories that deal with mental illness focus on violence" (Corrigan et al., 2005). This study found 39 percent of newspaper stories on mental illness relate to dangerousness and violent crime—most of these appearing in the front pages. The authors noted that a comparatively tiny percentage of stories discuss mental illness as a factor in being victimized by acts of violence, even though statistics suggest it's a significant predictor, and 4 percent of stories focus on *recovery* from mental illnesses. Other common stories are equally familiar to news consumers: Mental illnesses are biological, biochemical diseases that require treatment with drugs, or else people will relapse and become more confused, distressed, and violent. The science of diagnosis and treatment has advanced tremendously and is constantly progressing. Stigma and poor funding prevent too many people from getting the help they need.

Meanwhile, knowledgeable researchers are aware of what's rarely being reported. Presentations of the enormously diverse points of view of people who've been labelled mentally ill are few and far between. Average North Americans rarely learn of the staggeringly poor long-term outcomes for most people taking psychiatric drugs, or of the toxic withdrawal syndromes that precipitate many so-called intense *relapses* when people try to get off these chemicals (Whitaker, 2010). Few have heard about the frequent civil and human rights abuses going on in our psychiatric system (Melinda, 2005). And the insidious but increasingly demonstrable links between violence and reactions to certain psychiatric medications are still flying largely under the radar (Moore, Glenmullen & Furberg, 2010).

I'll leave it to the academic researchers to continue to analyze such findings on the grand statistical scales and opine about what it all means about our society. But what I can elucidate, as a long-time professional journalist, is how and why this is actually happening on a day-to-day operational level in most newsrooms. And I can provide reflections on how to help change this situation. Along the way, perhaps we'll also get a glimpse into what it all means about our society.

How News Is Pitched

Let's begin by briefly examining the way most ideas become stories and get into the news. Step one is usually what professional journalists refer to as *the pitch*. The pitch is an oral summary or written outline of a story. News pitches are brief. A journalist may describe the story basics in a minute or two, or write up a few lines to several hundred words for the editor or producer. Some back and forth may then ensue depending on the complexity of the story, time pressures, and working relationships between the researchers, writers, reporters, editors, or producers. For ease of reference, I'll refer to all of these people together as *news producers*. Then, the story is either a "go" for development, or not.

News stories themselves are generally divided into *hard news* and *soft news*. Hard news typically involves extremely timely reports about, for example, an important government decision, a major crime, or a natural disaster. Soft news stories are usually less time-sensitive explorations of health, the arts, people, community issues, lifestyle trends, and other such topics. The pitches and ensuing discussions for both categories often include many similar elements:

- The hook: What's interesting, important, engaging, exciting, new, or different in this story?
- What's the main drama or conflict?
- Is it timely?
- Who will be quoted?
- What experts or research will provide background or broader context, if necessary?
- Why would our audience care?

In theory, anything can make the news. In practice, the pitch is a powerful filter. Consider this story idea: The auditor general has found that a prominent politician used public money for personal expenses. Any news consumer instinctively knows there's a good chance that this story will be covered, even without further explanation. We can already picture interviews with the sober auditor general, the evasive politician, and the outraged critics. Likely there will be some background on how the politician previously pledged his righteousness, and any politically concerned audience will lap up this seamy story. But notice something else very important that goes unspoken: This story is based on innumerable shared values and beliefs. What are some examples of those unspoken shared beliefs? Money is important. Tax dollars shouldn't be wasted. The auditor general's work can be trusted. Stealing from others is bad. Politicians shouldn't be hypocritical. Essentially, there are many strong beliefs underlying this one-sentence pitch, which can go largely unspoken but are generally shared amongst the people in the newsroom. And that's why it doesn't require much more than a single sentence for everyone to *get* what this story is about and why it should be in the news. Similarly, these underlying beliefs won't have to be explained in the news report itself: We know our audiences also *get,* for example, without explanation, that tax dollars shouldn't be wasted.

We should not misunderstand the importance of unspoken shared beliefs in news production. Modern news is dominated by quick-turnaround coverage that must be attention-grabbing, brief and fast-paced, entertaining, and easy to understand— therefore, it generally has to reflect such mainstream beliefs and values. Otherwise, it would have to slow down all the time to explain and critically argue its own premises, and would morph from entertaining mainstream news into, for example, a lengthy feature in an intellectual magazine, a book, or a documentary. And pitching stories in newsrooms is that kind of modern, high-speed information processing—on amphetamines. Virtually everyone has to *get it,* virtually immediately. Unspoken, unquestioned, shared beliefs therefore comprise the crucial underlying foundation for the vast majority of what gets into the mainstream news.

That's utterly problematic when it comes to generating quality news stories about our mental health system. This is because the minds of most news producers are filled with shared beliefs but, in this case, most of them are misinformed, deeply prejudicial beliefs. That's why news stories about mental illness in North America are the way they are. In this limited space, I am not setting out to definitively prove all the countervailing arguments to dispel all of news producers' false, prejudicial beliefs. Readers can go to other chapters of this book, or to the resource lists, for more thorough investigations into specific issues. My purpose is to outline the main false beliefs most news producers operate under, and to explore how and why they're seemingly immutable even in the face of overwhelming evidence. I'll then suggest some approaches for concerned, knowledgeable people to more effectively engage news producers in developing better reporting on mental health issues, especially with regard to psychiatric survivor perspectives and civil rights concerns. I have chosen civil rights as a thematic focal point but, as we shall see, that issue connects to every other major mental health issue. Indeed, it's those complex interconnections that are the whole problem.

Untangling the Knot of Beliefs

In a proverbial metaphor about complicated conceptual frameworks built from lies and false beliefs, the "house of cards" symbolizes utter fragility: All the parts are so intimately connected to each other that, if you pull out even one card anywhere, the entire structure comes crashing down. However, consider another analogy: A knot of wires. When many long wires are tangled together, the totality can be extremely difficult to undo. All the elements are so tightly intertwined, that to untangle such a mess, every wire has to be loosened before any one can be extracted. And if you mistake the knot of wires for a house of cards and try to yank out one wire on its own, your effort recoils: the harder you pull, the more tightly the whole knot locks. The beliefs of most news producers about psychiatric issues are interwoven in exactly such a mess of knots.

Consider a news story the likes of which I've pitched: *A man was caught yelling and naked in the street by police. He says he was then given drugs and electroconvulsive therapy against his will at the psychiatric hospital. He claims he now has permanent parkinsonian motor dysfunction from the drugs and memory loss from the electroshock.* This story has a powerful human-interest angle along with scandalous, tragic dimensions and immense social importance, and events not unlike it happen frighteningly frequently. Yet few stories like it ever get into major news outlets in North America. Why? Pick a wire, any wire …

The Beliefs about Civil Rights

We begin with the issue of this man's civil rights being breached. The typical news producer has heard psychiatric treatments described by countless reputable sources as the equivalent of insulin for diabetics. He's under the impression that emergency mental health interventions are like rushing car-crash victims by ambulance to hospital. How, then, is this naked, yelling man being taken to hospital a *civil rights issue*, except perhaps insofar as he didn't or couldn't get into treatment soon enough? If he indeed suffered in any way from the intervention, obviously, it would've been even worse for him without the helping hospital.

When it's suggested to the news producer that everyone should nevertheless have the right to refuse psychiatric drugs and electroshock, he pictures countless unconscious car-crash victims bleeding to death as doctors try to get their written consent before performing surgery to save their lives. The suggestion seems patently ridiculous. Evidently, then, to be able to grasp that mental health treatment without consent might seriously undermine some people's civil rights, the news producer's mind first has to be free of at least one different belief first: his faith in psychiatry and psychiatrists. He has to be already doubting the medical effectiveness and scientific legitimacy of mainstream psychiatric treatments—which he isn't.

The Beliefs about the Science of Mental Illness

Most psychiatrists deny electroconvulsive therapy causes brain damage or permanent memory loss, and rarely publicly discuss tardive dyskinesia or other serious, debilitating effects of psychiatric drugs except under very probing, specific, informed questioning. Psychiatrists instead commonly tell journalists that hundreds of thousands of studies have established the biochemical basis for mental illnesses and the overall efficacy and relative safety (and necessity) of modern psychiatric treatments.

Under "What Causes Schizophrenia?" the US National Institute of Mental Health (NIMH) website has two headings: "Genes and Environment" and "Different Brain Chemistry and Structure" (National Institute of Mental Health, n.d.(a)). Under "What Causes Depression?" NIMH describes neurotransmitters being "out of balance," genes acting together, and MRIs showing that "the brains of people who have depression look different" (National Institute of Mental Health, n.d.(b)). The Public Health Agency of Canada's website answers the question "What is Schizophrenia?" with quotes from *The Broken Brain—The Biological Revolution in Psychiatry*: "It is quite clear that multiple factors are involved. These include changes in the chemistry of the brain, changes in the structure of the brain, and genetic factors" (Public Health Agency of Canada, 2011).

All of these assertions are boldly out of sync with actual levels of scientific understanding. In a less public venue, the American Psychiatric Association's Research Agenda for the fifth edition of the *Diagnostic and Statistical Manual of Mental Disorders* admits that, to date, "not one laboratory marker has been found to be specific in identifying any of the DSM-defined syndromes" and "lack of treatment specificity is the rule rather than the exception" (Kupfer, First & Regier, 2002). So in layman's terms, we cannot scientifically identify any mental illness, and our treatment strategies are guesswork. However, consider the picture these contrarian facts paint in the news producer's mind: We're tying vulnerable people up in chemical straightjackets and delivering severe electrical shocks into their brains, without any clue as to what we're really doing? The news producer struggles to imagine how that interpretation of the facts could possibly be accurate. It seems too "insane," too nightmarish, too overwhelming to believe.

To raise into question this predominant narrative of "medically safe, scientifically sound" psychiatry, then, the average news producer has to first be able to pose and answer another question: How and why could it possibly be that all these reputable scientists would be misleading everyone? That is to say, she has to first free herself from her belief that mainstream psychiatrists could not possibly have any reasons for being *that* completely corrupted and dangerous. Science is self-correcting, right? And so we must follow our way around the tangles to try to loosen a different wire first …

The Beliefs about Corporate Influence

Any news producer can certainly conceive of bias and corruption created by big dollars. And some may be aware that pharmaceutical companies' enormous public relations initiatives, and their advertising dollars, could be influencing their news teams directly. However, the sheer scale and magnitude of the actual bias and corruption at work in modern psychiatry are wildly out of proportion to anything with which most news producers are accustomed. Imagine, for instance, what the current state of public understanding of climate change would be if, rather than the current tiny percentage beholden to the oil industry, over 95 percent of climate scientists were employed by, on retainers from, taking speaking fees from, accepting kickbacks from, or being directly funded in their research by oil companies. That's close to the actual situation we have with modern psychiatry's relationship to pharmaceutical companies. One example: In 2001, the *New England Journal of Medicine* announced new conflict-of-interest policies as part of an effort to rein in the epidemic of bias caused by pharmaceutical company influence over drug studies (International Committee of Medical Journal Editors, 2001). By 2002, it was loosening its conflict-of-interest policies more than ever before, because it was no longer obtaining any new drug therapy studies at all (Drazen & Curfman, 2002). And here we need to remind ourselves that psychiatry, as generally more rooted in soft psychology than hard neuroscience, is from a purely scientific standpoint exponentially more susceptible to bias or corruption than medical research generally.

However, the news producer, like many of these well-intentioned researchers themselves, struggles to believe that the funding sources could be *completely* corrupting the science and reputable scientists. It's too far-fetched; it seems disrespectful. Pull too hard at that belief of theirs and you could start to sound like a "nutty" conspiracy theorist. Besides, it only raises another question in his mind: What about the family members of the mentally ill, and the responsible, caring, committed workers at mental health organizations, and all the people with no financial stake in any of this? Are they, too, implicated in this vast, paranoid conspiracy? So the news producer isn't able to accept the depth and breadth of the influence of corporate money, because he still believes in something else: He believes in the independence and scientific integrity of independent mental health organizations.

The Beliefs about "Independent" Organizations

The American Civil Liberties Union website lists over 60 issues it's dealing with, including entire sections on immigrants, women, gays and lesbians, and prisoners. Yet there's no mention of civil rights for the mentally ill—except with regard to situations where people may be denied access to treatment (ACLU, n.d.). It's the same for the Canadian Civil Liberties Association (n.d.).

They're following the lead of the major mental health organizations. Most of North America's largest mental health organizations, while often declaring themselves to be *independent patient advocacy* groups, tend to support mainstream psychiatry, and engage in activities diametrically opposed to protecting the civil rights of psychiatric patients (although they'll often spin it differently; for example, arguing that "compulsory treatment will usually restore someone's freedom of thought from a mind-controlling illness" (Shone & Gray, 2000, p. 5)). Examples of these groups include the Schizophrenia Society and its branches, the Canadian Mental Health Association and its branches, and the US National Alliance on Mental Illness. There are a variety of reasons for this. Many mental health organizations are run by mental health professionals, while empowering few people who identify as consumers or survivors. Many get funding from pharmaceutical companies or through government psychiatric programs. Many involve fearful and frustrated family members of people diagnosed with mental illnesses. For example, the British Columbia Schizophrenia Society (n.d.) describes itself as a "family support system" and it intervenes in cases to help ensure involuntary treatment laws survive court challenges (*Mullins v. Levy*, 2005). The Canadian Mental Health Association is often contracted by governments to administer involuntary treatment in communities (Fabris, 2011, p. 98). The US National Alliance on Mental Illness finally revealed during recent Congressional investigations that the bulk of its millions in funding annually is coming from pharmaceutical companies (Harris, 2009), and the Schizophrenia Society of Canada (n.d.) similarly counts pharmaceutical companies amongst its primary funders.

But even upon learning this, an average news producer is not ready to abandon all confidence in the mainstream psychiatric system. That's because there's another belief that endures in the news producer's mind, even if she comes to an understanding of the cozy relationships between major mental health organizations, government legislators, psychiatrists, and pharmaceutical companies. "Surely," she thinks, "all of these people are still genuinely trying to help the mentally ill, right?" She believes psychiatry is a support system.

The Beliefs about the Social Welfare System

Mental health professionals and researchers have worked hard to connect mental health issues in our society today with other social issues of homelessness, addiction, afford-able housing, welfare, employment insurance, health care funding, job training, etc. Consequently, our entire mental health system, including the psychiatric system, has been made to seem like an important element of our social safety net—the opposite of an infringement on anyone's civil rights or endangerment to anyone's physical well-being.

There are, of course, important differences between being provided with supportive housing or low-cost counselling, and being electroshocked against your will. However, most social service groups have picked up the "mental health safety net" refrain without trafficking much in those distinctions. There are several reasons for that. Once again, mental health professionals are involved in running many social service agencies. Fundraising requirements often make these agencies reluctant to be seen as antagonistic to mainstream beliefs. And perhaps most importantly, many, like emergency shelters, family and child welfare agencies, and seniors homes, frequently fall back on the involuntary incarceration and forced treatment powers of mental health laws to help restrain, sedate, or control their more challenging clients (Wipond, 1999). But the average news producer knows none of this and, significantly, who's left to tell him about it? Out of all these compromised people and groups, who's left to try to explain to a news producer that the psychiatric system resembles more closely a policing operation than a social welfare support? For the most part, there are only protesting (ex-)patients remaining to provide this alternative point of view: people, of course, who are by definition "crazy." And there are a lot of beliefs about crazy people that a news producer will not easily let go.

The Beliefs about the Crazy Person

People labelled with mental illnesses are not considered good sources by news producers. First of all, any ordinary, isolated individual simply does not generate instant credibility in the newsroom in the way that someone with links to expert titles, respectable degrees, and institutions and organizations does. Then, as far as organizations of Mad people go, there are usually two accessible groups: "consumers" and "survivors." These are often thrown together with a simple slash as *consumer/survivor groups* for the benefit of building organizations, working on issues, and facilitating public communications; however, while people who identify with either of these two groups generally agree on basic issues of empowerment for patients within the psychiatric system, they often have radically diverging points of view on all the other major issues, like the reliability of psychiatric science, the effectiveness of psychiatric treatments, and the value of involuntary committal (MindFreedom International, n.d.; National Network for Mental Health, n.d.). Unless he investigates all these issues thoroughly himself, this baffles the news producer and he doesn't know what to do with the information. He defaults back to the mainstream, educated, trained, professional, recognized mental health experts—and we've already seen where that leads.

Furthermore, the person who's been diagnosed with a mental illness is not trusted as much as the person who hasn't been. The news producer's distrust often grows substantially if the labelled person has any sort of quirky or unusual personality traits, or does not always communicate clearly and succinctly. This type of "sanism" is a form of discrimination, and it's very real in our society. How many would vote for a candidate who wore a silly red cap during the televised presidential debate, pondered questions for minutes before answering, and had once been diagnosed as schizophrenic? So unless their claims are easily verifiable and do not contradict every other expert available to the news producer, the perspectives of the Mad person will simply not be trusted, or consequently used as a basis for a news story. And there's a yet deeper reason for that. The news producer has to deal with something else first, before he's willing to truly open up to spending time with, hearing and trusting people diagnosed with mental illnesses: He has to deal with his own beliefs, and fears, about insanity. He has to be ready to consider the possibility that madness may not be by definition completely distorted, terrible, untrustworthy, unreliable, and in need of nothing other than prompt suppression. This particular wire is wrapped around his head, and twists its way into his own heart of darkness.

The Beliefs about Going Mad

Ours is a society addicted to quick fixes and technological solutions, and there's obviously widespread cultural buy-in to the biochemical model of mental illness and the promise of pill-popping cures that come with it. Part of the reason for that is reflected in our news media's portrayals of mental illness: Many of us have a primal fear of our own grotesque portraiture of "the madman," the agitated schizophrenic, the self-loathing depressive, the mentally unstable criminal whose violence against self or others explodes without reason or rationale, and so can never be predicted, reasoned with, or logically defended against. Many also have archetypal fears of "going insane" ourselves, of plunging into never-ending depression and dysfunction, of losing all bearings without hope of ever reaching understanding or clarity, or of descending into a permanent hell of pain and delusions. Understandably, then, these feelings produce resistance when we're asked to bring madness closer to ourselves in any way.

And so now we've reached the beliefs that hold all the wires and knots together most tightly—in a grip of metaphysical terror. To loosen and untangle these beliefs requires profound and persistent critiquing of cultural norms and social expectations, deep self-questioning, and confrontations with archetypal fear. Yet why would anyone question any of this so deeply? What would be the motive? Why would anyone want to understand madness intimately, or consider respecting it, even loving it? Why, indeed. Unless, of course, we already have experience with, and profound respect for, unusual states of consciousness and unconventional behaviours, in ourselves and in others. This is where we find ourselves, then, after our long journey following all of these twisted wires: back at the beginning of our knot of beliefs. It's now clear that a news producer is likely only going to be able to grasp how involuntary psychiatric treatment could be a fundamental attack on human and civil rights if she has ventured into her own inner craziness and experienced oppression herself. But then, if that happens and she does have this revelation, who's going to believe her?

Where Will Real News Break Through?

Trying to get quality hard news coverage about specific mental health-related events or issues is risky, then, because it's as likely to tighten the knot as loosen the wires, due to news producers' hasty reactions based on preconceived beliefs. An apt example is the way the *National Post* turned what could have been straightforward hard news coverage of the Toronto 2010 PsychOUT conference into a diatribe against "the crackpot" minds behind it (Brean, 2010b, p. A8). The *Toronto Star* provided fairer coverage, but they diverted the story to a soft news article by a disability columnist (Henderson, 2010). Soft news coverage does at least provide slightly more opportunities for news producers to take time, develop unusual stories, explore diverse opinions, and question their own and their audience's beliefs. It's useful, then, to review a few areas of improving awareness and coverage, because these can be incorporated into public teaching/learning strategies.

Anti-stigma and anti-poverty education have generated sympathy for goals that coalesce with some of the desires of psychiatric rights activists. These pre-established sympathies and understandings can be used, then, to pitch ideas for stories to news producers about, for example, the right of people who've been labelled with mental illnesses to obtain flexibility in employment settings or access to more affordable housing. Similarly, the issues surrounding corporate influence are relatively easy for news producers to understand. Some have already been conducting more critical examinations of the money behind pharmaceutical companies, scientific research and drug promotion, and politically driven mental health initiatives such as depression screening days. High-profile lawsuits, where lawyers have already done the research, are particularly prized by news producers. And two of the most significant developments are the dramatic increases in prescribing of psychiatric medications for young children and for the elderly in long-term care facilities, with sometimes concomitant use of coercion or force. Eight million children in the US take one or more psychiatric medications (Morris & Stone, 2011), and up to half of the elderly in Canadian long-term care facilities are being given antipsychotics (Wipond, 2011). This is exposing a much broader swath of our population to a range of psychiatric issues and to the extraordinary coercive powers of the psychiatric system on particularly vulnerable groups, and more people are putting sharper questions to politicians, health authorities, and news media alike. So if any of these topics connect to a story you'd like to see covered, it can be helpful to make that connection for the news producer.

For Activists: Tools for Change

The best way to get stories into the news is to write the pitch yourself: Show the news producers what the story is and how to tell it, in a way that they instantly *get*. The point-form outline in "How News Is Pitched" (on page 255) provides a basic guideline for writing up a one-page press release or email to a news producer about an event or issue. Clarity and conciseness are the drivers. After that, the higher the stakes, the more timely and provocative the story, the more reputable the sources, and the more understandable the context, the better. Note, however, that if talking to a news producer, never assume you're being "interviewed." Most journalists rarely have the time or interest to truly discuss issues, research them, and reflect critically. Instead, they're usually mining you for clear or provocative quotes that can be quickly understood by virtually anyone and could fit into a very small space—so prepare some quotes ahead of time.

In my opinion, though, attempting to access the mainstream media is not the best first-line approach to achieve change in news coverage for the reasons already discussed in this chapter. Investigative reporting is no longer a common feature of mainstream news, so the media tend to follow rather than lead on most issues requiring research or social critiques. First, then, it would be valuable to educate those who work with people statistically more likely to be subjected to the coercive powers of the mental health system. This would include groups providing services to youth, the elderly, the poor, single parents, immigrants, First Nations, and those with learning or physical disabilities. Bringing prominent civil rights groups up to speed on the issues would be a good step, and anything consumers and survivors could do to identify common ground and deliver common messages would be effective.

Finally and most importantly, there are three key groups that news producers generally regard as credible, and that could be doing much more to help elucidate criticisms of and alternatives to our dominant psychiatric system. These include some non-medical and alternative mental health workers and their professional associations, lawyers who understand the rights issues, and academic researchers who critique the psychiatric system. Anything that can be done to more consistently unite these voices with those of psychiatric survivors would be groundbreaking. It would be groundbreaking because there is a civil war going on out there for control of our minds, but most people don't even know it.

There are extremely passionate, committed teams of people, with enormous funding, working with religious fervor to promote psychiatric treatments and suppress the rights and points of view of psychiatric patients. Psychiatric rights activists can't out-muscle those armies. But we actually don't have to. We don't have to win that war. All we have to do is make the broader public aware that there *is* a war, that there are other, dramatically different, legitimate points of view and possibilities. All of the power of biological psychiatry is built on the widespread illusion it's rooted in such solid science that the ideological war is long over. And of course, it isn't over. Biological psychiatry cannot lay claim to the definitive explanations of what it means to be wholly, healthfully human. Still today, vast territories of our psyche remain unconquered and uncharted in all their vital, beautiful multifariousness. That's a message the world needs to hear, because it liberates everyone.

PART V Social Justice, Madness, and Identity Politics

Part V concludes the book with five chapters canvassing some of the key emergent issues in the field of Canadian Mad Studies—issues that are almost certain to generate intensifying critical dialogue and strategizing through the coming years. These final chapters are concerned particularly with the fashioning of a Mad political agenda for the 21st century; with how Mad activists might engage with the structured oppression experienced, and identity politics practised, by allied communities including First Nations and other racialized people, LGBTQ people, women, the poor, seniors, and youth; and with questions of pursuing grassroots recovery and empowerment projects, by and on behalf of psychiatrized people, under and beyond the imposing shadow of mainstream mental health. Integrating these themes diversely, the five contributors to Part V address, in turn, the dilemmas of identity in the building of Mad nationhood, the prospects for indigenizing survivor and antipsychiatry scholarship and praxis, the constitution of queer "in/visibility" within mental health contexts, the psychiatrization of youth violence in the province of Ontario, and the appropriation of the recovery paradigm under neoliberalism.

Interrogating the "Mad nationalism" inherent to essentialized identity politics within the Mad movement, Rachel Gorman (Chapter 19) cautions us all to attend to both the hazards and promises associated with the emergence of Mad Studies, including the "danger that Mad identity ... will be absorbed into white, middle-class narratives of disability." With eloquence and dedicated scholarship she addresses questions such as: "What are the implications of this identity politic for anti-oppression organizing?", "Who benefits from this reformulation, and who is still excluded from this discourse?", and "What are the implications of this shift for psychiatric survivors?" In this analytic process, Gorman effectively demonstrates the privileged articulation of Mad identity, given the racialized and classed relations of its emergence. She challenges us to critically analyze the "co-organization of colonialism and psychiatry" by drawing on transnational and postcolonial theory. The decentring of whiteness in Mad Studies and radical activism, as well as examining the connections between the regulation of migration, indigeneity, and racialized bodies with the psychiatrization process, are articulated as priorities in this regard. As such, Gorman contends that "transnational theoretical approaches allow us to understand disability as an assemblage of racialized and gendered narratives, national and postcolonial politics, and global capitalism." This represents an important strand of thought that may enable Mad Studies to undo its implicit lack of focus on race and the global within its analysis of psychiatric oppression.

Acknowledging the importance of critiquing Mad Studies itself, in order to continue to evolve and deepen our understanding of oppressive institutional relations and systemic resistance, Louise Tam (Chapter 20) provides a sophisticated analysis of the ways in which "race-thinking" constitutes psy knowledge as well as the necessity of decolonizing, rather than indigenizing, Mad politics, Mad cultural production, and Mad Studies. This analysis is framed through a textual analysis of an Icarus Project manifesto (McNamara and DuBrul, 2006) and a reflection on MindFreedom International's Occupy Normal campaign, which demonstrates colonialist white settler entitlement and domination in the form of the appropriation of Indigenous spirituality as well as complicity in (re)dispossession and "deculturation," amongst other aspects of racial governance that are reinforced within Mad politics. Tam argues convincingly that "fostering progressive critique and systemic resistance within the Mad movement is paramount because it makes us, as activists, writers, and cultural producers accountable to our politics by attuning ourselves to the varying effects of the political economy of 'madness' on different populations." Using the notion of conviviality, Tam demonstrates the ways in which race and madness are connected not only through intersecting aspects of multiple identities, but also through their material and discursive production. Moreover, she challenges all of us in her charge that "limited intervention has been taken by Mad-affiliated scholars and activists against psy discourse as a knowledge and institution that has everything to do with race in the origins and constitution of pathology."

In Chapter 21, Andrea Daley details a conceptual framework for understanding the experiences of queer women within psychiatry. Based on findings from an exploratory qualitative research project, women's negotiations of queer in/visibility are revealed as complex and as "constituted by three intersecting spaces: body space (self), intersubjective space (between service providers and women), and 'real' space (organizational)." Through attention to Daley's conceptual framework, we are confronted with "the things that drag upon queer women" within the intersecting spaces inherent to psychiatrization. Daley convincingly relates these issues to symbolic violence or more precisely "symbolic gendered, lesbophobic, biphobic, and homophobic violence" that is inherent not only to the psychopathologizing and regulation of sexuality and gender within psychiatry, but also within the ongoing fear and hatred towards non-normative sexuality and gender expression as experienced in the general public.

In "Rerouting the Weeds: The Move from Criminalizing to Pathologizing 'Troubled Youth' in *The Review of the Roots of Youth Violence*" (Chapter 22), Jijian Voronka offers a textual analysis of that weighty 2008 report that had been commissioned by the Ontario government in the immediate aftermath of a notorious yet isolated incident of "spectacular youth violence" (the shooting death of a Grade 9 student in a Toronto high school). Through her critical reading of *The Review*, Voronka uncovers the "stories about madness, race, and violence [that] are created and maintained through this text." As Voronka piercingly shows, the authors of *The Review* weave a compelling narrative of a province under siege from alienated children and adolescents who have been rendered unruly by their individual experiences of poverty and disadvantage. Lurking behind this chronicle of troubled youth in crisis are scarcely cloaked subtexts of racialized violence, of a "white settler society" imperiled, and of "spaces of exception" (read: inner-city slums) desperately in need of expert overview and self-governance. Couched in the language of benevolence and common sense, *The Review* embraces a theory of youth violence that is oblivious to class structure and systemic racial oppression, and which instead focuses on the undisciplined bodies and damaged mentalities of individual "at-risk" youth. For its authors, contradictorily, the blunt force of criminal law is no panacea for the problem of disaffected violent youth (in this respect, they part ways with the federal Harper government and its gratuitously punitive Safe Streets and Communities Act). Instead, *The Review* promotes a soft, restorative, community-based, knowledge-driven praxis—one that calls on the psy disciplines and other "helpers" to (ad)minister (to) these distressed communities, deploying risk assessments and "early interventions," singling out young people at risk, invoking technologies of therapy and surveillance, and "educating" disadvantaged citizens on how to manage their mentally wayward children (and, not coincidentally, themselves). That such a "mental health services" agenda wholly launders out the systemic oppressions perpetrated by biopsychiatry, that it fails to problematize "mental illness," and that it speciously conflates madness with violence goes (literally) without saying. Most insidiously, these normalizing state and psy accounts of pathological youth in need of fixing become internalized, and in consequence they multiply and endure. Observes Voronka: "These problemed children and youth, through the psy disciplines, come to understand their trouble in individualized, often biomedical frameworks that decontextualize the role that structural oppressions play in the constitution of their personhood."

Finally, Marina Morrow's Chapter 23 on the recovery concept analyzes this development within the context of political reform and reaction in contemporary

Canadian mental health policy. She discusses tensions around recovery between those who have promoted it as a way towards personal growth and autonomy from conventional psychiatric treatment, and a medical model approach that seeks to co-opt it within the mental health mainstream. Morrow critiques in particular the point that "what is often overlooked within discussions of recovery is an explicit recognition of the role of the social, political, cultural, and economic context in which people become mentally distressed and recover." Thus, social inequities relating to gender, class, race, and disability are highlighted as essential to integrate into an analysis on the location of recovery in people's lives. Morrow stresses how recovery can be used to buy into the neoliberal agenda of cutbacks to the welfare state by individualizing the experience of madness and further removing the state from providing well-funded social supports. She also notes it can lead to further "dialoguing" among psychiatrized people about the supports they want both at local and national levels. As her chapter shows, this conversation and tension continues between social justice imperatives and public policy retrenchment.

CHAPTER 19

Mad Nation?
Thinking through Race, Class, and Mad Identity Politics

Rachel Gorman

This chapter is motivated by reflexive questions about how Mad-identified activists/scholars can remain accountable to, and in solidarity with, larger, variously identified consumer/survivor communities. In particular, I will focus on the hazards and promises of "Mad nationalism"—that is, the articulation of the Mad movement through identity politics—and on psychiatrization and incarceration as issues for the "Mad citizen." Mad Studies takes social, relational, identity-based, and anti-oppression approaches to questions of mental/psychological/behavioural difference, and is articulated, in part, against an analytic of mental illness. With the emergence of Mad Studies, there is a danger that Mad identity—historically a product and cultural extension of the consumer/survivor movement—will be absorbed into white, middle-class narratives of disability. Emerging questions include: What are the implications of this identity politic for anti-oppression organizing? Who benefits from this reformulation, and who is still excluded from this discourse? What are the implications of this shift for psychiatric survivors? Through theoretical, narrative, and quantitative analysis of madness in relation to racialized, colonized, diasporic, and working-class communities, I will suggest ways in which Mad identity is being articulated as a position of privilege. I will argue that current challenges for Mad-identified activists include: uncovering culture- and class-specific relations through which Mad identities emerge; and articulating solidarity with, and recognizing privilege in relation to, people who have complex, ongoing, and involved experiences of legislative, institutional, and carceral oppression. I will highlight the potential of anti-racist Mad subjectivities, and hazard against the solidification of an "essential" Mad identity.

Citizenship in the Mad Nation

"Mad" signals an identity more expansive than psychiatric consumer/survivor identities—more expansive in its move past the expectation of aligning "for" or "against" psychiatric treatment; and more expansive in its possibility of including people who have been caught up in psy labelling beyond psychiatric hospitals and doctor's offices. Indeed, the etymology of "mad" comes from outside of medical and scientific discourse,

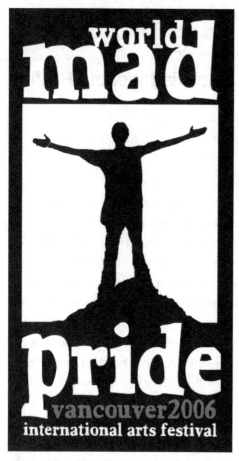

FIGURE 19.1: World Mad Pride

Every year on Bastille Day, July 14th, psychiatric survivors and activists around the world commemorate and celebrate their Mad pride with a cavalcade of cultural events and political activities. In Vancouver, Gallery Gachet, a survivor-oriented centre of art and culture, has been centrally involved in organizing Mad Pride festivities.

Source: Gallery Gachet, 2006.

implying both radical and conservative political possibilities. Through this shift, at least two contradictory political possibilities emerge for Mad identity and Mad ontology. First, Mad identity might be based on self- or community-defined histories and experiences, rather than on medical diagnoses. Second, through an appeal to an interpolated history, Mad identity might be based in claims of an essential ontology. The tendency towards identitarian origin stories has its parallels in early feminist, queer, trans, and disability rights movements, and their accompanying theoretical fields. While these tendencies have been widely critiqued in gender and sexuality studies, they are still rampant in the field most closely allied with Mad Studies—disability studies. The appeal to an imaginary historical subject reproduces a particular ontology in the political present, and vice versa. This disabled origin story has led to profound theoretical, political, and ideological distortions in the globalized, Western-dominated disability rights movement, and its companion area of academic interest, disability studies. My purpose in this chapter is to highlight the pitfalls of an identity-based Mad movement that reproduces a white, Western Mad subject. At stake is both who the movement will speak for, and what the movement will demand.

As an example of essentialist distortions in disability studies, I quote from a recent article discussing psychiatric disability in the context of Australian immigration detention centres. The authors avoid engaging in a critique of detention centres as part of a global system of racialized labour apartheid by focusing on what they call the "intersection" of race and disability. They note:

> The disabling effects of detention on adult asylum seekers have been well documented. The effects of detention on children have been extensively examined, including by Australia's Human Rights and Equal Opportunities Commission

(2004). A recent paper by psychiatrists Mares and Jureidini noted that almost all incarcerated children develop major depressive disorders, including "recurrent thoughts of death and dying," and that many "fulfilled the criteria for major depression with suicidal ideation." Little research, however, has been undertaken into the impact of Australia's immigration policy on people with disabilities and even less on lawful residents with a disability who have been held in Australia's immigration detention centres. (Soldatic & Fiske, 2009, p. 290)

This bifurcation of disabled subjects into "disabled already" and "disabled because of" leads to an implicit assumption of disability as a fixed ontological state (rather than a social relation), and defines the "deserving" or "innocent" disabled over and against those harmed through violence, poverty, and incarceration. In part, this bifurcation echoes and reinforces a preoccupation in white-focused disability studies with proving that disabled people (read as white) are "as oppressed as" racialized people, or colonized people (read as non-disabled). Indeed, psychiatric survivor literature has relied heavily on narratives of colonization and slavery (see Tam, Chapter 20).

Emergent critiques around the absence of critical race and transnational frameworks within disability studies collectively represent an "intellectual crisis for disability studies" (Meekosha, 2011). Current online debates within the US-based Society for Disability Studies focus on the need to bring both a discussion about race and a diversity of researchers to the field. This debate has resurfaced several times in the past decade, with little movement (Erevelles & Minear, 2010). The ongoing lack of critical race analysis within disability studies is striking, considering that the field has a significant history of engagement with social theory (Goodley, 2010). My doctoral research uncovered the ways in which positive representations of disability in the disability rights and culture movements have disallowed a focus on disablement caused by war, imperialism, and environmental destruction (Gorman, 2005). Meanwhile, attempts to research disability in global contexts have been hampered by an inattention to political economies of colonization (Meekosha & Soldatic, 2011). Bringing a transnational framework to the field of disability studies will allow us to move past the deadlock of a simultaneous inattention to race and under-theorization of the global in relation to disability. In the Canadian context, Mad Studies scholars drawing on transnational and postcolonial feminist critiques of multiculturalism and Canadian nation-building have produced important concepts that can help us think critically about the co-organization of colonialism and psychiatry. Roman et al. (2009) develop tools for thinking about "medicalized colonialism," while Howell (2007) traces the expansive regimes of ruling implicated in the narration of the racialized "terrorist."

Activists who identify as, or are allied with, Mad people of colour met as a caucus in Toronto over the spring and summer of 2010 in order to begin to articulate and problematize questions of madness and race.[1] We identified thematic priorities around examining the organization of Mad identities and/or psy labelling in relation to processes of migration and the regulation of indigeneity, as well as a decentring of whiteness in Mad politics and organizing. We noted the importance of knowledge produced by clients and staff of ethno-specific health agencies, in order to map ways in which the social relations of madness are caught up in processes of migration, detention, and settlement. We also noted the danger of further exposing communities living under matrices of social work, psychiatric, and juridical surveillance. How then to decentre whiteness in Mad politics if people of colour cannot afford to take on the identity? More importantly, what is the purpose of Mad political organizing if it further exposes people of colour to risk of institutional violence? Whose interests are being served by the expansion of political identities afforded by the shift to mad organizing? The answers to these questions lie in part in careful institutional mapping of the psychiatric "core" in order to trace how power relations play out on the periphery. For example, in his analysis of the implementation of Community Treatment Orders (CTO), through which outpatients of Toronto's Centre for Addiction and Mental Health are forced to comply with their medication orders, Erick Fabris (2011) uncovers a case of a refugee claimant who cannot be deported due to his CTO, yet wishes to be in order to escape forced psychiatric treatment.

My framing of madness and disability in the context of transnationality emerges from my synthesis of three contemporary strands of disability studies theory. The first strand emerges from ongoing calls to decentre whiteness in disability studies (Ejiogu & Ware, 2008) and to develop approaches to disability studies that can address the reality of Southern contexts, rather than transplanting theory and politics to analyze disability in the global south (Singal, 2010). While still theoretically undeveloped, these calls can gain much from both whiteness studies and recent developments in phenomenology (Ahmed, 2007). The second strand emerges from critiques of neoliberalism developed within queer theory and cultural studies, and brought to bear on disability theory, exemplified by recent work by Robert McRuer (2010) in which he applies Jasbir Puar's (2005) critique of homonationalism to his analysis of Western-focused disability politics as enacting a kind of disability nationalism. McRuer's approach echoes my own recent work on the erasure of disabled women's bodies via the articulation of postcolonial nationalisms (Gorman & Udegbe, 2010). Puar (2009) herself has recently begun to engage questions of disability in relation to neoliberal nationalisms in her work on "debility." The third strand informing my articulation of transnational approaches to disability emerges from the recent "postcolonialization" of the disability studies canon. Postcolonial literary theorists have begun to read and contribute to disability studies literature as they more closely investigate themes of disablement, environmental devastation, and trauma described in tri-continental literatures.

For several years, I taught in a gender studies program, which took transnational feminist theory as its major subject and theoretical base. Along with transnational, postcolonial, and critical race theory, I trained my students in feminist institutional analysis. Following this theoretical/methodological approach, students were able to pursue broader questions about embodied and affective consequences of racism they encountered in education, social work, health care, housing, immigration and settlement services; as well as ongoing histories of political violence, colonialism, slavery, and genocide.[2] Transnational theoretical approaches allow us to understand disability as an assemblage of racialized and gendered narratives, national and postcolonial politics, and global capitalism. For Mad Studies, a transnational approach can move us past the deadlock of a simultaneous inattention to race and under-theorization of the global in relation to psychiatric disability and psychiatric surveillance. One advantage of teaching gender studies, however, was that there was no requirement for students to understand their experiences of labelling, surveillance, and distress in relation to disability politics, Mad politics, or consumer/survivor politics. From my current position teaching in a disability studies program, it's a lot more difficult to persuade students that the field enables an exploration of experience that centres people of colour. As one South Asian and equity studies student noted recently, "I theorize disability and psychic trauma from a postcolonial perspective. I don't do disability studies" (Siva Sivarajah, personal communication).

Same Institutions, Different Stories?

Deconstruction of the role of narrative in cultural understandings of disability has been central to disability studies work in the humanities, and has been best articulated in the work of David Mitchell and Sharon Snyder (2000). This deconstructive approach has had enormous impact on how disability studies is done in the social sciences disciplines, with narrative coming to the fore in helping us understand the social relations of disability oppression (Smith & Sparkes, 2008). There is a dialectical relationship between psychiatric survivors telling their stories and the deconstruction of oppressive narratives of psychiatric disability. For example, Prendergast (2008) traces the reduction of tropes of "schizophrenia" used in postmodern theory to the mass emergence of psychiatric survivors telling their stories in the 1990s. Recently, activists have called for a critical evaluation of the ways in which stories are increasingly appropriated into institutional success stories, anti-stigma campaigns, and academic and community-based research (Costa, 2012). As I will argue below, institutionally based storytelling around race and disability is overwhelmingly organized around narratives of race as stigma, or race as trauma. In his field-changing work, Ghanaian literary theorist Ato Quayson (2007) has re-theorized disability narratives in the global field of analysis through his articulation of "aesthetic nervousness." Through his rereading of the historical narrative of a South African Mad woman, Quayson identifies ways in which racialized women, especially those who are interpreted as culturally and racially hybrid, are narrated as having an "inarticulable insight." In the following section, I will work deconstructively with my own madness narratives in order to explicate class and race relations.

I first used the narrative of my childhood diagnosis as "hyperkinetic" as an example of one possible entry point into the ruling relations of disability (Gorman, 2005, p. 42–52). I was trying to find ground on which to situate the disability-impairment dialectic. Trying to situate this dialectic in relation to madness can be fraught—we can deconstruct the ruling relations through which categories of madness are organized (the psy discourses), yet still be left with questions about embodiment, experience, and consciousness. These conceptual difficulties are reflected in our social movements, through a range of pro- and antipsychiatry positions, and through a range of identity positions—consumer, survivor, ex-patient, mentally ill, psychiatrically disabled, and Mad.

> In the context of this relational/reflexive social analysis, how must we under-
> stand the experience and subjectivity of the knower who is also a political
> actor? This can only happen if we cut through the false polarity posited
> between the personal/the private/the individual and the mental, and the social/
> collective/the public and the political, and find a formative mediation between
> the two. (Bannerji, 1995, p. 85)

As we discover how particular experiences are mediated through social relations, we can connect the "immediate" experience we started with to the larger social organization. Describing experiences that are marginal to objectified knowledge is not the end of this project, but the beginning. A deeper discussion about the dialectic of experience and consciousness shows that ontologies of madness cannot be separated from epistemologies of madness. That is, we cannot divorce our embodied experiences of madness from the social relations through which our consciousness about our embodiment is organized.

I narrate the story of my childhood diagnosis in my doctoral dissertation in a way that highlights the ambiguity and historical contingency of the *Diagnostic and Statistical Manual of Mental Disorders* (DSM) (Gorman, 2005). I have since re-narrated the story in order to highlight gender—it is an unusual diagnosis for a girl (Gorman, 2009a); and again to highlight the ways in which my mother was caught up in class imperatives towards scientific parenting (Gorman, 2009b). However, taking a transnational approach to the story reveals that I have yet to narrate the dialectics of race and class through which ADHD evolves. I was a mixed race girl in a working-class immigrant neighbourhood at the time of my diagnosis in 1974. In the evolution of *hyperkinetic reaction of childhood* into *attention deficit disorder* and then *attention deficit hyperactivity disorder*, a DSM-organized transformation concurrent with my childhood and adolescence, there is also an evolution from connotations of class degeneracy and eugenic delinquency, towards the consolidation of a biological impairment that acts as a double-edged sword, as "hyperactive" children of colour are segregated in special ed, while "attention deficit" middle-class youth are provided with specialized computers and tutors. In her study of Canadian immigration law, Ena Chadha reveals the race and class dimensions of the diagnosis of "moral imbeciles," who were "turbulent, vicious, rebellious to all discipline; they lack sequence of ideas and probably power of attention" (Alfred Binet, 1905, cited in Chadha, 2008). When re-narrated in the context of histories of "moral insanity" (Martens, 2008) and "cultural deprivation" (Sleeter, 1987:2010), race and class dimensions of my diagnosis emerge.[3]

In her 1978 essay "K Is Mentally Ill," feminist sociologist Dorothy Smith deconstructs the narrative through which K comes to be known as mentally ill—and more importantly, the framework through which the narrator knows, and expects the listener to know, that K is mentally ill. Later in my dissertation I narrate experiences from my early adulthood as difficulties rather than differences.

> In 1988, I went to university to study astrophysics. I arrived during "frosh week" in my first year to a campus under siege by drunk, aggressive, male engineering students. I started class to find that I was one of two women in a class of sixty physics majors. By the end of first year, I was convinced that I was not smart enough to do physics, so I dropped it and switched to soil sciences. In the fall of my second year, in an incident that ended up making international news, male students at my university used the length of their residence to post signs advocating rape (see DeKeseredy & Schwartz, 1998, 126–127 for an account of this incident). In December of that same year a man shot and killed fourteen women in their engineering classroom in nearby Montréal. During the following summer, I did a placement at an engineering company as a soils technician, where I was excellent at my job, and where I was also subjected to daily harassment. By the end of my third year I had dropped out completely, one and a half credits short of a degree. I stayed in town for one more year, which I devoted to activism. (Gorman, 2005, p. 73)

Here I narrate through a feminist analytic approach, which assumes the traumatic effects of patriarchal violence.

I left the psychic experiences of this time out of the story, hazarding *in a footnote* only those references that would add up to learning disability and associated stress. Even as I acknowledge my concern about psychiatric intervention, I continue to manage the risk within the narrative itself, sticking to symptoms more commonly acknowledged in popular culture, and highlighting the "reason" up front.

> These events took a toll on me. I was unable to focus. I could not read to the end of a sentence without my mind drifting off. I felt dizzy and sleepy during

lectures. I decided not to consult disability services. Having already a brush with a diagnostic label regarding these symptoms, I was unwilling to subject myself to this process. I was also sure that the positivist, measurement-based approach to learning disability in higher education (for example, extra exam time, and a spell-checking computer) would not help me. Having read Sylvia Plath's (1966) *The Bell Jar*, and listened to a lecture by Kate Millett, I must admit I was also more than a little fearful of more severe diagnostic intervention. After I had dropped out of school and settled into full-time feminist activism, I heard there was a feminist counsellor in town, but her time was all booked by others in my leftist cohort. (Gorman, 2005, p. 73)

Part of our resistance to violence was organized through our understanding of the psychic impact of gender violence—and very clearly we understood psychiatry itself as part of the organization of this violence. Yet despite our collective approach, our understanding of embodied experience was organized through appeals to feminist psychoanalysis.[4]

Years later, having access to a Mad identity allowed for the interpretation of my experiences as alternative ways of knowing.[5] Other moments of psychic "difference" emerged as narratable—moments beyond the narratives of diagnosis, trauma, and escape. It became possible to narrate these moments in relation to my awareness of being mixed race. Amina Mama (1995) shifts feminist psychoanalysis' primary focus on gender to account for ways in which women of colour repress racialized identifications. And while her description of repression may work to explain my experiences, and generalized experiences of racism in a binary culture, understanding experiences of race as "repression" expands the category of "traumatized" (and ultimately stigmatized and individualized) subjectivities.[6] Despite its inadequacies, the narration of race as trauma extends the hope that the *privileges* some people gain through the process of labelling may become available to others:

Which aspects of a person's way of being are seen as inherent, and which are seen as changeable depend[s] on the social context. During my twenties I worked on-call, rotating and night shift schedules, while parenting step-children, living in crowded, run-down apartments, and moving frequently due to rent increases and disputes with room-mates and landlords. During this time I was confused, easily distracted, and had difficulty focusing. As discussed earlier, this way of being is called ADHD in middle class North American children, and "learning disability" in North American university students. Among lesbian social services workers and union activists—that is, in a working class context—it is called "struggling," or just "life." What might be diagnosed as a treatable disorder in someone with relative access and privilege may be thought of as an inherent characteristic of someone in a different social location. (Gorman, 2005, p. 75)

The same diagnoses may organize racialized "othering" in primary school, or "whiteness" in secondary and higher education. They may lead to surveillance and institutional violence, or specialized services and support; or be narrated as "just life," and remain outside of the institutional frame.

Whiteness and Its Others

In 2009 I completed a reflexive inquiry into the experience of being a faculty member with a "hidden" disability.[7] As part of my commitment to best practices in universal design, and a social model approach to educational inclusion, I had archived four years of my teaching practice. I analyzed this data source for three trends: the evolution of my overall classroom practices, as I modified my practical understanding of universal design; the hidden labour of student accommodation; and the evolution of specific negotiations with students who presented themselves to me for accommodations. Because several of the courses I taught were in disability studies, because I took a disability-focused approach to teaching, and because I was known for this kind of work and research, many students with disabilities enrolled in my courses. I began with the hypothesis that universal design may be more effective at accommodating white, middle-class disabled students, while further marginalizing students of colour. Like my narrative above, students of colour would describe their problems to me as socially contextualized difficulties (or "just life") while white-identified students would describe themselves as having a disorder (anxiety or depression being the one most commonly described to me). My analysis of my hidden labour revealed more about who felt entitled to seek out the support of the professor than it revealed about how marginalized students survive the higher education experience. Mostly it threw into relief the extent to which feelings of empowerment towards accessing support coincided with taking on identities of learning disability and mental illness.

Most surprising, however, was my finding that the institutional petition process was reproducing particular "ideal types" of disability narrative. Based on a record of petitions to complete course work after the end of the course, I had a sample of 17 students who were accommodated, in difficulty, or who identified as disabled—15 from the main campus of the university, and two from the satellite campus. According to a comparison of my teaching practices to a pamphlet circulated by the disability services office of the satellite campus of the university, I apparently employ all of the recommendations of universal instructional design—whereby a professor modifies the course materials and delivery in order to make a course more inclusive, usually by building in a diversity of approaches to accommodate different learning styles. It is therefore significant to look at students who still had to negotiate with me or appeal to their registrar at the end of the course in order to submit course work after departmental and college deadlines for submitting marks. This sample of 17 includes

13 students who had to negotiate and/or petition at the end of the course. Of these 13, eight negotiated with me directly (six were able to negotiate ways to complete the assigned course work or alternate course work). Two went through the petition process on my advice (one was successful and one was not) and three went directly through the petition process without my having to advise them of their right to do so. Of the three who went directly through the petition process (all of them successfully), two were confident the process would work, and one engaged in it as a last resort.

Of the 13 students in difficulty, nine were already registered with disability services and were receiving or had received some form of accommodation at some point in their undergraduate careers. Six of the nine registered students were students of colour. The four students in difficulty who were not registered with disability services would have had a case for going through a diagnostic process that would enable them to register with disability services. Three of the four non-registered students were students of colour. Two of these students of colour were the two students from the satellite campus whom I included in my sample of 17. On the downtown campus, about half of my students were students of colour while on the satellite campus about 80 percent of my students were students of colour. In order to get a sense of students who identify as disabled and/or who are registered with disability services and who *did not* report difficulties at the end of term, I included three white students who were registered with accessibility services, and one student of colour who identifies as disabled but who was not registered with accessibility services. All of these students negotiated with me throughout the term and frequently emailed me and visited my office hours to discuss their course work. These students seemed comfortable expressing their needs, spending time with the professor (an average of four hours of individual time per student per semester), and accessing appropriate campus services as needed. From the archive of four years of teaching records, it appeared that white students were more comfortable requesting services, and requesting more of my time.

The petition process reproduces raced and classed narratives about who is disabled, who is unusually burdened, and who is genuinely deserving of help. The process of documenting a disability also reproduces raced and classed narratives about who is to blame for their difficulties and who deserves help. It is often during times of crisis when students are sent forward to go through the process of registering for disability services— through the diagnosis of either a learning disability or mental distress/illness. Racialized narratives of who is understood as having a diagnosable disorder, and who is understood as attempting to manipulate the system, are evident in the petition process and in parallel institutional processes that assist with emergency bursaries and housing.[8] The fact that two of the four non-white, non-registered students are from the satellite campus is significant. The satellite campus has more accessible, integrated, proportionately better-funded disability services. They also have engaged in successful campaigns to educate professors about universal instructional design—a campaign that followed a Teaching and Learning for Diversity project that focused on culturally inclusive curriculum and ESL students, as well as disability. Students of colour with evident physical and sensory disability are duly registered with disability services; however, white students are more likely to be registered with disability services than students of colour who report comparable emotional and academic difficulties. Similarly, students of colour on the downtown campus reporting emotional and academic difficulties are more likely to be registered with disability services than students of colour on the satellite campus, reflecting the spatialization of race and class in the city.

There is a bifurcation between students who are narrated as being disadvantaged by race and class on one hand, and by disability on the other. In the end, students who are affected by racism, poverty, and violence are the ones against whom the successfully accommodated disabled student is articulated. An analysis of universal design reveals the ways in which the university is organized around time and stress management—equity and access in a university context are limited to expanding the skills of rationality, self-care, and self-management through individualized support. Students who come to understand themselves as having mental illnesses that can be individually treated, and additional needs that can be individually accommodated, may also come to understand themselves in relation to an essential identity. These processes must be understood as being central to how Mad identity gets organized, who may become politicized through Mad identity politics, what political demands are made, and what kinds of alliances and solidarities are forged. As Mad politics become more visible, and mental health agency anti-stigma campaigns become more ubiquitous, more students come to identify themselves as Mad. Like any political identity (for example, "woman" or "queer,"), Mad identity can be associated with a range of political leanings and epistemologies. One might identify as Mad and individually unique, or as Mad and part of a history of anti-oppression struggle, or both.

Conclusion: The Pitfalls of Identity

The political economy of mental health services, the coordinating of services, and the bidding for project-based health care dollars has extended the reach of psychiatric hospitals into corners of the community they could not access in the past. Based on their progressive disability politics, and their activist connections to marginalized communities, several former students have been recruited by large agencies who have been funded to recruit queer youth and youth of colour into their client base—a move that is generating critique from these activists turned mental health workers (Udegbe & Vo, 2013). Meanwhile, more people who are thinking and organizing from critical transnational and Indigenous perspectives are asking questions about intergenerational and collective effects of war, colonialism, and political violence. Psychiatric hospitals, which prompted the psychiatric survivors' movement, are now linked with community-based agencies. Anti-stigma campaigns and the framing of psychiatric treatment as a health care right mask the coercion at the heart of psychiatric treatment regimes (Wipond, 2008). Psychiatric profiling and drugging occur in prisons and detention centres (Howell, 2007; Kilty, 2008), and psy technologies are expansive through education, social services, policing, and immigration and settlement services. In this local and global context, it becomes increasingly urgent to refuse the separation of Mad identity and a critical Mad politics—politics that are historically rooted in the anti-oppression and class struggles of psychiatric survivor movements, and currently striving to connect to the anti-racist and anti-colonial struggles of racialized and Indigenous communities.

Notes

1 Participants in this series of strategic conversations towards a politics of race, migration, and madness included Peggy-Gail Dehal-Ramson, Erick Fabris, Kevin Jackson, Nadia Kanani, Jenna Reid, Rick Sin, Louise Tam, Onyii Udegbe, and Onar Usar. I am also grateful to Lucy Costa for ongoing conversations about madness in relation to cultural exclusion and immigration status.

2 My former undergraduate and graduate students at the University of Toronto who have taken up the challenge of engaging complex questions around race, disability, madness, trauma, and embodiment include Mariam Aslam, Darcel Bullen, Sadia Ferdous, Deana Kannagasingam, Chantal Persad, Thijiba Sinnathamby, Louise Tam, Onyii Udegbe, Edward Wong, and Annie Kashamura Zawadi.

3 Jijian Voronka's (2008b) study of the Queen Street Asylum begins the work of untangling narratives of race and class within an institutional monolith.

4 See Bonnie Burstow (2003) on the politics and limits of understanding the effects of gender violence as "trauma."

5 I finished my doctoral work and started teaching in 2005, which coincided with the emergence of the Coalition Against Psychiatric Assault and the Mad Students Society. Doing political work with Mad activists Jeremiah Bach, Lucy Costa, and Erick Fabris exposed me to possibilities of developing Mad epistemologies. Being surrounded by an activist community reduced the risk of speaking about my diagnosable experiences, yet as I spoke, I framed them in the context of "avoiding or outwitting psychiatry," in the style of what Linda Morrison refers to as "heroic survivor narrative" (Morrison, 2006).

6 Both Frantz Fanon and Achille Mbembé locate the individual psychic effects of colonialism in larger social narratives. Fanon (1963, 1965) argued that narratives of persecution "delusions" shifted as the anti-colonial war in Algeria progressed, and emphasized the role of torture in the development of thoughts of persecution. Mbembé (2002) discusses larger trends in African postcolonial thought through which loss, theft, and colonial genocide are occluded or repressed.

7 I presented this research at the 2009 Disability Studies in Education conference at Syracuse University.

8 In a study of gender persecution cases heard by the Canadian refugee hearing board, Sherene Razack (1998) found that "stories of race" determined whether women are understood as being at risk, or whether they are understood as trying to manipulate the refugee system to escape poverty.

CHAPTER 20

Whither Indigenizing the Mad Movement?
Theorizing the Social Relations of Race and Madness through Conviviality

Louise Tam

The Mad movement and Mad Studies have arrived where they are today from more than five decades of resisting against "psy" knowledge (destabilizing diagnostic categories, naming psychiatric violence, resisting pathologization, and creating countercultures). Users, survivors, Mad people, and their allies attempt to discuss the significance of race, racism, and racialization for Mad people's oppression through using various frameworks for analysis, including analogy, intersectionality, and trauma. For example, Roman et al. (2009) argue psychiatric disenfranchisement is a new form of colonialism. Contesting previous accounts of the birth of British Columbia's first insane asylum, Roman et al. (2009) argue the Woodlands School (formerly the Public Hospital for the Insane) was an example of juridical medicalized colonialism from 1859 to 1897. The authors use this term to describe the conditions experienced by majority "white" inmates at Woodlands (Roman et al., 2009, p. 36). Inmates, regardless of race, are characterized as colonized. This rhetorical move is risky in the context of settler colonialism seizing Indigenous land, which differently positions the stakes of settlers from those of First Nations people.

As a metaphor, colonialism is used by Roman et al. (2009) to represent how "actual people were horrifically abused, many losing their lives" and to claim that survivors of the Woodlands School require reparation from the Canadian government that mirrors Prime Minister Stephen Harper's 2008 "apology to all Aboriginal, Métis and Inuit former students of residential schools for First Nations" (p. 53). They state "[n]o such step has been taken with the survivors of Woodlands or any other residential school for people with developmental disabilities in Canada" (Roman et al., 2009, p. 53). Without explaining why they use the term "residential school" to describe disabled whites, the likeness the authors draw between the violence of colonial education and survivors of the Woodlands School construes Indigenous and disabled communities as two discrete populations, relatable only through comparison. Their choice of phrasing suggests that techniques and strategies used to justify Indian residential schools and later reconcile that history are not borrowed from, influenced by, or endemic to scientific constructions of normality/abnormality. It omits important questions, including the following: How does psychiatric commitment co-constitute the construction of the "Indian" as Other?

Where Roman et al. (2009) do concretely connect disability and race, they rely on an additive model of oppression. To elaborate, they only discuss race in Woodlands as an unfortunate marker of difference that justifies additional penalties—namely deportation for migrant Chinese inmates. Also known as the "invisible knapsack of privilege," this approach to analyzing social difference is sometimes endemic to theoretical applications of intersectionality. Feminist theorists (Crenshaw, 1991; Hill Collins, 2003; McIntosh, 1989) use intersectionality to analyze difference as axes of identity, in which gender, race, class, sexuality, and disability all interact with one another on different levels. Due to the framework's reliance on identity, users of intersectionality reify race and disability into entities and attributes, consistent across time and space, forgetting such discourses are often tethered together in their formation and enforcement as technologies of power.

In Mad Studies, Wolframe (2011) has advocated that educators teach privileged people about how to be allies through this concept of the invisible knapsack, in which "sane" people have privileges that are unique from other privileges. Although she adds that sometimes people without psychiatric patient histories cannot separate their privilege from race, gender, and class, she fails to elucidate the ways in which discrimination against Mad people can be inextricably bound up with institutions such as immigration, stymying applications for family reunification.

Conversely, Mad allies such as Titchkosky and Aubrecht (2010) reify madness as essential difference while simultaneously attempting to centre race through the concept of trauma, specifically "anguish." In their study of the World Health Organization's literature on mental health, Titchkosky and Aubrecht (2010) argue that the WHO "dichotomizes mental diversity into mental illness or not, and colonizes relations to anguish and to knowledge" (p. 180). They assert that mental health outreach is colonizing because it neglects traumatizing histories ("anguish"). By interpreting the WHO's actions as abstracting people from historical reasons for suffering, the authors substitute one explanation of mental illness for another by theorizing "mental difference" as a response to external stimuli. Their social analysis of disability remains steadfast to a material body that ends in the individual, in which mental illness names an observable disturbance to the mind. They implicitly adopt a trauma model and advocate diverse treatments based on diverse traumas. The argument of history-as-symptom is itself a mental health discourse used to racialize people. A positive representation of disability as "wounded soul" can still be used to prescribe social remedies, such as empowerment work and affirmative thinking—other forms of governing the self. In their effort to challenge "how disability is constructed as nothing but a problem," Titchkosky and Aubrecht (2010) prescribe a vague, overdetermining victim narrative (p. 181).

There remains a gap in mapping relations of race *to* and *in* madness. It is this epistemic gap that fails to account for how race-thinking inherently constitutes psy knowledge. For example, newcomer discourse, in the form of education for immigrants about culture shock, uses psychological tools such as self-help to encourage a colonial mentality among newly arrived people of colour. Newcomer literature promotes immigrant adjustment to the many benefits of Canadian multiculturalism and instills hope in non-Indigenous racialized people—the hope that they will eventually belong through accumulating national belonging. Strategies such as these help maintain Canada as a settler state and deny Indigenous nationhood. According to Lawrence and Dua (2005), without taking Indigenous sovereignty seriously, we remain complicit in a colonial order that continues to target Indigenous people for legal and cultural extinction and fail to recognize the differential terms on which we occupy this land. This is not to suggest that "all migrants are settler colonists" or that "'different' people should be in 'their own' places" (Sharma & Wright, 2008, pp. 123–124). An anti-capitalist decolonizing project also requires acknowledging the migration of people who have been colonized and dispossessed of their prior livelihoods, in which enslaved Africans, indentured Asian labourers, and First Nations people have more in common than not in their struggle for a global coexistence. "Many people have been brought together through historical relations of expropriation and exploitation, but at times they have connected with one another through a common struggle against these processes" (Sharma & Wright, 2008, p. 132).

Mental health institutions are part of the ongoing displacement and assimilation of migrant, Indigenous, and migrant Indigenous people over the last five centuries through their involvement in multiple projects of settlement. Unfortunately, Indigenous peoples make their presence in Mad culture predominantly through culturally appropriated non-medicalized practices of healing. The following critique focuses on how narratives connecting race and madness, specifically in representations of indigeneity, have so far occluded a relationship of critical dialogue and anti-colonial intervention. How can we decolonize rather than indigenize the alternative culture and health strategies advocated by Mad activists?

My objective is to challenge the relational terrain on which people with embodied experiences of mental/behavioural/emotional objectification (called madness) locate and interpret their biographies as Mad, so that decolonization is understood as necessarily a part of addressing madness as a systemic oppression. This paradigm shift I outline—from discrete intersections between race and psychiatrization to a framework of inter-institutional psy oppression, and from analogy to material relationships—is an attempt at fostering solidarity with Indigenous peoples who have survived the violence of institutionalization, incarceration, intellectual supremacy, and white supremacist behaviour policing. Without such a project of historical recovery that maps how the psy complex pathologizes and continues to manage different populations, Aboriginal people and people of colour cannot see themselves in a Mad movement that marginalizes their realities through a pluralist framework.

In this chapter, I examine the work of two influential user/survivor-led organizations in North America in order to identify general trends in the Mad movement. I am interested in these organizations' relationships to race and colonialism in their predominantly white claims of entitlement to particular practices and to the land. The Icarus Project is a New York-based radical mental health collective that resists narratives of disease and disorder and supports people living with "mad gifts" in "an oppressive and damaged world" (Icarus Project website, "About Us"). The collective was co-founded by Jacks Ashley McNamara and Sascha Altman DuBrul. Together, McNamara and DuBrul (2006) edited the book/zine *Navigating the Space between Brilliance and Madness*, a collection of stories and lessons from multiple members of the Icarus Project. Described as an "atlas of alternative maps to the particular breed of madness that gets called bipolar," *Navigating the Space between Brilliance and Madness* remains one of the most popular publications downloaded and distributed from the Icarus Project's website. The zine is a testament to the growth of the Mad movement through the collective's dissemination of resources over the Internet, resources that are also cross-posted on other psychiatric survivor forums such as MindFreedom International's website (Icarus Project website, "Resources").

With affiliate groups in at least eight states, the Icarus Project is second in size only to MindFreedom International, an international non-profit organization based in Eugene, Oregon, with over 100 sponsor and affiliate grassroots groups (MindFreedom International website, "About Us"). MindFreedom International organizes various human rights campaigns, protests abuses in the psychiatric drug industry, and supports self-determination for users and survivors of psychiatry. To initiate dialogue on the place of "race" in Mad cultural production, I open this chapter with a textual analysis of McNamara and DuBrul's (2006) zine. I trouble the editors' constructions of space, time, and spirituality. Subsequently I reflect on MindFreedom International's Occupy Normal or Boycott Normal campaign. The Occupy Normal campaign is an example of recent coalition-building efforts in the Mad movement.

Cultural Criticism for Co-existence

In "Dialectically Down with the Critical Program," hooks (1992) advises us against political organizing through feeling good or feeling bad when forming radical subcultures. Speaking to black critical thinkers, she warns that by merely feeling good as a community, through things such as material acquisition, we risk willingly participating in the commodification of blackness and perpetuating the existing social order. She argues that only through an ongoing, unsettling systemic resistance and oppositional work can we affirm ourselves as people and as individuals. For those of us working within anti-colonial, anti-racist, psychiatric survivor, and Mad movements, hooks' warning is one we might heed. Rigorous critique and thoughtful reflection are a part of systemic resistance and need not be viewed as antithetical to our movements. In our struggles to relate race and racialization to madness, we might consider how hooks' demands for systemic resistance are substantively relevant to the organizing goals of Mad activists. It is not in our best interests to celebrate any work by a Mad-identified person at the risk of passive consumption because rigorous critique is a gesture of respect and love. For this reason, I urge Mad cultural producers and their allies to examine what claims we make in our work about madness and who relates to those claims.

Along these lines of inquiry, I notice that a gap exists between Mad people's conceptualization of Mad people's oppression and anti-racist analysis of ongoing practices in (post)colonial and cross-cultural psychiatry. Too often, Mad artists and activists such as McNamara and DuBrul blame capitalism for devaluing "unproductive" Mad bodies without calling attention to how capitalism is a global system that helps to maintain gendered and racial lines. Consequently constructions of health, including mental health, are shaped by various racial projects, defined by nation-states and global policy frameworks. In particular, I notice the Mad movement extolling the virtues of culturally appropriated practices such as mindfulness meditation and shamanism, without disclosing their own relationship to Indigenous peoples, transnational or not.

Across socio-political, cultural, or material contexts, psychiatric oppression and sanism (Perlin, 2000) shape Indigenous communities in ways that dialectically position them differently from other racialized people. Andrea Smith (2006) offers a heuristic framework for conceptualizing how we are differently impacted by white supremacy, which affects how different communities organize against oppression. Smith (2006) outlines three different relationships people of colour have to white supremacy: slavery/capitalism, genocide/colonialism, orientalism/war. The first pillar concerns the slaveability and commodification of blackness, the second pillar refers to manifest destiny and the present absence of Native peoples—the belief that non-Indigenous people are "the rightful inheritors of all that was indigenous"—and the third pillar signifies how the East is continually perceived as a threat (Smith, 2006, p. 68). These pillars are not exclusive to particular communities: orientalism may impact Latino migrants, for example. Smith (2006) argues that if we are only subjected to one of these pillars, we are susceptible to being seduced by the other two. Likewise, mostly white social movements are susceptible to reinforcing all three logics.

In the context of the three pillars of white supremacy, fostering progressive critique and systemic resistance within the Mad movement is paramount because it makes us, as activists, writers, and cultural producers, accountable to our politics by attuning ourselves to the varying effects of the political economy of "madness" on different populations. Smith's (2006) framework demonstrates how comparative racialization functions to benefit a white nation-state. I argue that the delineation of our mental capacities—psychological explanations for racial/ethnic inferiority—help to justify the subordination of Native people and people of colour.

One theoretical tool for mapping how race and madness are not only connected through our multiple identities, but through their discursive and material co-production, is Jasbir Puar's (2009) theory of conviviality. "Conviviality," a word that traditionally means fond feasting and jovial company, is used by Puar (2009) to conceptualize social differences such as race, class, and sexuality as *happening* in real-time events, encounters, and activities rather than inherent attributes of people. From a conviviality perspective, gender, race, class, sexuality, and disability are unstable, shifting in their temporal-spatial constructions and articulations; futurity (the possibility of social change) is enabled through the continuous process of collectively reconstituting our social relations. To Puar, not only is sanity/insanity (ability/debility) an unreliable division, but a division that shifts based on the organization of other facets of social difference. "Madness" as a discourse changes based on the social. By social, I mean the convivial interaction of bodies in the dissemination of knowledge, the institutionalization of policy, and the creation of cultural artifacts. Experiences of imperialism, race, class, and disability are not fixed or compartmentalized objects, but a chain of interdependent events: "a tagging of where the body once was" shaping where it "continues about its perpetual motility" (Puar, Pitcher & Gunkel, 2008).

Conviviality draws attention to how disability, and by extension madness, is something we can have without identifying as such. It draws attention to the broader politics of debility in (post)colonial and transnational contexts, politics that are not about cultural perceptions of madness per se, but about the deployment of ability/debility in state governance. For example, quoting Livingston (2006), Puar (2009) cites the geopolitically specific normalization of disability in Botswana where newly impaired miners have access to a rigorous system for providing them with tools such as prosthetics to manage their anticipated bodily states. Here, disability can be understood as a product of Western biomedical interventions that sustain a system of neocolonial resource extraction reliant on the senescence of black bodies.

By attending to (post)colonial and transnational governing structures like those described above, I argue that racial oppression is sustained through "madness"—through people's encounters with psy knowledge. Race happens through complex socially organized activities and is not merely a fixed attribute, but a relationship constituted through legal regimes and state-based practices (Omi & Winant, 1994; Puar, Pitcher & Gunkel, 2008; Thobani, 2007). Many of these socially organized activities have to do with the management of our thoughts (feelings) and our actions (behaviour)—our psychology (Howell, 2011). In the following case study, Mad alternatives to recovery foregrounded on an objectifying Native exoticism serve as the substrate through which I further distinguish the solidarity-building capacities of madness as conviviality versus madness as personal identity. My hope is not to preclude community based on Mad identity, but to destabilize our identities by historically locating ourselves and our privilege, and to suggest anti-colonial and anti-racist strategies for creating subversive "Mad" narratives.

Cartographies of Madness: The Icarus Project and "Bipolar Worlds"

Despite their attempts to address a wide audience including youth and university students, McNamara and DuBrul (2006) empty out their life experiences of North America's colonial histories in their homogenous leftist narratives of Mad identity and self-discovery in *Navigating the Space between Brilliance and Madness*. Personally removed from broader political and economic conditions of marginalization, McNamara and DuBrul suggest that deviance is simply "crazy behaviour" that resists generic "American norms" without qualifying those norms in terms of the politics of nation-building. Throughout the zine, contributors also describe Mad people's alienation from *mainstream* society one-dimensionally as the byproduct of their loss of productivity in wage labour, holding accountable a non-specific capitalist America. Capitalism is not explored in transnational contexts, in the form of temporary labour migration, or in colonial contexts, in the form of Native land dispossession. As such, in their analysis of madness as the transgression of labour regimes, the editors and contributors do not consider how race constitutes different desirable or undesirable capitalist subjects.

Map as Metaphor: *Remapping* Experience and *Hitchhiking* to Recovery

> All the moments of pain and elation carve into our terrain with the crooked grace of rivers and ravines.
>
> —McNamara and DuBrul (2006, p. 2)

McNamara and DuBrul (2006) use geography, in the form of roads and paths for travel, to describe mental health recovery as an exercise in mapping yourself to wellness. The figure of the forked road represents the numerous ways people are told "how to cope, and what is good" (p. 2). In this analogy, McNamara and DuBrul characterize resistance against mainstream recovery practices such as psychiatric assessment as a deviation from the path. Both editors use maps as a rhetorical device in their introductions, in which they provide their itinerant stories of survival. Missing from their intervention on acceptable "roads" to wellness is a reflection on their own relationship to the land.

As Jacks McNamara recalls:

The map they [psychiatrists] gave me was terrifying.... You will take psychiatric medication for the rest of your life. You will need to see a doctor constantly and always be on the lookout for side-effects. We will test your blood and your kidneys and your liver function every 3 months. You must have health insurance. You will need to live in one place.... You should try to have a steady job, but you might never be able to, because this is a serious disability.... The map those doctors had drawn for me did a very effective job of scaring me away from the whole mental health establishment and I had yet to meet anyone with flight patterns like mine. (McNamara & DuBrul, 2006, pp. 5–6)

McNamara then describes living an independent life in rural New Jersey, watching sunrises, working with horses, and eventually going to Greece, and then resettling again in San Francisco.

Although McNamara and DuBrul seditiously identify themselves as creatures branded with a contour map with rocky sunrises and "the fractal branching of so many threads of understanding" (McNamara & DuBrul, 2006, p. 5), their off-road map to wellness is complicit with colonial master narratives. The dream of an open road to no discernible destination, of empty land, of being naturally close to the earth and its animals, yet fleeing at will to the cityscapes of their desires, draws a picture of economic mobility and inheritance to space that can only exist through settler colonial myths of a frontier nation in which Indigenous nations are nowhere to be found. The sensation of being lost and never feeling at home runs McNamara and DuBrul's *maps* into a paradox twofold: on the one hand, true, they may never feel at home—as the land they live on is contested and stolen; on the other hand, their sensation of displacement unwittingly commodifies the narratives of diasporic racialized peoples. The violence through which migrant people of colour have arrived on this land and those biographies of asylum-seekers, by boat, and by plane, are not historically captured or even gestured to by McNamara and DuBrul (2006). Ultimately the use of natural paths such as rivers and ravines to instill in readers a liberating journey of recovery are hegemonic in their allegedly universal appeal, minimizing the historical power differences between white settlers, racialized migrants, and Indigenous peoples through the assumption that water and land carry the same symbolic meaning to every (labelled) individual (in distress).

McNamara and DuBrul (2006) do not acknowledge how knowing your future also relies on how you relate to your past: a past that extends further back than your early childhood development, a process of coming to know that requires tools like genealogy. Bannerji (2000) calls attention to how the insider/outsider status of people of colour is not merely the result of recent prejudice in society. Their feelings of exclusion are the result of a long history of being de-skilled and marginalized by decertification and force into the working class. Bannerji (2000) argues people of colour constitute "a reserve army of labour" that fuels the capitalist development of Indigenous lands, marked by such conflicts as Oka, Gustafson Lake, and Ipperwash (pp. 75–76). Consequently, liberation is a more complicated task of addressing multiple coordinated state-instituted practices of exploitation and exclusion and requires us to situate ourselves in relation to how our oppression connects to the struggles of other communities.

If McNamara and DuBrul (2006) want to transgress the maps created by mental health, they could take issue with the way social services have historically structured the mobility of racialized people as well as the relationships different racialized communities have to one another. Recently, a woman of colour I know shared her frustration over non-geographically specific narratives of people's madness experiences: for her, the marginalization of being "Mad" is invoked by the risk of her deportation due to her decision not to disclose her psychiatric diagnosis on her visa application. Policing of state borders through sanist measures controls the flights and roads taken by people of colour. Yet borders do not end at those enforced by the nation-state. A cartography of madness also includes non-borders. Consider how settlement workers encourage volunteer work to newcomers so that they can cope with their "culture shock"; now consider those volunteers enlisted to "help" impoverished urban Aboriginal users of the shelter system who are increasingly legislated out of existence and out of relevance to land claims through the Indian Act.

Wong (2008) warns Asian Canadians that beyond opposing white privilege, collectivist strategies must be taken to hold ourselves accountable to all those excluded by the state. In this present moment, she argues, little attention is paid to unpacking "the specific problematics of racialized subjects who have inherited the violence of colonization" (Wong, 2008, p. 158). A politics of oppositionality or *freedom from* the whiteness of psychiatry does not imply a politics of solidarity with Indigenous survivors of psychiatry and leaves us susceptible to a politics of *freedom to*. Anti-racism and decolonization, though not mutually exclusive, are frequently taken up as different political projects. As a racialized child of migrant parents, I could resist the medicalization of worker burnout in Asian communities (which normalizes brute meritocracy as a rite of passage to Asian economic ascendency) through calling attention to state-instituted practices of foreign labour exploitation and demanding citizenship rights. Yet, my experiences of pathologization are adjoined to those practices that construct Indianness as a deficit; together, narratives of Native alcoholism and Asian workaholism reify white supremacy. Demanding citizenship rights lends false legitimacy to the settler state (Walia, 2012). Collective remapping requires white settlers and settlers of colour to come to terms with the violences we can recreate if we remain invested in the self-interested strategies of liberal pluralism. Recognizing who is most impacted by institutionalization and therapeutic governance will transform how we collectively resist sanism and psychiatric violence.

Constructing Indigeneity as an Untapped Resource

Sascha DuBrul's alternative identity and off-road mapping is also reliant on seizing Indigenous knowledge and cosmology through his practice of journalling about time rather than space, or about space-time. He relates to indigeneity through language as artifact, describing himself as a time traveller as he reconstructs his fleeting memories to chart the rhythms and patterns in his pain. DuBrul relates to Hopi language, where

> there's no past, present, or future in the grammar structure—different objects and people have different "states of becoming." It's a way of conceiving TIME that is completely unlike the one with which we've all grown up. This idea has always resonated with me and captured my imagination—maybe it's because of the non-linear nature of my mind and the blessing or curse I carry of feeling things strong and synchronous. (McNamara & DuBrul, 2006, p. 7)

Drawn above this reflection are images of a railroad track, a scar, and a ladder, labelled with the words "tracks, movement," "scar, memory," and "ladder, hope," respectively. His relationship to Hopi culture, while offering a tool for him to meditate on how "bipolar" symptoms are constructed through a Western model of time, commodifies and detaches Hopi worldview from contemporary Hopi experiences with madness and the mental health system. Rather than positioning Hopi culture as the alternative for him to consume, which contributes to the racializing tendencies of cultural revitalization in liberal multiculturalism, a relationalist approach would be helpful for him to locate shared political realities.

DuBrul's connection to the Hopi in itself can begin to decolonize the practice of map-making: some 1,500 miles away from New York state and 100 years ago, Hopi women and children were among the multiplicity of Indigenous people incarcerated and sent by train to a federally funded program at the Hiawatha Asylum for Insane Indians in Canton, South Dakota (Yellow Bird, 2010). If DuBrul is going to engage with radical notions of temporality, historicizing psychiatry's intercultural narratives would simultaneously acknowledge his privilege and locate him as a potential ally alongside Indigenous communities that have endured the legacy of their ancestors being institutionalized as "Indian 'defectives'" (Yellow Bird, 2010, p. 7). For now, his sketches of railroad tracks and ladders point upwards, suggesting a spiritual ascension that borders on colonial fantasy.

In an article titled "The Freedom to Sit" (under the topic "Spirit and Mysticism" on the Icarus Project's website), Will Hall (2007) also reflects on madness and alternate relationships to time, advocating the accommodation of people with psychiatric labels at Buddhist meditation retreats. Positioning himself as spiritual as a result of his experiences labelled "mental illness," Hall (2007) asserts that people with *and* without psychiatric history find themselves unable to complete challenging retreats that disrupt daily routine and require long periods of stillness, an act that can be triggering or emotionally overwhelming (p. 35). He says, "[t]hose of us who have been through a 'psychotic episode' may be more equipped to deal with strong feelings and emotions when they arise" (Hall, 2007, p. 36). As a woman of colour, I have complicated feelings about the trendiness of Buddhist meditation because Buddhist ontology was displaced by Protestantism and Catholicism in my family history. My father's alma mater was a Catholic missionary school specializing in science and technology that inculcated a sense of moral responsibility in its students to become international professionals. Many of his classmates migrated to North America and Australia.

While Mad people search for self-actualization and refuge from the rhetoric of neuro-determinism in psy knowledge, sometimes through new ageism and "going Native," diasporic Hong Kongers seek out Christianity as a tool of ascension, cultural supremacy, and white intelligibility in Canada. The only way I can honestly relate to Buddhism is by refamiliarizing myself with where I came from, and in doing so, understand where I am now and what possible connections I do have to Indigenous peoples (rather than beginning from disembodied spiritual beliefs).

Monoculture or White Supremacy?:
Qualifying the Dominant Culture as a "Consumer Culture"

So far, I have troubled McNamara and DuBrul's (2006) visions of a Mad utopia in their references to off-road maps and their appropriation of Indigenous beliefs. Part of their justification for building alternative mental health practices is their observation that normality is crazy. However, calling normality crazy merely places blame on the individual, rather than illuminating the privilege that is often required to "opt out." "Making sense of being crazy in a crazy world" is one catch phrase used by the Icarus Project (McNamara & DuBrul, 2006, p. 16). This phrase is the title of one section of their zine. Below the title, there are pictures of call centre employees, agricultural workers, and the military, accompanied by questions such as "What is normal? Who gets to decide?" (McNamara & DuBrul, 2006, p. 16). In this section, anonymous contributors argue that Americans live in a sick culture that has generated disease categories such as compulsive shopping disorder and oppositional defiant disorder; "mental illness" is "a convenient label for behavior that disrupts the social order" (McNamara & DuBrul, 2006, p. 17). However, such criticisms unwittingly reify the pathologization of people of colour, due to McNamara and DuBrul (2006) casting the survival jobs of racialized people into their version of the real loony bin. They also preclude a consideration of how disease categories such as oppositional defiant disorder are notoriously applied to inner-city impoverished youth of colour.

Pictures of farm labour and technicians in a call centre represent spaces of work frequented by black and brown people, ferried into survival jobs through structures such as the Temporary Foreign Worker Program in Canada. McNamara and DuBrul's

(2006) characterization of these workers as "crazy," unenlightened, oppressed people reduces white supremacist conditions for labour exploitation into a hermeneutic impasse, unwittingly reifying the commodification of working-class, racialized bodies. I argue that madness as a relation is produced not only through discourses of underproductivity or dysfunction, but also through hyperproductivity and worker burnout. McNamara and DuBrul's (2006) privileged standard accounts result in an Icarista subculture that contradicts the lived experience of those most marginalized by the white supremacist pillar of slavery/capitalism (Smith, 2006).

Occupy (Occupied): MindFreedom Boycotts Normal

McNamara and DuBrul's (2006) generic characterization of working- and middle-class America as a duped consumerist culture grossly limits a radical user-led analysis of psychiatric power and political economy. To illustrate my point, I look to a larger organization in their affiliate network. Like the Icarus Project, MindFreedom International (MFI) is a mainstay in the psychiatric survivor and Mad movement with multiple branches worldwide. On October 10, 2011, MFI launched a new international campaign called Occupy Normal or Boycott Normal (MindFreedom International website, "Occupy Normal"). On the same day in Eugene, Oregon, MFI coordinated guerilla theatre to "outcrazy" the Chamber of Commerce. As indicated by its namesake, Occupy Normal is an effort by MFI to "[link] mental health consumer/psychiatric survivor issues to Occupy and other movements" in the hope of initiating united actions in the future (MindFreedom International website, "Teleconference on Working with Occupy Movement").

Occupy Wall Street and other Occupy demonstrations are an ongoing movement organized against global structural inequality and corporate greed initiated by *Adbusters*, an anti-consumerist magazine based in Vancouver (NPR, 2011). One objective of Boycott Normal is to challenge the ongoing creation of psychiatric labels in the *Diagnostic and Statistical Manual of Mental Disorders*. The director of MFI, David Oaks, envisions users, survivors, and their allies joining the Occupy movement as providers of alternative mental health services such as peer support to protestors and the homeless in the public spaces in which demonstrations are being held (Oaks, Imai & Erickson, 2011). Oaks posits that if crazy exists, normal is reprehensible because it represents the current financial and climate crisis. Collaborating with Oaks is Aki Imai, a clinical psychology student leading a blog campaign to encourage people to share their experiences of hope after getting psychiatric labels, a campaign he likens to Dan Savage and Terry Miller's (2011) *It Gets Better*. Imai believes mental health users have an affinity with Occupy protestors based on his observation that increasing unemployment correlates with North America's increased psychiatric labelling.

Repeatedly during Oaks' October 8, 2011, web radio broadcast for the launch of Boycott Normal neither he nor his guests connect the American economy and mental

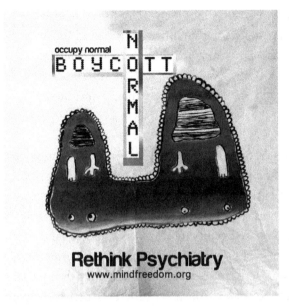

FIGURE 20.1: Boycott Normal

MindFreedom International, directed by David Oaks and centred in Eugene, Oregon, is one of the world's leading psychiatric rights organizations. MindFreedom's Boycott Normal campaign exhorts us to "peacefully occupy the mental health industry" and "unite in an international campaign to question how psychiatric corporations violate our human rights by trying to control us and our democracy through enforcement of 'normal,' with harmful labeling, forced drugging and electroshock."

Source: MindFreedom International

health to racial governance. For example, cross-disability leader and MFI board member Krista Erickson argues during Oaks' broadcast that "Normal has done what? Wrecked the planet and it's done a really good job of wrecking the economy ... maybe we should occupy it." By making class relations synonymous with normal, both Oaks and Erickson construct crazy subjects (Mad people) as a natural subversion of corporate greed and as the natural subject of Occupy. However, this double dichotomy between normal/crazy and rich/poor has played into the white liberal discourse of the Occupy movement. In alternative media and the blogosphere, there is increasing criticism of Occupy. Desjarlait (2011) argues that Occupy has only understood financial inequity through white and black and argues red and brown peoples of the Americas have suffered financial inequity "ever since the oppressors first invaded our shores" (para. 3). He further states that

the core message seems to be that corporate America and the wealthy need to share the profits. Certainly, one can't argue with that. But the question is—how are these profits made? The profits of the wealthy are made through industries they own. These industries fuel and generate profits. And they create jobs and programs. The mining, oil, and energy industries generate enormous profits. And those profits come at a cost to Indian Country, to say nothing of the environment in general. (Desjarlait, 2011, para. 14–15)

Desjarlait's observations leave us asking ourselves: How can we occupy land that is already occupied?

Echoing Desjarlait, Shiri Pasternak (2011) has drawn attention to the political economy of Indigenous dispossession in Canada, stating:

There are over 2,600 Indian reserves across Canada today. This forced resettlement resulted in a unique spatial phenomenon that unwittingly placed Indian reserves on the frontier of vital national and regional boundaries: frontiers, for example, for natural resource extraction, suburban development, military training grounds, oceans and in-land waterways, state borders, and energy generation. (para. 12)

If demarginalizing Indigenous peoples is relevant at all to MFI, rather than "occupying" normal, psychiatric survivors and Mad people need to consider how we are variously oppressed and at times complicit in each other's oppression. It behooves us to reflect on how psychiatry, psychology, and related disciplines have not only dehumanized us with labels or forced treatment, but also structured rights to citizenship and to land, with profound effects on the racial consciousness of Canada. Besides the inherent trouble with the term "occupy," black queer writer and activist Kenyan Farrow criticizes the rampant comparisons to slavery in the Wall Street protests: "What's the difference between saying these young white kids are slaves to banks and Michele Bachmann saying slavery wasn't so bad for black families?" (Sterling & Farrow, 2011, October 15). Desjarlait, Pasternak, and Farrow all suggest that we are called to the task of "doing our homework" so that our demands for economic justice are historically specific and comprehensive.

Imai's inspiration from Savage's It Gets Better campaign also returns my discussion to the politics of feeling and my call for a progressive critique of Mad cultural production. Jasbir Puar (2010) suggests that the It Gets Better campaign has worked to generate sympathy for reinstating the privilege of whiteness lost in queer sexuality and sidelines the present-day struggles of people of colour. The expectation of getting better is foregrounded on the expectation that we are still normal, too. Savage recommends that queer youth pursue happiness through achieving white gay normalcy: buy a condo, travel, have a family. Ironically, this is probably not Imai's message to psychiatric user-survivors, but Puar's (2009) point illustrates how we need to carefully consider the movements we choose to appropriate, let alone build solidarity with. Erickson and Imai's resistance against diagnostic representations of people's lived experiences also marginalizes other forms of "psy" interventions on the lives of people of colour, such as cultural competence.

Building a Lateral Consciousness

Frequently racism is understood by users, survivors, and Mad people as an additional oppression superimposed onto the conditions of mental health service users. Within sanist institutions, racism is conceptualized as a personal affect, or everyday attitude held individually by medical staff that further marginalizes the dehumanizing experiences of institutionalized patients. Racism is also understood to contribute to the conditions that "add up" to arriving or being indefinitely held at an asylum, perhaps through "factors" such as literacy. A pluralist approach to intersectional analysis of race and madness, while a heuristic tool for understanding how multiple oppressions can deepen day-to-day discrimination, neglects a dialectical reading of psy discourse as a set of knowledges that inherently articulate racist and colonial ideologies through biopower—the scientific impetus for the nation-state to make live and let die, or in other words, control quality of life on a mass scale (Foucault, 1997, p. 239). Race-thinking is constructed "in" psy discourse. Limited intervention has been taken by Mad-affiliated scholars and activists against psy discourse as a knowledge and institution that has everything to do with race in the origins and constitution of pathology. I end this chapter by comparing theoretical frameworks used by Indigenous scholars and psychiatric survivors as a relationship-building practice.

Solidarity in Revisiting the Standard Account(s)

Chrisjohn, Young, and Maraun (2006) warn that the turn to "tackle present manifestations of existing, unintentional injuries [from Indian residential schooling] with all the armamentaria of modern social science" is an extension of the total institution of Indian residential schooling (p. 20). The imposition of the colonizer's methods for "healing" their own consequences continues to support white supremacy and "deculturation" (estrangement from your own history). One such continued destruction of inner life through symptom-naming and after-effect-finding is the diagnosis of residential school syndrome (RSS). A relational analysis that locates residential schools and psychiatric disorders within the same violent logic of settler colonial domination, I suggest, radically shifts the standard account of psychiatry critiqued and opposed by Mad culture. Chrisjohn, Young, and Maraun (2006) join two ostensibly different problematics—one that poses the consequences of genocide as an Aboriginal problem, and another that poses mental illness and behavioural dysfunction as everyone's problem—in their observation that "everyone, it seemed, wanted to be a psychologist … [w]hen it came to understanding Indian Residential School[s]" (p. 20). Taking RSS as our fulcrum looking out into the social relations of *madness,* it is possible to see how psychological practices are not only a product of historical context, but a tool for governing different populations in conditions of social unrest. Chrisjohn, Young, and Maraun (2006) explore how RSS is used to pathologize anger and convert public outcry for accountability into survivors being accountable to themselves as traumatized patients. As Puar (2009) describes, "[f]ear of the social—that is, any notion of illness as a form of social unrest or dis-ease—becomes muted through the production of fear of one's own body" (p. 168).

The hegemonic structures Mad activists wish to resist necessarily open up into psychiatry's complicity with genocide(s). Critical medical histories reveal how pathology is articulated in a multitude of racial projects. Jonathan Metzl (2009) asserts that the 1968 revision of the diagnostic criteria for schizophrenia, from problems of emotional disharmony to problems of intellect, was a historically codified way of controlling blackness catalyzed by the Black Power movement. Metzl's (2009) work is relevant to decolonizing resistance due to his analysis of the schizophrenic symptom of "projection," in which patients blame others for characteristics they cannot accept in themselves—a symptom used to depoliticize struggle, specifically black civil rights.

Solidarity through Historicizing Healing

Wastasecoot (2000) contends that Western helping practices oppose her knowledge as a Native woman who adopted and learned from Anishnawbe practices of healing and cleansing, such as the sweatlodge. She supports this critique through comparing and contrasting the practice of sedation and seclusion by psychiatric hospitals against anger work in Native workshops Wastasecoot has facilitated. Wastasecoot (2000) frames anger work within Native teachings that posit all human beings are in harmony with the universe and disharmony occurs through what happens in life. Wastasecoot's (2000) advocacy of alternatives arises from suspicion of labels such as schizophrenia not only because they "sum [Native youth] up into a category from which they were never expected to move," but because such diagnostic trajectories ultimately discourage and further pathologize mental health users for releasing pain (p. 128). Her resistance against mainstream mental health services and her focus on Indigenous healing practices are motivated mainly by the need to listen to people's rage so that they may live, and in living, restore community relationships. Wastasecoot's (2000) desire for an alternative does not begin at preventing the damage mental health practices can do, but at remedying the pattern of lifelong dehumanization that has happened and is still happening to many Indigenous people—a pattern with which Western mental health is complicit.

If people who have experiences being labelled *mad* seek to authenticate their identities outside of mainstream mental health services and wish to find a language to express their pain, this process needs to begin through locating where their unease with the psy knowledge arises. We must ask ourselves: How might my story differentiate from other people's histories within the psy complex? From there, nurturing an identity with integrity may begin with a lateral political consciousness. The use of race as an analogy in the constitution of collective identity is embedded in how social movements relate to one another. Smith (2006) warns that the commodification and slaveability of blackness are perpetuated through the appropriation of Civil Rights discourse without movements fundamentally forming relationships with black people in activist organizing.

During a 2010 keynote address at PsychOUT: A Conference For Organizing Resistance Against Psychiatry, the first global conference of its kind, David Oaks of MindFreedom International described the growing community of survivors by employing phrases such as "like the Civil Rights movement." Likewise, antipsychiatry activists in the Toronto context have referred to indigeneity and colonialism as "similar, but not the same" in reference to psychiatric oppression. What is disconcerting about such comparative analyses is the simultaneous increasing popularity of appropriating spiritual practices such as shamanism in the Mad movement as self-help alternatives, some instances of which I've explored in this chapter, without acknowledging the fight for the ongoing cultural survival of Indigenous spirituality and healing and without contextualizing such non-Eurocentric praxis within multiple ongoing struggles for Indigenous sovereignty. New ageism has had the unsavoury effect of deepening the assumption that Native people are always disappearing and dying, and that their practices can be easily co-opted. New ageism promotes the white settler myth of human kind being universal proprietors of mother earth—a narrative emptied out of histories of displacement. Theorizing psychiatric violence as being like racism or like colonialism writes out the existence and relevance of colonial gender violence in the foundations and ruling organization of mental health services.

CHAPTER 21

Spaces in Place:
Negotiating Queer In/visibility within Psychiatric and Mental Health Service Settings

Andrea Daley

Introduction

In this chapter I present a conceptual framework that depicts the complex and layered processes of negotiating queer in/visibility within psychiatric and mental health service settings. The framework emerged from qualitative research that explored the psychiatric and mental health service experiences of queer women, and is constituted by three intersecting spaces: body space (self), intersubjective space (between service providers and women), and "real" space (organizational). The conceptual framework directs attention to the things that drag upon queer women as they move through psychiatric and mental health services, and that allow and delimit their performances of queer. The conceptual framework implicates the productive effect of intersecting body, intersubjective, and "real" spaces on performances of "queer" while complicating these performances as dynamic, subtle, tentative, complex, and layered.

I will advance this chapter in a series of steps. I begin by providing a backdrop to the conceptual framework, which includes a brief description of the women that informed its development, and an examination of the notions of space that undergird the framework. Next, I provide an overview of the framework by describing its structure (surfaces) and content (elements) as well as elucidate the language of "negotiating in/visibility." I conclude the chapter with a summary of ideas, thoughts, and implications as generated by the conceptual framework.

Background
A Queer Informed Framework

The conceptual framework presented in this chapter emerged from research that explored psychiatric and mental health services in relation to women's queer sexuality. Women informed the development of the conceptual framework through their participation in individual interviews based on their experiences as women who self-identified as lesbian (18), bisexual (2), two-spirited (1), and not subscribing to sexual identity labels (1) and who have been extensively involved with psychiatric and mental health services. A total of 22 diversely situated women participated, based on sexual orientation/identity, race/ethnicity, age, diagnoses received, employment and professional status, income, and experience and knowledge of hospital- and community-based mental health service settings. These women's experiences occurred over a period of 5 to 20 years of involvement with psychiatric and mental health services, and within a range of general and population-specific services (e.g., women, ethno-cultural, and lesbian, gay, bisexual and transgender).

Intersecting Spaces

This conceptual framework is premised on two concepts related to the materiality of women's bodies and the notion of space—body space and material space. The notion of "body space" is defined by Butler and Parr (1999) as including the "immediate envelope of space which the body occupies in moving around and 'doing things'" (Butler & Parr, 1999, p. 13). In this sense, "body space" includes culturally located discursive meanings, which frame and inscribe women's bodies (Butler & Parr, 1999). Conceptualizations of materiality developed by Bordo (1998) and Brown (2000) resonate with Parr and Butler's (1999) notion of "body space." For Bordo (1998), attending to the materiality of bodies means retaining a notion of the reality that hegemonic gender and sexuality discourses of society create a substantial reality for gendered and sexualized bodies—a reality in which bodies suffer (Hekman, 1998). Thus, Bordo (1998) argues that what it means for a body to be gendered and sexualized must be contextualized in space and time, and suggests that this meaning shifts across time and space.

Similarly, Brown (2000) directs attention to the immediate context as a powerful structuration of performativity by juxtaposing "real" (material) space with the notion of space as metaphorical. As a metaphor, space is conceptualized as a sign that alludes to certain kinds of locations, distance, accessibility, and interaction. For example, a common spatial metaphor associated with queer sexualities—"the closet"—has come to signify both the psychological and social dimension of alienation as a broad effect of homophobia and heterosexism (Brown, 2000). Similarly, with respect to women and madness, the spatial metaphor of the "Madwoman" is often invoked by feminist literary theorists to signify women's anger and protest or submission and surrender (Caminero-Santangelo, 1998). Either way, the "Madwoman," as a spatial metaphor, signals women's relations to a social position (Openheimer, in Caminero-Santangelo, 1998), as well as women's rejection of the social order and the inscription of gender and sexuality norms.

Alternatively, "real" space is conceived as substantially more than metaphor—it is concrete and dynamic. "Real" space does not simply represent power, it materializes it—that is, space is realized as a dimension of all social relations by which knowledge/power gets materialized in the world (Brown, 2000). In this regard, "the closet" also signifies the material production of heterosexism (ibid). Similarly, the "Madwoman"

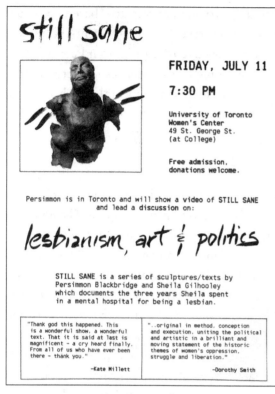

FIGURE 21.1: Still Sane

The 1985 book *Still Sane* by Persimmon Blackbridge and Sheila Gilhooly is a lacerating account of Blackbridge's three-year psychiatric confinement following the divulgence of her lesbian identity to a psychiatric professional. The exhibit advertised here (re)presented these experiences through an innovative multimedia forum of artwork and text.

Source: Psychiatric Survivor Archives of Toronto, 1985.

does not simply signify women's rejection of the social order but signifies the material (re)containing of women who transgress gender and sexuality norms, and hence, signifies the material production of heteropatriarchal discourse.

The usefulness of the construct of "real" space is its strength to capture the interactions between questions of the performative construction of gender and sexuality and questions of institutions. Implicit in this statement is an understanding of space as both produced by and productive of identities and broader social relations (Brown, 2000; Curran, 2005; Probyn, 1995). As such, the conceptual framework presented in this chapter locates women's queer bodies within the "real" heteropatriarchal space of psychiatric and mental health service settings. While it is not within the scope of this discussion to provide a full exploration of psychiatric and mental health spaces as heteropatriarchal space, I will suggest that a) heterosexual epistemologies and research discourses; b) historical and contemporary psychiatric discourses on women (gender), sexuality, and "mental illness"; and c) heteronormative health and institutional sexual behaviour policies constitute conditions that produce heteropatriarchal psychiatric space (Daley, unpublished). Heterosexual epistemologies and psychiatric and mental health research discourses are implicated in the relative absence of queer sexualities in research and/or the production of a unitary, singular queer subject. Psychiatric discourses on women (gender), sexuality, and "mental illness" interact with lay public discourses to reify the cultural norm of compulsory heterosexuality (Butler, 1999). Similarly, through an adherence to "non-specificity," health and institutional sexual behaviour policy (re)produces heteronormative notions of gender and sexuality (Daley, unpublished).

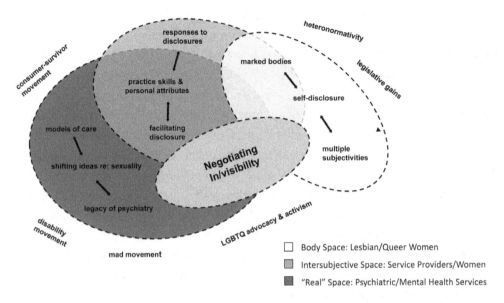

FIGURE 21.2: Negotiating In/visibility

This conceptual framework, depicting the complex and layered processes of negotiating queer in/visibility within psychiatric and mental health service settings, involves three intersecting surfaces of body space, intersubjective space, and "real" space.

Source: Andrea Daley

The Conceptual Framework: Negotiating In/visibility

The conceptual framework (Figure 21.2) represents the culmination of women's lived ideas, opinions, and experiences. It also reflects the richness and depth of queer women's experiences and knowledges related to psychiatric and mental health services. Importantly, the ideas, opinions, and experiences of women that constitute the framework are not constrained to a particular psychiatric and mental health service time and space, but rather represent a culmination of ideas, opinions, and experiences across time and space. The women who participated in the study recalled stories and experiences emerging from their extensive involvement with the psychiatric and mental health system as consumers/survivors and/or mental health service providers over time, and within a variety of hospital- and community-based mental health settings. Their experiences are not representative of all queer women involved with the psychiatric and mental health system; nevertheless, they offer depth and breadth towards an understanding of the psychiatric and mental health service experiences to performances of queer.

The Surfaces and Associated Elements

The conceptual framework depicts the complex and layered process of negotiating in/visibility by drawing together various elements within three intersecting surfaces represented as body space, intersubjective space, and "real" space. Body space refers to the material bodies and subjective experiences of queer women. Intersubjective space includes mental health service providers; however, it refers more specifically to the space in which service providers and queer women interact/exchange/share "subjective states" (Scheff et al., 2006). "Real" space refers to institutions, organizations, and agencies where mental health services are provided. Importantly, the size and location of each surface does not correspond with its significance, rather each surface has a productive effect towards the materialization of queer identities and broader social relations, and thus, influences women's subjective experiences of queer sexuality.

The three intersecting surfaces representative of queer bodies, mental health service providers/women interactions, and psychiatric and mental health services are constituted by particular elements. The interconnectedness of elements within and between the three intersecting surfaces is depicted by the broken circles that demarcate their boundaries and the two-headed arrows that connect the elements. Each element will be explored in turn.

Body Space—Lesbian/Queer Women

The elements enclosed within the surface (on the right side of the figure) representing the material bodies and subjective experiences of queer women—*body space*—include marked bodies, self-disclosure processes, and multiple subjectivities. The term "marked bodies" refers to women's understandings of their sexuality; the heterosexist myths, stereotypes, and beliefs about queer sexuality to which they have been exposed; and their experiences of self-disclosing to family and friends. The notion of marked bodies suggests that queer women enter into relationships with psychiatric and mental health services from particular standpoints and as particularly inscribed bodies based on life experiences related to self-understandings, the violence of lesbophobia, biphobia, homophobia and heterosexism, and the support and affirmation—or not—of family and friends. In addition, the term "marked bodies" acknowledges that the intersection between sexuality and age, race, relationship status, and gender performance inscribes women's bodies in particular ways. "Marked bodies" is closely associated with "self-disclosure processes." Women articulated an understanding of self-disclosure processes in relation to their understanding and self-affirmation of queer sexuality. This was determined, in part, by the extent to which they internalized and/or navigated/resisted negative and disparaging stereotypes and beliefs about queer sexuality, as well as their range of experiences of support and affirmation from family and friends.

The element "multiple subjectivities" represents women's experiences, suggesting that subjectivity based on sexuality, although significant, is only one aspect of self that must be negotiated within the context of psychiatric and mental health services. In addition, "multiple subjectivities" refers to women's recognition that some queer women will be required, or will "choose," to subjugate a sexualized subject position some of the time in order to prioritize other subjectivity-related concerns including those related to race and class.

Intersubjective Space—Sharing Subjective States

The elements enclosed by the circle in the middle of the figure include those that are associated with service provider interactions with queer women—*intersubjective space*. These include service provider responses to women's self-disclosures, general practice skills and personal attributes, and facilitating self-disclosure processes during their interactions with queer women. Women described relevant service provider-related factors that influence self-disclosure including: a) responses by service providers that pathologize and problematize their sexuality/desire, b) microaggressions practised by service providers, and c) providers' ability to "pick up" nuanced expressions of lesbian/queer sexuality (Daley, 2011). While the elements within the surface are differentiated from one another, women described the elements as intersecting and reinforcing one another in ways that convey overt and/or covert messages of recognition/non-recognition, acceptance/non-acceptance, and affirmation/non-affirmation (Daley, 2010).

"Real" Space—Psychiatric and Mental Health Services

The elements that constitute the surface on the left side of the figure are representative of agency, organizational, and institutionalized philosophies and practices related to equity, gender and sexuality, and understandings of madness and associated treatments—*"real" space*. Included on this surface are: models of care (i.e., medical, feminist, cultural); the legacy of psychiatry in regulating and pathologizing women's sexuality and "homosexuality"; and shifting ideas and beliefs about women (gender), sexuality, and madness. The elements that constitute this surface contribute to the characterization of the range of psychiatric and mental health services as an uneven terrain that must be skillfully negotiated by queer women.

Beyond Three Intersecting Spaces

Circulating outside of the intersecting body, intersubjective, and "real" spaces are social forces that bump up against and shape the experiences of queer women, service provider interactions, and psychiatric and mental health services. The broken lines enclosing the various surfaces imply an intersection and interaction not only between the surfaces but also between beliefs, attitudes, and practices related to women (gender), sexuality, and madness within the broader social and structural context. These beliefs, attitudes, and practices are represented by: consumer/survivor/ex-patient, disability, and Mad movements (e.g., challenging normative psychiatric discourse); legislative gains in civil rights for lesbian, gay, bisexual, transgender, and queer (LGBTQ) communities (e.g., same-sex marriage); and LGBTQ health-related advocacy and activism (e.g., challenges to institutionalized practices related to "gender identity disorder" and proposed DSM-5 revisions related to sexuality and gender-related disorders).[1] Importantly, the broken line enclosing the surfaces allows for a circling back to the beginning of this narrative that identifies the impact of women's understandings of their sexuality; the heterosexist myths, stereotypes, and beliefs about queer sexuality to which they have been exposed; and their experiences of self-disclosing to family and friends. More specifically, the broken line around the "real" space surface allows for the possibility that the beliefs, attitudes, and practices outside of the immediate "real" space of psychiatric and mental health services impact the subjective experiences of queer women and processes of negotiating in/visibility.

Coming to Terms: "Negotiating In/visibility"

"Negotiating"

The conceptual framework centres "negotiating in/visibility" in relation to the intersecting surfaces, and as a primary organizing theme of queer women's experiences during their interactions with psychiatric and mental health services. The choice to use the term *negotiating* was made in consideration of two factors. First, it was chosen based on women's descriptions of self-disclosure as processes characterized by the presence of dialogue and exchange, or rather, "conference, discussion, and compromise" (Hawker, 2003, p. 409), either with themselves (i.e., resisting reconstructions based on service provider responses and microaggressions; prioritizing subjectivities) and/or service providers (i.e., general practice skills and personal attributes; interpreting nuanced expressions of queer sexuality; facilitating disclosure through a sequence of subtle and tentative strategies). The term *negotiating* may be contrasted with the term *managing*. The term *managing*, defined as "to handle or direct with a degree of skill" (ibid, p. 376), seemed appropriate in terms of representing women's expertise in their decisions to engage, or not, in self-disclosure processes. However, it implies a unidirectional process in that one would direct, control, or lead. This fails to capture self-disclosure processes as dynamic and fluid exchanges that occur within, and are influenced by, intersubjective space and the "real" space of psychiatric and mental health services. Second, the term *negotiate* was also chosen based on its meaning, "to successfully travel along or over" (ibid, p. 409). In this regard, the term *negotiate* aptly depicts women's experiences of travelling within and between the uneven terrain of recognition/non-recognition, acceptance/non-acceptance, and affirmation/non-affirmation as experienced within intersubjective and "real" spaces (Daley, 2010).

"In/visibility"

The term *in/visibility* recognizes that queer women embody gender and sexuality differently, and consequently are seen as differently gendered and sexualized subjects contingent upon the intersection between body, intersubjective, and "real" spaces.

Women who described performing normative gender (i.e., normative performances of femininity based on dress, hairstyle, mannerisms, etc.) within (heteropatriarchal) psychiatric and mental health service spaces and during their interactions with mental health service providers often described feeling "unseen" or invisible as queer women (e.g., assumed to be heterosexual/straight). Conversely, women who described transgressing normative gender roles (i.e., performed masculinity through dress, hairstyle, and mannerisms) within similar spaces and interactions often described feeling very "seen" or visible as queer. As such, both groups of women describe an experience of only ever being "seen" or visible as a singular subject, that is, visible or invisible as a sexualized subject. In terms of queer subjectivity, the range of experiences described by women, which are based on a heteronormative assumption of a coherence of relationship between gender and sexuality (Butler, 1999), might be cumulatively represented through the term *in/visibility*.

The use of the term *in/visibility* is also an attempt to capture the effects of women's use of multiple mental health services in relation to intersecting identities based on sexuality, race/ethnicity, and class. Women's insights and experiences suggest that they negotiate their in/visibility differently across various psychiatric and mental health service settings. Women indicated that they experienced a greater level of safety, and likelihood of, performing "queer" within community-based, LGBTQ- and women-specific mental health services as compared to hospital- or institutionally based services. They described being more likely to be subjected to signifiers of heteronormativity within hospital- or institutionally based contexts and associated interactions with service providers. For example, they were more likely to be asked questions that assumed heterosexuality (e.g., explored their interest in men only) and subjected to reassurances of "normality"—"someday you will get married [to a man] and have children." Importantly, within these contexts similar differences were described by women in relation to their experiences across programs within a single institution. Thus, the term *in/visibility* functions to represent women's experiences of simultaneously being "seen" and "unseen" as contingent on space.

This is not to say that women described the practices of community-based, LGBTQ- and women-specific programs as absolute in their performances of queer. In fact, some women described relative silence in relation to sexuality compared to gender and race within some community-based and women-specific programs. However, it was not suggested that community-based and women-specific programs necessarily rendered queer sexuality visible through pathologizing and problematizing discourses. Rather, given the foregrounding of gender and race within these contexts, women were as likely to be pulled into a "matrix of intelligibility" (Butler, 1999) as gendered and/or raced subjects while subjectivity based on sexuality was subjugated. As such, the term *in/visibility* is responsive to women's experiences of negotiating multiple subjectivities beyond that of a singular queer subjectivity.

Implications: "Out" in Space/"Out" Space

The conceptual framework directs attention to the productive effect of intersecting body, intersubjective, and "real" spaces on women's experiences of in/visibility in relation to queer sexuality. In this regard, Dyck (1995) states:

> Attention to the body in the material ["real"] context provides the potential for exploring the involvement of dominant discourses, concrete practices, and power relations in the construction of gendered and sexualized subjectivities. (p. 308)

This statement resonates with Probyn's (2003) call for a knowing of the things (ideologies, institutions, bodies, distances, emotions, noises, smells) that "drag … upon us as we move through space" (p. 291), and which allow and delimit performances of self. The surfaces of the conceptual framework represent the spaces that women occupy—or that occupy women—including the material space of body, the intersubjective space of service providers and service users, and the "real" space of psychiatric and mental health services. The elements that constitute the surfaces represent those "things" that queer women must come to know, evaluate, and negotiate as related to their performances of "queer."

Conceivably, from the perspective of queer women the conceptual framework may represent a kind of collective safety map produced from their aggregated experiences. Von Schulthess (1992) offers the concept of "safety maps" to describe how members of sexual minority communities (LGBTQ) assess potential danger or risk to personal safety associated with their visibility as sexual minorities. Safety maps are described as

> an ever-changing, personalized, yet shared, matrix of attributes and relations that individuals employ to make their way in public and private space. In constructing these maps individuals draw upon their knowledge of the ways in which specific variables render them vulnerable to personal danger. (Mason, 2001, p. 29)

Mason (2001) suggests that the ways in which safety maps are produced are influenced by the type of violence to which people believe they are vulnerable. What is particularly relevant to this exploration of queer women's experiences in relation to the spaces of psychiatric and mental health services is the notion of symbolic gendered, lesbophobic, biphobic, and homophobic violence. Mason (2001) emphasizes that violence does not have to be experienced to have repercussions, but rather we must consider the "symbolism of homophobic violence" (p. 30). She states:

> The symbolism of homophobic violence is contingent upon the extent to which an individual first recognizes his/her own vulnerability in the victimization of others with similar identities or lifestyles, and second, interprets abusive, hostile and violent acts within a continuum of possible interconnected dangers. (Mason, 2001, p. 30)

The notion of symbolic violence is particularly significant to the psychiatric regulation of gender and sexuality. As such, the implications of symbolic violence are not confined to those queer women who experience only the violence itself. Rather, women's articulation of the historical and contemporary violence caused by lay public and psychiatric pathologizing and problematizing of women's non-normative expressions of sexuality and "homosexuality" suggests that they are acutely aware of the symbolism of lesbophobic, biphobic, and homophobic psychiatric violence. Women expressed an acute understanding of the precarious position they held within institutions that have been conferred with the symbolic and material power to regulate gender and sexuality. For example, women were subjected to service provider responses to self-disclosure processes that pathologized and problematized their performances of "queer." These responses may be conceptualized as representing the symbolic power of psychiatry to (re)configure and (re)contain women who transgress normative performances of gender and sexuality—as well as those who do not (Daley, 2011). A focus on symbolic power does not negate the very real violence and harm inflicted through such processes; this very real violence and harm was clearly evidenced by women's responses that valorized self-disclosure and service provider responses that recognize, accept, and affirm queer sexuality in relation to women's well-being and recovery (Daley, 2010).

From the perspective of mental health service providers and psychiatric and mental health services, the conceptual framework may comprise a planning map towards the development of "out" space—that is, foster understandings/approaches, policy, and practices that facilitate the possibility, or probability, of supporting women's own representations of queer. I make this statement with recognition that the power of service provider responses and institutional forces to reconstruct or reconfigure women as queer is simply one half of the interaction between the "practices and schemas" (Crossley, 2004, p. 162) of lay public discourses—those "things" beyond the three intersecting spaces—and psychiatric and mental health discourses on women (gender), sexuality, and madness.

Bartlett, King, and Smith (2004) offer an example of the interactive effect between lay public and psychiatric discourses in their report on the experiences of professionals who administered and evaluated treatments for "homosexuality," such as aversion therapy with electroshock and psychoanalysis, in Britain since the 1950s. Bartlett et al. suggest, based on qualitative interviews with various types of mental health clinicians, that an interaction between public morality (i.e., sex/gender and sexuality norms) and professional authority led to a naturalizing of cultural norms that pathologized "homosexuality." For example, one clinical psychologist stated:

> With hindsight I look back and say that's just part of the horror stories of the 1950s and 1960s of general homophobia. The fact that it had a theoretical underpinning was true but essentially an element. *Nobody would have thought of using that theory to treat homosexuals had there not been this great big kerfuffle about homosexuality that was still existent.* (Bartlett et al., 2004, p. 2, emphasis mine)

In terms of the conceptual framework then, consideration must be given to how body space, the already inscribed material bodies of queer women as an outcome of public morality, intersects with service provider responses (the intersubjective space) and the heteropatriarchal space of psychiatric and mental health services ("real" space) to impact queer women's negotiation of in/visibility. For example, women suggested that the reactions of family and friends to their self-disclosures that associated their sexuality with "illness" or "cause of illness" were similar to those of service providers reactions that subtly, and not so subtly, pathologized and problematized queer sexuality.

This suggests that one of the tasks of psychiatric and mental health services and service providers is to understand how professional and institutionalized practices and policy reflect and reproduce heteropatriarchal lay public metaphors and psychiatric discourses on women (gender), sexuality, and madness. A second task is to understand how heteropatriarchal lay public metaphors and psychiatric discourses on women (gender), sexuality, and madness intersect within the spaces of psychiatric and mental health services to impact how queer women negotiate in/visibility. And finally, and importantly, psychiatric and mental health services and service providers must begin to identify and implement practice and policy changes in response to these understandings.

Conclusions

I have presented a conceptual framework that suggests that to know the experiences of lesbian/queer women requires the placing of women's queer bodies in the context of mental health service provider interactions and psychiatric and mental health services. The conceptual framework implicates the productive effect of intersecting body, intersubjective, and "real" spaces on performances of "queer" while complicating these performances as complex and layered. The chapter contributes to existing theorizing on space and the performance of subjectivity based on women's gender and sexuality with its specific focus on psychiatric and mental health service settings.

Note

1 The American Psychiatric Association (APA) is in the process of revising the current version of the *Diagnostic and Statistical Manual of Mental Disorders* (DSM-IV-TR) towards the publication of the DSM-5 in 2013. At the time of writing, the proposed DSM-5 will include a range of diagnoses that include an exclusive focus on sexuality (e.g., paraphilias) and gender (gender dysphoria) that continue to rely on heteronormative constructs of gender (e.g., femininity and masculinity) and expressions of desire. As such, these diagnoses may have a disproportionate negative impact on LGBTQ people and communities.

CHAPTER 22

Rerouting the Weeds: The Move from Criminalizing to Pathologizing "Troubled Youth" in *The Review of the Roots of Youth Violence*

Jijian Voronka

During the summer of 2007, following the shooting death of a Grade 9 student in a Toronto high school, Premier Dalton McGuinty commissioned former Chief Justice and Attorney General Roy McMurtry and former Speaker of the Legislature Alvin Curling to investigate the epidemic of "youth violence" in Ontario. A panel of inquiry was put in place to "help identify and analyse the underlying causes contributing to youth violence and provide recommendations for Ontario to move forward" (McMurtry & Curling, 2008b). As a result, in November of 2008, *The Review of the Roots of Youth Violence* (hereafter referred to as *The Review)* report was released to the public. This chapter will examine what knowledge is produced through this report, in the province's attempts to understand and prevent the roots of youth violence. Specifically, I want to inquire, through a textual analysis of *The Review*, what stories about madness, race, and violence are created and maintained through this text. Ultimately, the provincial narrative that emerges from this review has a productive function that works to solidify notions of Ontario as a white province, and allows for the construction of actionable policy recommendations aimed at "caring, curing, and controlling" Mad racialized bodies in Ontario (Hanafi, 2009b, p. 8).

Premier McGuinty launched the inquiry because he felt that "no parent should ever have to worry about losing their child to violence," and that as a province we have a responsibility to do everything we can to "make children, schools and communities safer ... and help young people make good choices" (McMurtry & Curling, 2008a, p. 7). Triggered by an incident of youth violence, the inquiry produced, in little over a year, an extensive five-volume report that totals just under 2,000 pages of text. In order to narrow the scope of my analysis, I have concentrated solely on *The Review of the Roots of Youth Violence: Volume 1, Findings, Analysis and Conclusions*—a 400-page text that works as the main body of *The Review*.[1] The stated intent of *The Review* is clear: the province wants to discover what are the "roots" of the problem of youth violence. Those roots are immediately identified as resulting from what the report calls disadvantage: from racism, from poverty, emerging from sites of disadvantaged exception. It is this "disadvantage" with which *The Review* concerns itself. From this inquiry, *The Review* blossoms into a document that acts as a reparation to itself: we are told what is broken, and how the province is to be made whole again.

I start my analysis by looking at how the province of Ontario is framed as a benevolent white settler space, paternally concerned with its "disadvantaged" children. I show how, through the establishment of white settler space as imperilled by raced violence, *The Review* legitimizes its right to intervene. I then examine *how* and *what* racialized subjects are considered in the document, and argue that the approach *The Review* takes disappears the history of white settler colonial violence. I then consider recommendations that *The Review* advances to cure the problem of raced violence, many of which ask for an increase in mental health services for children and youth in targeted sites of exception. I end with a critique of *The Review*'s proposal to solve over-criminalization in racialized inner-city slums by substituting such governance with mental health services. I understand this shift as a move away from overt policing through the criminal justice system, to a more subtle system of self-governance that asks racialized communities to individually pathologize the problem of collective systemic oppression.

Province-Building: Ontario, Ours to Discover

The Review begins at the same site that I want to begin: in the grounded territory of the province. From the first page, and repeated throughout the text, we are informed that "Ontario is at a crossroads":

> While it is a safe place for most, our review identified deeply troubling trends in the nature of serious violent crime involving youth in Ontario and the impacts it is having on many communities. Those trends suggest that, unless the roots of this violence are identified and addressed in a coordinated, collaborative and sustained way, violence will get worse. More people will be killed, communities will become increasingly isolated and disadvantaged, an ever-accelerating downward cycle will ensue for far too many, and *our social fabric as a province could be seriously damaged.* (McMurtry & Curling, 2008a, p. 1, emphasis mine).

We, as a suddenly imperilled province, have hit a fork in the road: how we proceed will determine our future. The image of a crossroads acts as a literal dividing practice that informs us what is at stake: we can either confront, contain, and cure raced violence, or we can succumb to it. As the review imagines for us, "we believe that Ontario is at a crossroads. One of the two main roads leading from that crossroads will, with strong leadership and sustained commitment, lead us towards an ever-safer society with increasing security and opportunity for all. The other will lead to an entrenched cycle of violence, which could plague this province and limit its potential for years to come" (McMurtry & Curling, 2008a, p. 83).

We stand at a crossroads, and we are being asked to choose what road to take. Through the tropes of haunting and racial paranoia, our social fabric is being torn at by the notion that "nits make lice" (Smith, 2005, p. 80). Stemming from one particularly high-profile act of spectacular high school gun violence, the province has determined that the goodness of our respectable white settler province is in jeopardy, and it is now that we must intervene. Ruth Gilmore talks about how moments of spectacular violence are used to harness interventions on problematized bodies: "The 'terrible few' are a statistically insignificant and socially unpredictable handful of the planet's humans whose psychopathic actions are the stuff of folktales, tabloids (including the evening news and reality television), and emerging legislation.... The media, government officials, and policy advisers endlessly refer to 'the public's concern' over crime and connect prison growth to public desire for social order" (Gilmore, 2007, pp. 15, 17). Through this moral panic, we make demands on our nation to act, and the province has responded through *The Review* by unveiling to us knowledge that all is not right with the province's "disadvantaged." Spectacular violence, when harnessed by state administration, has the productive value of allowing us as a province justified access and opportunity to collect and produce knowledge on those who are "at risk," and who pose a risk to us (for further reading on moral panics and "at-risk" youth management, see Barron & Lacombe, 2005; Wotherspoon & Schissel, 2001).

As a nation, and more locally as a province, *The Review* documents that we are in jeopardy. To paraphrase Andrea Smith, Canada is not at war; Canada *is* war. For the system of white settler supremacy to stay in place, Canada must always be at war (Smith, 2005, p. 69). Through *The Review*, we are confirmed in our fear that our (read: white) province is under constant threat by unpredictable raced violence, and *The Review* works to allow us to know, intervene, and discipline the racialized bodies that pose threats to our civility. Our province is at a crossroads, under threat by those outside the core of our social fabric, and our white supremacy must be defended at any cost. As Martinot and Sexton note:

> Owing to the instability of white supremacy, the social structures of whiteness must ever be re-secured in an obsessive fashion. The process of re-inventing whiteness and white supremacy has always involved the state, and the state has always involved the utmost paranoia.... White supremacy is not reconstructed simply for its own sake, but for the sake of the social paranoia, the ethic of impunity, and the violent spectacles of racialization that it calls "the mainte-nance of order." (Martinot & Sexton, 2003, pp. 179–180)

One productive value of *The Review* is its construction of white settler supremacy as being under threat, in the process offering a multitude of interventions that will recreate and maintain the status quo. The specific focus of *The Review* on "disadvantaged" populations (poor racialized inner-city bodies) adds and sustains a discourse that demonstrates "a specific obsession with those denigrated that characterizes the socius of white supremacy, its demands for allegiance, its conditions of membership … derogation comes in many forms—as stories, aphorisms, discourses, legal statuses, political practices. The reputation of derogation becomes the performance of white supremacist identity, over and over" (Martinot & Sexton, 2003, pp. 174–175). *The Review* calls not only on those who are under threat by the Other to be vigilant, but also depends on those "at risk" to identify, know, and come to discipline themselves through the tools, training, education, methods, recommendations, and resources that are identified and offered throughout this report. In this very crucial way, Ontario's spaces of exception come to be permeable through benevolent interventions, and "slum administration replaces colonial administration. The city belongs to the settlers and the sullying of civilized society through the presence of the racial Other in white space gives rise to a careful management of boundaries within urban space" (Razack, 2002, p. 128).

We are told in *The Review* over and over that we must act in order to prevent further trauma to our social fabric. In a particularly telling passage on why we must act now against the terror of youth violence, the analogy of a disease outbreak is invoked to illustrate how we cannot risk being careless:

> If these trends and impacts are seen as akin to a public health issue, then it makes no more sense for those not immediately affected to blame those who suffer from them, and otherwise ignore them, than it would to ignore an infectious disease outbreak in one community or neighbourhood. We know infections can spread and, even if they don't they can weaken other parts of the body and its systems, with regrettable mid- to long-term consequences. Therefore, we deal with the problem collectively and cure it, because ignoring it will simply make matters worse for ever-increasing parts of our body politic. (McMurtry & Curling, 2008a, p. 102)

Likening both raced youth violence and the problem of "disadvantaged" inequities to a plague is a rhetorical tool that turns socially produced structures of oppression into scientific facts that can be mediated through the impartial reign of biomedicines. No one is implicated, it is all just fact, and it makes common sense to spatially attack the bodies and sites in which this problem resides. There is no room in this account for the non-reasonable pain that leaks out of these interventions, that permeates *The Review*. There is no language for "the haunting," for the racism that exists beyond words. Rather, *The Review* depends on and harnesses "the language of common sense, through which we bespeak our social world in the most common way, [and which] leaves us speechless before the enormity of the usual, of the business of civil procedures" (Martinot & Sexton, 2003, p. 172). *The Review*, in calling on common sense and the common good—and on unveiling the story of raced youth violence—becomes the hero that is equipped to intervene on the racialized incivility that is erupting in corners of this clean province. Further, while always ignoring structural violence, it is white settlers who come to suffer from the sight of it, and must be called in on the adventure to stop it.

Before delving into what *The Review* says, I just want to mark *who says it*. The proverbial "we" that penetrates the text is a white settler "we," and the assumed readers and writers are always unraced whites. Indeed, the text thoroughly understands race to be a problem of blackness, and occasionally of aboriginality.[2] But the might that is white that thoroughly structures the text is unquestionably universalized. Despite *The Review*'s constant emphasis on incorporating critical race theory, culturally appropriate and sensitive services, governances, and so on, the entry point to this topic is always through the lens of unraced whiteness. Statements such as "we were taken aback by the extent to which racism is alive and well and wreaking its deeply harmful effects on Ontarians and on the very fabric of this province" (McMurtry & Curling, 2008a, p. 39), and "recent instances of racial profiling and other related matters of course kept the issue [of racism] alive for us as it did for many, but perhaps hid the depths to which racism is ever more embedded throughout our society" (McMurtry & Curling, 2008a, p. 39), illustrate that the standpoint that the provincial "we" speaks from is one that is unquestionably that of the white bystander, surprised and unaffected by racism.

Thus, *The Review* as a body replicates that too familiar journey that respectability constantly engages in, creating an "us" through exploring a "them." The task of producing knowledge on the Other once again leads white settler subjects to "learn who they are, and, more important, who they are not. Moving from respectable space to degenerate space and back again is an adventure that confirms that they are indeed white men in control ... [and] have an unquestioned right to go anywhere and do anything" (Razack, 2002, p. 127). "We" have a right, a duty in fact, not only to protect Others from themselves, but in doing so, work to create ourselves as the harbingers of civility.

(A)voiding Colonial Context

To begin to understand what is sustained through the discourses of *The Review*, I want to start with how racialized bodies are understood as to have *arrived* here. White is of course naturalized, and diasporic immigration is understood within the neoliberalist context of choice:[3]

> Canada and Ontario, in particular, are blessed by their many and diverse immigrant communities. People from around the world have chosen to make Canada their new home and embraced their adopted homeland with affection, passion and energy. People immigrate here for a number of reasons, primarily because they want to succeed and because they want their children to succeed. (McMurtry & Curling, 2008a, p. 74)

Void from this sunny, polite, and welcoming take on multiculturalism is the resolute absence of the historical, structural, and contextual ways in which whiteness is implicated in the forced migration of racialized bodies. I want instead to forefront how racialized bodies dwell on this territory because of white "histories of domination and subordination for which we [as Canadians] are accountable" (Razack, 2002, p. 128). Further, the constant referral to this land as "ours" solidifies white settlers as non-immigrants and indigenous to this land, while denying honest engagement with white settler practices towards Aboriginal peoples.

The disavowal of our genocidal practices towards Aboriginal peoples is exemplified through the stunning statement that *The Review* makes about where Canada stands as a nation in relation to severe violence:

> We need to note that Ontario is in the relatively early phases of this degree and kind of violence. Some of those we met referred to Ontario experiencing the first generation of violence driven by economic disadvantage and racism, compared to the United States and the United Kingdom, which they considered to be more deeply mired in second or third generations of this kind of violence. (McMurtry & Curling, 2008a, p. 103)

The notion that Ontario has only recently begun to engage in racialized and economic violence critically emphasizes where *The Review* is willing to begin the story of violence on this land that is now called Canada. That story in *The Review* largely begins in the 1970s when raced crime statistics began to be harvested to investigate crime divided along race lines. The structural and collective violence that was enacted to secure this province as a white settler territory is rendered invisible through this account. While *The Review* lays claim that it is committed to considering systemic issues, our colonial legacy is completely ignored in this account. Not only does this quote mark us as only beginning to enter into a phase of severe violence, but it also positions us as a less implicated, less violent, middle power nation when compared to the US and the UK: maintaining an understanding of ourselves as the compassionate nation in relation to superpowers (Razack, 2004, p. 26).

The disappearing of the reasons why "multiculturalism" and "First Nations" issues are understood as problems in this province decontextualizes the true "roots" of our own implications in violence: that of systemic oppressions both at home and abroad. With this in mind, the approach that *The Review* takes to First Nations peoples is that there is no room in this report to consult or speak directly to their needs. The act of excluding First Nations from a report that concerns itself with youth violence (which certainly pertains to Aboriginal peoples as their youth are subjected to all forms of violence, and are among the most over-criminalized populations in Canada) effectively treats Aboriginals as a dead culture: a culture beyond hope, and beyond benevolent intervention. Aboriginality is understood as a disappeared culture in the imagination of this province, a culture "that must *always* be disappearing, in order to allow non-indigenous peoples rightful claim over this land ... Native peoples are a permanent 'present absence' in the [Canadian] colonial imagination, an 'absence' that reinforces, at every turn, the conviction that Native peoples are indeed vanishing and that the conquest of Native lands is justified" (Smith, 2005, p. 68).

Aboriginals in *The Review* are a present absence: present, because they are identified as a population that is racially marginalized within the province—but decidedly absent because they are excluded from the immediate conversation that *The Review* engages, however noting that "having regard to the practical and jurisdictional reasons why our review did not seek to study violence within First Nations in Ontario, the Province should meet with First Nations leaders to consider the potential applicability of our advice to those communities" (McMurtry & Curling, 2008a, p. 379). *The Review*, in choosing to disengage from the Aboriginal "problem," circuits itself away from having to confront our own colonial legacy and implication in our violence against them. It allows us as a province to remain unhinged to "white people's historic participation in and benefit from [the] dispossession and violence" that we depend on in order to maintain the myth of our province as a benevolent one (Razack, 2002, pp. 126–127). Focusing on raced violence is a more facile strategy, since these bodies are framed in *The Review* as people who have chosen to move here (and we welcome them). But to engage with First Nations peoples in *The Review* runs the risk of forcing the inquiry to confront our own colonial history, and in turn re-centre what we are willing to locate as "violence." Thus, in *The Review*, Aboriginal bodies are understood to be implicated in "a problem of violence," but that problem is left as vague perpetrators of violence, and "the over-policing, incarceration, and high suicide rates of Aboriginal peoples were not brought to bear on the details, [and thus] the stain that is Aboriginality could not be seen as socially constructed" (Razack, 2002, p. 129).

From System to Subject

The main intervention that I want to analyze is one that permeates the core of *The Review*. While the report makes a plethora of structural and system change recommendations, and insists on understanding itself as a report that is invested in structural amendments, I want to show how structural oppressions (or systems of disadvantage, as they are referred to) are moved into troubled communities; and how, in turn, those "disadvantages" land on targeted individualized bodies, to be assessed, understood, and fixed. This practice, this business-as-usual of localizing structurally embedded oppression on individual bodies, continues the process of solving social violence on the bodies of degenerate subjects, instead of the work of dismantling the structures that cause such harm.

One of the main problems identified in *The Review* is the over-criminalization of racialized youth in the province. *The Review* recognizes that "the criminal justice system, while generally used to good effect, can nonetheless also be used in counterproductive ways when the exercise of its power leads to the inappropriate treatment of youth and to over-criminalization" (McMurtry & Curling, 2008a, p. 267). The violence of the criminal justice system is understood to land on racialized bodies in particular, and this heightened policing and intervention on racialized bodies are understood as producing *more* raced crime, as they produce subjects that become enraged with the system. Ultimately, they produce risk for "us": rightfully angry youth who are more likely to become unpredictably violent, which can lead to "association with youth gangs" (McMurtry & Curling, 2008a, p. 269), or "alienat[ed] and disaffected youth [who] walk our streets and enter our schools carrying loaded handguns" (McMurtry & Curling, 2008a, p. 362). The problem of over-criminalization poses a threat to the province, and as such, other methods of discipline must be enacted to counter this constantly burgeoning potentiality of risk.

To counter the over-criminalization of racialized youth, *The Review* proposes strategies such as lenient punishment for nonviolent offences, and using approaches such as restorative justice to punish young offenders (McMurtry & Curling, 2008a, p. 358; see also Harris, 2000). Alongside such structural shifts to criminal enforcement, *The Review* emphasizes "a community approach to individual interventions." Instead of relying on the prison system, which can "stigmatize a youth in their own minds and others, disrupt their education or employment, label them as a serious criminal, expose them 24/7 to many youth who are a danger, and destroy their self-esteem and sense of hope" (McMurtry & Curling, 2008a, p. 269), *The Review* calls on problemed communities themselves to identify and intervene on youth who are at risk. Thus, problemed communities must learn to act on their own, to identify, intervene, discipline, and cure their own troubled individuals in their communities. In this way, structural violence becomes, yet again, an individualized issue that must be weeded out at the source: a spatialized, racialized practice of self-governance.

This self-governance must be done in localized settings, to allow for the weeds to be rooted out. This "approach to violence prevention locates the more proximate risks of youth violence in local communities. A local community might be defined as a block, a neighbourhood, a housing project or an ethnic enclave" (McMurtry & Curling, 2008a,

p. 355). The subjects of these racialized slum spaces must come to harness their power over their communal children and intervene on them before the police do. Services within slum spaces must be made available to concerned citizens and "at-risk" youth alike, services that offer ways of disciplining them outside of the criminal justice system: services that are accessed through educational, community, and social services hubs.

In this way, we are shown how *systems require one another.* In moving away from over-criminalization, *The Review* offers other, more seemingly benevolent systems of service that will take the place of the criminal justice system. The more interventionist of these services are to be made available to those who have already succumbed to their criminality: services such as cognitive behavioural therapy, and core rehabilitation services (including anger management training, cognitive skills training, sex offender treatment, and substance abuse treatment) (McMurtry & Curling, 2008a, p. 359). But more importantly, *The Review* wants communities to target youth who have yet to give in to their potentiality as violent perpetrators, but who exhibit "at-risk" symptoms, as a preventative measure to ensure community safety. This classic rhetorical tool reconstructs collective systemic oppression as a problem that is graphed onto racialized inner-city bodies, and a problem to be sorted out in kind. As *The Review* proposes, it becomes "necessary to identify specific children from a community (typically from 7 to 14 years of age) at particularly high risk of engaging in criminal or violent behaviour in the future. After being identified, these youth can be provided with additional services including intensive mental health counselling, behaviour modification, family therapy and adult mentorship" (McMurtry & Curling, 2008a, p. 355). In this way, the systems shift that *The Review* makes is one that moves away from a criminal justice system that overtly governs a problemed community, to one that uses mental health as a system of internalized self-governance: as Hanafi notes, "society is governed much less by law and order but more *through [self-] administration and management*" (Hanafi, 2009a, p. 116, emphasis in original; see also Hook, 2007; Rose, 1990).

Benevolence Is Not Benign

This rerouting of "troubled youth" from the criminal justice system to mental health systems is one that *The Review* argues strongly for, as a way of solving the stigma and damage that early criminalization can impose on "the disadvantaged." I want to argue here that this move, in recognizing the structural issues inherent in the criminal justice system, is being solved through the shifting of systems of governance from the power of criminalization onto the powers of pathologization. It is a system shift from the structural powers of criminalization (that are understood as problematic in race relations) onto the individualizing powers of pathologization (which are understood to be benevolent and problem-free). *The Review* understands that the criminal justice system does harm to racialized youth, and thus proposes that we instead offer preventative and interventionist measures through the goodwill of the psy disciplines (Rose, 1990). Martinot and Sexton ask: "How can one critically discuss policing and imprisonment without interrogating the very notions of freedom, citizenship, and democracy?" (Martinot & Sexton, 2003, p. 177). They answer that question, and *The Review* enacts how, rather than disassembling systems of structural violence, instead "remedies can always be found *within* liberal capitalism: from psychological counselling, moral and scientific education, legal prohibition, or even gene therapy …" (Martinot & Sexton, 2003, p. 178, emphasis in original). Evident here is how the structural problems inherent in the criminal justice system are seen as being solved by drawing on another system of power, that of mental health, that *individualizes* this structural violence as personal pathology. Moving "troubled youth" into being managed by psy disciplines not only masks how this disadvantage is structurally rooted, but also localizes the problems that "at-risk" youth face into the core of their bodies: the structures of their biomedical souls.

This relocation of the violence of criminalization into the violence of pathologization is one that I want to bring forward. This "tactic of pathologizing these individuals, studying their condition, and offering 'therapy' to them and their communities must be seen as another rhetorical manoeuvre designed to obscure … the moral and financial accountability of Euro-Canadian society in a continuing record of Crimes Against Humanity" (Chrisjohn et al., 2006, p. 22). That *The Review* clearly recognizes that the criminal justice system is a troubled system that produces and maintains systems of disadvantage within targeted populations is clear. However, the solution offered—to increase youth mental health services in Ontario by $200 million— completely overlooks the violence that is inherent in psychiatric pathologization. *The Review* offers to solve the violence of criminal justice systems by strengthening the power and violence of mental health services. The fact that mental health services remain untroubled in this report (unlike racism, poverty, immigrant integration, etc.) demonstrates how entrenched the dividing practices of the psy disciplines remain in this province. Denied is how mental health systems "are implicated in the reproduction of hierarchies and in the structural violence against which they claim to offer protection" (Harris, 2000, p. 800).

The common sense argument *The Review* offers is that in order to prevent the stigma and rage that occurs when "disadvantaged" youth are criminalized, the province must increase its spending on child and youth mental health services (from its current $444 million annual budget) to "catch at-risk" youth before they erupt into criminality. What this common sense line of thinking ignores are the discrimination, rage, damage and worse that pathologization enacts on young bodies when they are marked as mentally ill. Is it really better to be labelled insane than a criminal? Further, these problemed children and youth, through the psy disciplines, come to understand their trouble in individualized, often biomedical frameworks that decontextualize the role that structural oppressions play in the constitution of their personhood. Needless to say, *The Review* also unquestionably links madness to criminal behaviour. Ultimately, individuals are asked to fix themselves, instead of acting on and resisting the systems of oppression out of which violence arises.[4] Again and over again, the problem begins within.

Criminality to Pathology

With this call to self-governance in mind, the recommendations that I want to highlight from *The Review* are those that work to increase psy monitoring within racialized inner-city slums. Both recommendation numbers 15 and 28 (the latter of which is marked for priority implementation) ask for increased child and youth mental health services in "disadvantaged" communities. As recommendation number 15 suggests:

> The province must take steps to bring youth mental health out of the shadows. The province should enhance prevention through programs that promote health, engagement and activity for youth. It should also provide locally available mental health services that afford early identification and treatment for children and youth in the context of their families and schools, that are culturally appropriate and that are integrated with the community hubs we propose. (McMurtry & Curling, 2008a, p. 377)[5]

I want to start by saying that *The Review* engages with mental health and illness in purely biomedical terms, and never considers madness as a socially constructed and mediated model. Unlike race and racism, which are understood as being *created*, madness simply *is*, in existence and in need of identification, isolation, and eradication. Culture and difference are understood as in need of understanding and cultivation: madness is to be killed. It is never imagined that different ways of thinking, experiencing, interpreting, or being in the world could ever be of value (see Voronka, 2008b). Eradication of madness is always the rule. Normalization is always the goal.

Madness as a rampant problem in need of a cure is postulated *ad nauseum* throughout *The Review*: statistics circulate, facts concur, experts agree.[6] Further, perpetrated violence is attached to Mad bodies, in claims such as "In the age group committing the most violent incidents, individuals with mental disorders account for a considerable amount of violence in the community. Retrospective studies have shown that more youth with mental health disorders are arrested for violent offences than are youth who do not meet the diagnostic criteria for mental disorder" (McMurtry & Curling, 2008a, p. 69). Thus, *The Review* not only manages to reinforce discourses on raced violence, but also continues the belief that those diagnosed as mentally ill are more likely to be violent perpetrators. It is never considered here, as it is with racialized bodies, that "more youth with mental health disorders are arrested for violent offences" because they too are an over-criminalized body (ibid.). In this way, *The Review* has the productive function of marking madness, and not psychiatric interventions, as where violence's "roots" occur.

I want to consider how *The Review* works to solidify biomedical notions of madness within communities that are understood as operating outside of common sense knowledge about mental illness. The cultural move—and mental health move—to educate racialized inner-city slum communities about the biomedical approach to mental illness is marked as work that must be undertaken by the province. Psy professionals must be culturally competent, able to relate and translate to culturally diverse populations (who may have an understanding of madness outside of Western medical dominance), and to convert them to the "right" (read: white) ways of approaching madness as biologically embedded. This work of educating deficient cultures about how to think properly about madness requires "skilled and sensitive outreach, effective 'navigators' to help youth and their families sort out options and align services and creative, culturally conscious mechanisms to break down parents' reluctance to have their children use [mental health services]" (McMurtry & Curling, 2008a, p. 247). Respectable professionals must enter slum spaces and educate racialized peoples about biomedical understanding of madness. Others must submit themselves and their families to the precarious truths that operate through the psy disciplines, and open themselves up to scrutiny. Once social oppressions are biocultured, racialized slum spaces can move from over-policed spaces to sites of exception that learn to police themselves.

Finally, of great concern in *The Review*'s recommendations is how it asks to increase the level of surveillance within racialized inner-city slums. *The Review* moves away from increasing police/population ratios in these sites of exception, but counters with increasing psy monitoring within these racialized spaces. Parents, teachers, mentors, coaches, police officers, and so on are asked to identify "and recognize the signs of mental illness so that they can recommend interventions" (McMurtry & Curling, 2008a, p. 247). Mental health practitioners are called to be integrated throughout social institutions, ready to intervene on any youth who is identified as outside of normal. Of particular concern is just how early these interventions are to be enacted. Over and over again, "early interventions" are stressed (ibid., pp. 70, 246). Statistics inform us that "70% of childhood cases of mental health problems can be solved through early diagnosis and intervention," although it is forebodingly noted later that "there is no end date on mental illness" (ibid., pp. 70, 156). This "early intervention" is identified as needing to begin within school settings "starting at *age five, or even earlier*" (ibid., p. 246, emphasis mine), and that "*preschool and younger* school-aged children who suffer from mental illness be given higher priority than at present" (ibid., p. 70, emphasis mine). That *The Review* seeks to counter systemically "disadvantaged" youth by increasing pathologization among small children should strike fear, anger, and strong resistance in communities that have already been problematized to death.

Conclusion

The Review as an analytical tool shows us how an everyday neoliberalist government-produced text can work to solidify white settler supremacy through common sense and benevolent discourses and policy recommendations. It shows us how systems use one another to offset and relocate the powers of governance. The good intent as it runs through *The Review* under the guise of helping racialized slum spaces manage their violence works to further entrench the right that is white settler and psychiatric supremacy in this province. By upholding the credo of the inherent goodwill of our systems of governance, regardless of the talk of systems of "disadvantage," the change that must be made continues to land on individual bodies: those that have borne the legacy of our collective violence. To that end, I would like to conclude by reasserting Chrisjohn et al.'s reminder that "Present-day symptomology found in Aboriginal Peoples and [and all Othered] societies does not constitute a distinct psychological condition, but is the well known and long-studied response of human beings living under conditions of severe and prolonged oppression" (Chrisjohn et al., 2006, p. 21).

Notes

1 Much could be said about the other four volumes of *The Review*: *Volume 2, Executive Summary*; *Volume 3, Community Perspectives Report*; *Volume 4, Research Papers*; and *Volume 5, Literature Reviews*.

2 Racism (but not race or racialization) garners a lot of attention in the text. To give the reader a sense of how racism is understood to work in *The Review*, I offer this quote that exemplifies how racism is understood as an individual belief, even when structurally manifest: "Racism is manifested in three ways. There are those who expressly espouse racist views as part of a *personal* credo. There are those who *subconsciously* hold negative attitudes towards black persons based on stereotypical assumptions concerning persons of colour. Finally, and perhaps most pervasively, racism exists within the interstices of our institutions. This *systemic racism is a product of individual attitudes and beliefs* concerning blacks and it fosters and legitimizes those assumptions and stereotypes" (McMurtry & Curling, 2008a, p. 238, emphasis mine).

3 "A variety of scholars and activists have critiqued the choice paradigm because it rests on essentially individualist, consumerist notions of 'free' choice that do not take into consideration all of the social, economic and political conditions that frame the so-called choices that [immigrants] are forced to make" (Smith, 2005, p. 99).

4 Psy disciplines are often used as a way of quelling resistance to social oppression. An example of this in *The Review*: "The Behavioural Monitoring and Reinforcement Program is another school-based intervention that has shown positive results among juvenile populations. It targets students in the seventh and eighth grades from low-income, urban, racially mixed neighbourhoods and is *designed to challenge youth cynicism about the outside world* and related feelings of hopelessness and alienation" (McMurtry & Curling, 2008a, p. 180, emphasis mine).

5 Recommendation number 28 reads: "*Children's Mental Health*: This issue affects many aspects of the roots: the stability of families and the ability of parents to work and parent, how youth develop with their peers, how they do in school, how they interact with the justice system and

their life chances overall. We believe that one or more associations with expertise in youth mental health should be retained immediately to prepare a plan for universal, community-based access to mental health services for children and youth for the earliest possible implementation. They should also prepare plans for all interim investments that are feasible within the limits of the available professional expertise in Ontario. In a province with a health budget of $40 billion and a youth incarceration budget of $163 million, we believe that the $200 million estimate of the cost of providing universal youth mental health services is manageable within this government's mandate" (McMurtry & Curling, 2008a, p. 380).

6 Scientific and statistical truths are continually called upon to justify the need for psy intervention in *The Review*: "One in five of Ontario's children and youth experience[s] a mental health or behavioural disorder requiring intervention. ... However, only one in five young people who need mental health services receives them" (McMurtry & Curling, 2008a, p. 70).

CHAPTER 23

Recovery: Progressive Paradigm or Neoliberal Smokescreen?[1]

Marina Morrow

Introduction

Despite a well-established research literature that illustrates the ways in which mental distress is intimately tied to social inequities such as poverty, homelessness, racism, homophobia, and sexism, the social and structural determinants of mental health continue to be marginalized in research, policy, and service provision even as debates in Canada about the failings of the current mental health care system abound. Using the resurgence of recovery paradigms as my example, as well as recent empirical research that engaged mental health services users, policy actors, and practitioners in a World Café dialogue on recovery (see Morrow, Jamer & Weisser, 2011), I argue that this marginalization can be attributed to the continued dominance of biomedical paradigms, which in turn determine resource allocations that favour psychiatric over social care in mental health.

The neoliberal policy context, which has resulted in massive spending cuts to social welfare services, further bolsters approaches and discourses that individualize and medicalize mental health problems. Recovery as a concept and a paradigm is poised to either disrupt biomedical dominance in favour of social and structural understandings of mental distress or to continue to play into individualistic discourses of "broken brains," "chemical imbalances," and "self-management," which work against social change. In this vein, I ask the questions: What happens to recovery frameworks when they are implemented in neoliberal political regimes? And, do recovery frameworks have the potential to redistribute power in the mental health care system? I conclude with a discussion of the challenges and possibilities of the recovery paradigm and the role of "recovery" dialogues for advancing social justice in mental health.

Recovery and Social Inequities[2]

Over the last number of decades, reforms in mental health, in particular the shift from institutional-based to community-based care, have led to new models of mental health care. It was in this context that the concept of recovery emerged out of two distinct sectors—psychiatric survivor and professional. The former used the notion of recovery in ways that challenged the medicalization of mental health and the power of psychiatry to define people's lives and experiences (e.g., Deegan, 1988), while the latter has shaped the concept to reflect the needs and concerns of mental health service providers (Anthony, 1993; Cleary & Dowling, 2009; Collier, 2010; Davidson & Roe, 2007; Davidson, Rakfeldt & Strauss, 2010). The tensions arising from these differing origins of recovery are evident in contemporary debate and reflected in the ways in which psychiatric survivors themselves understand their own recovery. For example, the Toronto-based Mental Health "Recovery" Study Working Group (2009), in their research with psychiatric survivors, found three conceptualizations of recovery: 1) recovery as personal journey, 2) recovery as a social process (including access to jobs, income, housing, safety, and education), and 3) recovery as critique—that is, wresting recovery from the hands of professionals in order to put it back in the hands of people who experience mental distress.

Although the concept of recovery in mental health began circulating in the 1980s and 1990s and undoubtedly began a revolution for many people who had been psychiatrized and institutionalized in terms of how they understood their lives and possibilities, it has been taken up unevenly in policy and practice in mental health care (Adams, Daniels & Compagni, 2009; Piat & Sabetti, 2009). This arises, in part, from the fact that recovery as a concept is understood in myriad ways with no agreed-upon definition or framework for supporting people. Further, the fact that mental health care practitioners struggle to foster recovery from within service systems that place constraints and controls on people diagnosed with mental illness (e.g., involuntary committal and mandated treatments) makes fostering the underlying philosophy of recovery, which includes supporting autonomous decision-making, difficult if not impossible (Fabris, 2011; Morrow, Pederson, Smith, Josewski, Jamer & Battersby, 2010). Given this lack of consistency, considerable barriers, and the absence of an overarching framework for delivering mental health care,[3] shifting how we think about and actualize recovery is a complex task. In the Canadian context, where mental health care planning and delivery are decentralized and mostly regionalized, the response to the fragmentation of services and the lack of an overarching framework for mental health has been to establish the Mental Health Commission of Canada (MHCC). One of the key roles of the MHCC has been to develop a mental health framework and strategy for Canada. It must be noted that the MHCC itself is constrained in that in the context of Canadian federalism and the division of powers it is not able to mandate how services are delivered, but in its unique role can only attempt to foment change through national consultations and moral suasion. It is in this particular context that the concept of "recovery" is currently being used in Canada to promote a paradigm shift in mental health. It behooves us then to look at how the MHCC in its framework for a mental health strategy (2009b) describes recovery. That is, as "a journey of healing that builds on individual, family, cultural and community strengths, and enables people living with mental health problems and illnesses to lead meaningful lives in the community, despite any limitations imposed by their condition" (p. 8).

Not only has the concept of recovery been slow to catch on in contemporary policy and practice in mental health, but particular understandings of recovery have come to predominate. With few exceptions (e.g., Jacobson, Farah & The Toronto Recovery and Cultural Diversity Community of Practice, 2010; Mental Health "Recovery" Study Working Group, 2009; O'Hagan, 2004b; Piat, Sabetti & Couture, 2008), the conceptualization of recovery suffers from its individualistic framing as a personal journey, which has neglected a wider analysis of social and structural relations of power in mental health (e.g., racism, sexism, homophobia, and the power of psychiatry to define experience) that signal systemic discrimination, on people's experiences of mental distress and how these interact at an individual and social level. So, despite some definitions of recovery that include social components, like access to housing, income, education, etc., and others that focus on system transformation (e.g., Adams et al., 2009; Mental Health Commission of Canada, 2009b; Piat & Sabetti, 2009; Ramon, Healy & Ranouf, 2007), what is often overlooked within discussions of recovery is an explicit recognition of the role of the social, political, cultural, and economic context in which people become mentally distressed and recover.

At issue here are several interconnected points, including that experiences of mental health and mental illness, regardless of their origins, take place in a wider social, cultural, and historical context (e.g., Hacking, 2002; Porter, 2002; Watters, 2010), which includes environments of discrimination and oppression that are played out in distinct ways for different groups. Several examples here will help to illustrate my point. There is now an established literature documenting the ways in which psychiatry historically and contemporarily continues to pathologize women and racialized groups, and specifically how psychiatry has been used as a form of social control to contain and constrain individuals who are seen to be disrupting the social order. For example, with respect to gender, psychiatric diagnostic practices continue to medicalize both normal reactions to living in a sexist culture—such as the effects of violence on women—and normal female life transitions, including menopause and the perinatal period (e.g., Chesler, 1972; Penfold & Walker, 1983; Ussher, 1992, 2011). Ussher's (2011) work is illustrative of the ways in which the "myth of women's madness" continues to be perpetuated within contemporary research and practice as she carefully untangles what Foucault (1980) calls "regimes of truth" about women's mental health, that is, the values, mores, belief systems, and assumptions that society uses to prop up its scientific enterprises. With respect to racialized groups, the literature in the UK and US shows that black men and poor people are more frequently diagnosed with schizophrenia and other mental illnesses (Baker & Bell, 1999; Delahanty, 2001; Van Os, Kenis & Rutten, 2010). Metzl (2009), for example, in his careful historical analysis shows how this diagnosis was used during the rise of the civil rights movement in the US to contain black men. Both Ussher (2011) and Metzl (2009) carry on an important tradition of scholarship dedicated to making visible the ways in which race, gender, and sexual orientation get written into definitions of mental illness, often with devastating consequences for disenfranchised communities.

Other researchers have focused their attention on documenting the effects of social inequities on mental health—for example, the dire consequences of colonialism on the mental health of First Nations, Inuit, and Métis populations, especially with respect to suicide, violence, and substance use (Health Canada, 2000; Kirmayer, Brass & Tait, 2001; Ross, 2009). The particular effects of colonialism on the lives and mental health of First Nations women have also been documented (e.g., Browne, Varcoe & Fridkin, 2011). Other researchers have recorded the effects of racism and the stresses of acculturation on immigrant and refugee people's mental health (Boyer, Ku & Shakir, 1997; Canadian Task Force on Mental Health Issues Affecting Immigrants and Refugees, 1988; Morrow, Smith, Lai & Jaswal, 2008), as well as the ways in which heterosexism and transphobia result in heightened suicide attempts (Bagley & Tremblay, 2000; D'Augelli, Hershberger & Pilkington, 2001) and the experiences of multiple forms of abuse and violence that affect the safety and mental well-being of these populations (Courvant & Cook-Daniels, 1998; Eyler & Witten, 1999). Further, much attention has been given to the links between mental distress, poverty, and homelessness (Patterson, Somers, McKintosh, Shiell & Frankish, 2008; Standing Senate Committee on Social Affairs, Science and Technology, 2009). What this tradition of scholarship illustrates is the very concrete ways in which inequity negatively impacts emotional well-being.

Another way of thinking about the intersections between social inequities and mental distress can be found in the ways in which stigma and discrimination resulting from a mental illness diagnosis act on disenfranchised groups. So, for example, women, First Nations peoples, substance users, people living in poverty, racialized groups, and individuals with disabilities all experience stigma and discrimination differently, in ways that compound their experiences of mental distress (Gary, 2005). Pregnant substance-using women, for example, are demonized in the media and subject to harsh social and policy interventions (Greaves, Varcoe, Poole, Morrow, Johnson, Pederson & Irwin, 2002).

Finally, still others point to the ways in which Western conceptualizations of the "self" and the psyche are inadequate for peoples from cultures that emphasize collectivity and holistic ideas about health (Ross, 2009; Watters, 2010). An example here would be Watters' (2010) descriptions of the ways in which Western biased ideas about psychiatry have been exported internationally, in ways that ignore local histories and understandings of mental distress, often with unintended and disastrous consequences. In Canada, First Nations communities have worked hard to influence

Eurocentric ideas about mental health, in order to bring into focus Indigenous ways of knowing (Ross, 2009).

Despite the richness of the literatures that address, from a variety of angles, the links between mental health and social inequities, the discussion in more medically oriented mental health literature has focused on the association of gender and other social inequities with poor mental health outcomes and with differential access to services and supports. That is, the argument that is advanced is that many people are mentally ill and not receiving treatment and services, and that this is particularly true for certain marginalized, "vulnerable," or "at-risk" groups. Often in these literatures the language of epidemiology ("at-risk populations") is imported as a way of individualizing the social problems underlying the experience of distress. What is typically ignored in such scholarship is that the ways in which services are designed, and the assumptions that they operate under, may reproduce the very inequities they purport to ameliorate. Further, in the push to develop *magic bullets* to treat mental illness, society has ignored the scientific evidence that reveals the iatrogenic effects of psychotropic medications, which are most often the primary response to illness (Whitaker, 2010, p. 47). Counter to this, a critical and feminist body of literature and practice has arisen that illustrates the ways in which diagnoses and labels of mental illness result in stigma and discrimination and constitute a form of inequity—this is referred to as "sanism" (Birnbaum, 2010; Fabris, 2011; Ingram, 2011a; Perlin, 2000). This has led to a deepening analysis of the ways in which the "psy" sciences[4] shape our understanding of human behaviour and, in so doing, often reinforce oppressive practices (e.g., Chan, Chunn & Menzies, 2005; Ussher, 1992, 2011). The question remains, then, as to whether the move in the Canadian context towards implementing recovery models and frameworks in mental health opens up a space for a larger dialogue on the role of social and structural inequities in mental health and people's recovery, or whether it is in danger of reinforcing the medical dominance it is purported to attenuate.

The Neoliberal Context

Neoliberalism can be understood as a form of governmentality (Foucault, 2010) and as constitutive of discursive practices that influence the understanding of our social world. The tension between biomedical frames and the discourses surrounding the social determinants of mental health is intimately tied to structures of power where psychiatry has the most resources and where people (and women and marginalized groups, in particular) are limited with respect to their choice of treatments and supports in a public health care system that covers only certain kinds of care. Biopsychiatry is tied ideologically to neoliberalism, which promotes individualistic understandings of complex social problems (Morrow, Wasik, Cohen & Perry, 2009;

Ramon, 2008; Teghtsoonian, 2008). Foucault's (1980) concept of "bio-power" and Rose's (1990, 1998, 1999) work on the neoliberal self are useful here to underline the ways in which disciplinary practices such as medicine intersect with neoliberalism by responsibilizing us and urging us to take charge of our bodies and minds.

When translated into policy and practice, neoliberalism favours welfare state retrenchment and the increased use of managerialism (market mechanisms) in the delivery of health and mental health services (Morrow, Frischmuth & Johnson, 2006; Morrow, Wasik, Cohen & Perry, 2009; Shera, Aviram, Healy & Ramon, 2002; Teghtsoonian, 2008), and does not overly concern itself with ties between the pharmaceutical industry and the health care system. Neoliberalism shifts the emphasis away from the collective rights of citizens to policies that emphasize the individual and his/her economic independence regardless of social circumstances (Morrow et al., 2009; Teghtsoonian, 2008). For people experiencing mental distress, who in the course of "treatment" may lose certain citizenship rights and who may rely on and off on the social service system for most of their lives, the emphasis on private solutions to social problems is particularly reprehensible.

What are the consequences of inserting the concept of recovery into neoliberal policy contexts, especially conceptualizations of recovery that emphasize recovery as a social process and a critique of power? Following this, how might the discursive strategies used by neoliberalism undermine social and collective ideas about recovery? Finally, given this context, is recovery as a concept and framework capable of informing progressive social change?

What Happens When Recovery Frameworks Are Implemented in Neoliberal Political Regimes?

Neoliberal policy reform over the last number of decades has resulted in social welfare state restructuring with particular implications for the mental health care system (Cohen, Goldberg, Istvanffy, Stainton, Wasik & Woods, 2008; Morrow, Frischmuth & Johnson, 2006; Morrow et al., 2009). For example, British Columbia over the last 15 years has suffered the most severe cuts to social welfare supports in Canadian history and has undergone significant policy shifts, which included changes to base funding and eligibility thresholds for social assistance and new requirements for disability benefits, including for people diagnosed with mental illness (Morrow et al., 2006; Morrow et al., 2009). Some community-based mental health services have been cut and funding for anti-poverty work, legal aid, and women and immigrant serving organizations remains unstable and inadequate, resulting in decreased advocacy and support for people (Morrow et al., 2010). These shifts at a policy and service level have arguably intensified the resource split between acute/medical care over community-based supports in mental health. A concrete example of this development in the context of British Columbia is that during the process of deinstitutionalization few new government monies have gone to community-based supports; but rather as people are transferred out of Vancouver's Riverview Psychiatric Hospital money is transferred primarily to new and existing psychiatric tertiary care facilities (Morrow, Pederson, et al., 2010). Notable in the Canadian context is that the Kirby Report,[5] in its final recommendations, called for a mental health and housing transition fund that would have had the federal government transferring funds to the provinces and territories, specifically to fund housing and community supports (Kirby, 2006). The fact that the federal government did not act on this recommendation, and to this day has provided no new core funding for housing and community supports, means that the philosophy of recovery is exceedingly difficult to actualize and power in mental health remains in the hands of psychiatry.

Dwindling resources at the state level to address poverty and homelessness have, over time, led to the framing of social justice and human rights issues as health problems. Thus, housing is garnered not by activists resisting poverty, but by experts who demonstrate that it is people with mental illness and addictions who populate our streets and must be housed because of their severe health problems. Meyer and Schwartz (2000, p. 1189), writing about homelessness, document what happens when "social problems are refracted through a public health prism" including an undue focus on the individual, the institutionalization of research paradigms and findings (i.e., epidemiology), and the prioritization of social problems based on their health consequences. This "healthification" of social problems fits neatly into the agenda of neoliberalism with implications for the ways in which the concept of recovery is poised to being taken up as an individual journey requiring the "manpower" of the individual to create a healing environment, and his or her family and social support network to provide the engine of hope, devoid of any analysis of the social context in which mental distress occurs and is managed.

Indeed, neoliberal policy change is accompanied by discursive strategies that emphasize the individual, and individual responsibility for mental health. An example would be the recent proliferation of self-management strategies for mental illness (Teghtsoonian, 2008). Discursive strategies that cast mental illness as an illness like any other physical illness also play directly into the idea that "broken brains" can be fixed by individually oriented psycho-pharmaceutical interventions. Given that at a systems level these discursive strategies emphasize cost efficiencies, accountability, and tangible performance measures, it seems unlikely that recovery will stray far from the hands of the professionals who are tied to these exigencies.

Do Recovery Frameworks Have the Potential to Redistribute Power in the Mental Health Care System?

Given the current economic and political landscape, and the ongoing power of bio-psychiatry to define mental distress and circumscribe treatment and responses, it is difficult to imagine the emancipatory potential of recovery frameworks. Nevertheless, here I argue that recovery has potential in two specific ways. First, in the hands of individuals who have experienced mental distress and who began the dialogue about recovery in its early days, recovery has transformative potential. This potential has been documented in the many stories of individuals who describe their experiences of mental distress and their resistance to psychiatry and/or critical uptake of mental health care in ways that work best for them, and in the stories of individuals who make clear links between their experiences and poverty, racism, sexism, and sanism (e.g., Blackbridge, 1997; Blackbridge & Gilhooly, 1985; Capponi, 1992, 1997, 2003; Danquah, 1999; Ingram, 2005; Shimrat, 1997). In these testimonies are the seeds of change that have spawned numerous psychiatric survivor networks and given rise to Mad activism and a whole host of critical historical and contemporary discussion about the ways of thinking about, and living with, mental distress (e.g., Chan, Chunn & Menzies, 2005; Everett, 2000; Fabris, 2011; Ingram, 2005; Reaume, 2006, 2011). Although many of these activities would not be specifically identified as "recovery," and the activists involved might even reject the terminology as too medicalized, they all share some of the central tenets of recovery—that is, that people have the right to more control over and autonomy in their own lives, and that people diagnosed with mental illness lead lives marked by discrimination. Collectively, the power of narratives about people's lived experiences of mental distress and the mental health care system, combined with activism to create alternative ways of thinking about and responding to mental illness, have the potential to begin shifting the way power is distributed in the mental health care system. Indeed, there is evidence that this is occurring especially with respect to psychiatric survivor-run initiatives and alternatives to psychiatry (Church and Reville, 2001; Morrow et al., 2009; Nelson, Ochocka, Janzen & Trainor, 2006a,b,c,d; Whitaker, 2010). This is evident in the tension apparent in the discursive practices used to describe people diagnosed with mental illness—that is, "psychiatric patient" versus "consumer" versus "psychiatric survivor" versus "person with lived experience" versus "mad identified." Each term used reflects different ways of thinking about people experiencing mental distress and specifically foregrounds the tensions between medical understandings and social and political understandings.

Second, neoliberal barriers notwithstanding, as a framework for mental health system transformation, recovery has the potential to shift the ways in which society thinks about and responds to people experiencing mental distress. That is, there is evidence across some jurisdictions that the push towards recovery-oriented systems, at least on paper and in emerging policy, is shifting the focus away from psychiatry and illness towards mental health promotion and a greater attention to the diverse needs of populations (Adams et al., 2009; Friedli, 2009; Piat & Sabetti, 2009; Victorian Government Department of Health, 2011). Although only some of these articulations explicitly address inequities (see Friedli, 2009), the sheer scope of policy frameworks and initiatives over the last decade focused on recovery-oriented principles and practices (Weisser, Morrow & Jamer, 2010) provides heft to the argument that the mental health care system is undergoing a paradigm shift. So what then can recovery offer and how can it be made productive for social justice?

Dialoguing about Recovery

In the spirit of Poole's (2011) work on critical recovery, which emphasizes the notion of recovery as rhetoric and manifest in different types of "recovery talk," I concur that the concept of recovery is an ever-changing set of ideas and beliefs about mental health and mental illness. Thus, one way forward is, as Poole (2011) suggests, continuing the dialogue on recovery. In 2010 a research team of committed advocates, policy actors, people with lived experience, academics, and mental health care providers came together to explore the ways in which recovery was being talked about and conceptualized by individuals with close connections either personally or professionally to the mental health care system in Vancouver, BC (Morrow, Jamer & Weisser, 2011).

Specifically, we were interested to find out whether people were talking about social inequities in mental health in the context of recovery. Using the methodology of World Café,[6] the research team brought together 24 people for one day, including mental health and social service front-line workers, mental health and addictions managers, policy-makers, people with lived experience of mental health issues, family members, and community leaders engaged in mental health work, to engage in a dialogue about mental health recovery, gender, and social inequities. The goal of the research project was to identify key components of a recovery model that could address social and structural inequities (Morrow, Jamer & Weisser, 2011). Although some people attending had more than one connection to the mental health field (e.g., some were both service providers and people with lived experience, or family members and policy actors), overall about half of the participants identified as having lived experience of mental health issues, and about half were service providers, managers, or policy actors in the mental health field.

Four key themes or areas of focus emerged from the World Café discussions: the language of recovery, a social justice approach to mental health, mental health and social policy, and the role of peer workers in recovery (Morrow, Jamer & Weisser, 2011). What was fascinating with respect to each of these themes was that participants simultaneously demonstrated an understanding of the underlying social and structural factors as they related to mental health, while at the same time the discussion frequently returned to talk about recovery that was focused at the individual level. So, for example, participants tended to see mental health through a social determinants lens, which included an understanding of the role that supports like income security, housing, and employment play in ameliorating mental health problems. Specifically, in their conversations, participants highlighted policies or practices (e.g., disability benefits, barriers to employment) that prevent people from realizing recovery fully.

However, despite enthusiasm for social frameworks of recovery rooted in principles of social justice, participants also frequently slipped back into discussions around individual aspects of recovery. So although participants sometimes gave examples of how sexism, heterosexism, or poverty might impact recovery or result in inequitable access to services and supports, the conversation typically returned to recovery as an individual journey. Adding to this was another kind of discussion, one that focused on the ways in which people with diagnoses of mental illness are pathologized, stigmatized, and discriminated against. Participants felt strongly that people were often reduced to their diagnostic label, which, they argued, obscured the complexity of people's lives and experiences. Here again participants were well able to articulate the connections between diagnostic practices, dominant modes of treatment, and the ways in which this disempowered and harmed people—so much so that many called for a social justice approach to mental health recovery.

Emerging from this dialogue, then, are tensions that have always been present in discussions about recovery (Poole, 2011), but may also be indicative of the ways in which dialogues, which use methodologies that intentionally help us deepen our understanding of an issue, may be useful for pushing the boundaries of the current dominant conceptualization of recovery.

Recovering "Recovery": Challenges and Possibilities

As the foregoing has illustrated, recovery as a concept and a paradigm is continually evolving and is poised either to disrupt biomedical dominance in favour of social and structural understandings of mental distress, or to continue to play into individualistic neoliberal political agendas and discourses that work against social justice in mental health. Ranged against recovery are some key challenges. First, the ways in which biomedicalism and neoliberalism are co-constitutive enhance and support each other ideologically, creating significant barriers to shifting society's understanding of mental distress. These barriers are both discursive and material. They are discursive in that the individualized notion of mental illness as a disease or disorder of the brain that can be alleviated through psycho-pharmaceutical interventions is showing no signs of abating. Indeed, media reactions in 2011 to the MHCC draft strategy suggest that at least some members of the general population and health opinion-makers are hostile to any kind of rebalancing of the mental health system towards the aims of mental health recovery and promotion (Brean, 2011a; Inman, 2011a,b; Picard, 2011). Second, neoliberal policy reform has meant real decisions about allocation of resources, which continue to favour acute and psychiatric care over social forms of care such as housing and income supports.

In favour of recovery are some key developments. The MHCC has opened up a space for a national dialogue on recovery and, in particular, a place to include social understandings of recovery in its work. Given the profile of the MHCC in the Canadian context this is an important development and, as documented above, it is already garnering attention and debate beyond its own process. Dialogue about recovery is one way forward. But perhaps most importantly, the critical work of psychiatric survivors, Mad activists, and their allies has continually pushed society to think beyond purely medical understandings of mental distress. This activism and writing harbours the most potential for a real paradigm shift in mental health that holds a place for recovery as a radical idea grounded in social justice.

Notes

1 I would like to acknowledge the team at the Centre for the Study of Gender, Social Inequities and Mental Health, www.socialinequities.ca (Brenda Jamer, Lupin Battersby, Julia Weisser, Susan Hardie, and Richard Ingram) for their many insightful and engaging conversations over the years on mental health and recovery and for their helpful review of this chapter.

2 By social inequities I mean differences between and among groups that are *systematic*, *socially produced*, and *unfair* (Whitehead & Dahlgren, 2007).

3 Indeed it has been noted that Canada is the only G8 country without a mental health strategy. See www.mentalhealthcommission.ca/SiteCollectionDocuments/strategy/ Mental%20Health%20Strategy%20framework%20release.pdf. Accessed September 28, 2011.

4 The term "psy professions" or "psy sciences" has its origins in the work of Foucault (1979) and Rose (1998).

5 The report, *Out of the Shadows at Last: Transforming Mental Health, Mental Illness and Addiction Services in Canada* (Kirby, 2006), was the culmination of a three-year nationwide study and consultation on mental health services undertaken by one of Canada's senators, Michael Kirby, and the Standing Senate Committee on Social Affairs, Science and Technology, during a period of intense public debate about Canada's health care system and health reform.

6 The World Café methodology involves concurrent round table discussions that are focused around a set of questions (Brown & Isaacs, 2005). This approach allows for multi-layered discussions that build upon one another and fosters the expression of multiple perspectives and kinds of knowledge (personal, professional, academic).

Glossary of Terms

Ableism: An assemblage of laws, policies, attitudes, words, and actions that privilege the able-bodied and disadvantage people with disabilities. Ableism stems from the time-worn discriminatory prejudice that disability is a "defect" that renders its bearers less capable than their able-bodied counterparts of contributing to society and participating as full citizens.

Adultism: The oppression experienced by children and young people at the hands of adults and adult-produced/adult-tailored systems. It relates to the socio-political status differentials and power relations endemic to adult-child relations. Adultism may include experiences of individual prejudice and discrimination as well as systemic oppression. It is characterized by adult authoritarianism towards children and adult-centric perspectives in interacting with children and in understanding children's experiences. Within child psychiatry, adultism and sanism may intersect in ways that are experienced as intolerable and resisted by children.

Akathisia: A movement disorder caused by psychiatric drugs, often accompanying the neurological syndrome called tardive dyskinesia (TD—see below), characterized by muscular quivering, restlessness, and an inability to sit still.

Anti-oppressive practice (AOP): A reaction to the "mainstreaming" of social work, and rise of neoliberalism, and part of a move beyond class, AOP is an approach to social work that began in the United Kingdom during the late 1980s. Part of the critical social work tradition, it addresses social divisions and structural inequalities, and embodies a person-centred philosophy as well as a focus on process and outcome. Key practice principles include critical self-reflection and critical assessment of users' experiences of oppression, empowerment, partnership, and minimal intervention.

Antipsychiatry: A set of beliefs and initiatives involving strategic and radical resistance to psychiatry; its fundamental goal is dismantling or abolishing psychiatry. See the website of the Coalition Against Psychiatric Assault, a grassroots political action organization, including its mandate—http://coalitionagainstpsychiatricassault.wordpress.com.

Assertive community treatment: A treatment model whereby mental health workers can invade a person's home in order to enforce coerced compliance with medication orders.

Big Pharma: The pharmaceutical industry, with particular reference to the giant multinational corporations that manufacture and market psychoactive drugs. Since the release of chlorpromazine by Rhône-Poulenc in 1953, the trade in neuroleptics, "anti-anxiety" drugs, "antidepressants," and other brain chemistry-altering compounds has generated profits to the tune of tens of billions of dollars for corporations like AstraZeneca, GlaxoSmithKline, Eli Lilly, Janssen, Johnson & Johnson, Pfizer, and Roche. For decades, Big Pharma has been the subject of widespread critique and resistance focusing on the damaging effects of its products, its questionable testing and marketing strategies, its collusion with biomedical psychiatry, and its targeting of vulnerable populations including children, seniors and, increasingly, inhabitants of the global south.

Biomedical psychiatry: Grounded in a century-long tradition dating to the work of German psychiatrist Emil Kraepelin, the biomedical model of psychiatry asserts that "mental illness" is a brain disorder caused by pathological genes, chemistry, or neural matter. In the 21st century, biomedicine remains the central paradigm of psychiatric theory and practice.

Bradykinesia: A movement disorder caused by psychiatric drugs, often accompanying the neurological syndrome called tardive dyskinesia (TD—see below), characterized by slowed or decreased movement.

Conscientization: A term popularized by Brazilian educator Paulo Freire—a form of consciousness-raising that prioritizes dialogue, reflection, and action. It is the attempt to humanize the world, to name the world in order to change the world.

Consumer: A euphemism for "mental patient." Many people feel that the use of this term is highly inappropriate because it implies such marketplace criteria as choice and customer satisfaction.

Consumer/survivor: A term used to encompass both those who have received psychiatric treatment voluntarily and those who have had it forced upon them.

Consumer/survivor advocates: Former or current mental health patients who take a critical human rights perspective on the mental health system and advocate within that context for the individual or collective rights of mental health consumer/survivors. This rise of rights-based ideas and practices has been an important aspect of the broader shift to community-based mental health services.

c/s/x community: c/s/x is an acronym for consumer, survivor, ex-patient, all of which signify particular identity politics or relations to the psychiatric system. It is a handy way of referring to people who are receiving or have received psychiatric treatment (see "consumer/survivor" above, and "psychiatric survivor" below). The "x" may stand for "ex-patient" or "ex-inmate."

Deinstitutionalization: Commencing in the 1960s, governments began to downsize and, eventually, to close down public "primary care" psychiatric institutions. Within 25 years, the number of long-term in-patient beds in Canada had plummeted by 50,000 (by the 1980s, about two-thirds of beds had been emptied). Trumpeted as an innovative venture in "community mental health," deinstitutionalization proved to be a catastrophic exercise in state minimalism, fiscal conservatism, and the privatization of the health and social service sectors. Countless thousands of psychiatrized people found themselves being "dumped" from hospital; consigned to survival existence in an inner-city world of chronic poverty, homelessness, and victimization; and "transinstitutionalized" from the mental health system into the criminal courts, jails, and prisons.

DSM: The *Diagnostic and Statistical Manual of Mental Disorders* of the American Psychiatric Association is the world's most influential compilation of psychiatric labels. Since the publication of DSM-I in 1952, the manual has undergone six revisions, with DSM-5 slated for release in May 2013. The DSM has come under widespread criticism—even by such former advocates as Robert Spitzer and Allen Frances—for its unscientific foundations, its entrenchment of cultural biases, its use as a profit-making instrument by biogenetic psychiatry and the pharmaceutical industry, and its pathologization of ever-expanding realms of human experience.

Electroshock: Also called "electroconvulsive therapy" or "ECT." A controversial psychiatric procedure in which electricity (usually 150–300 volts) is delivered to the brain in a series of "treatments." Immediate and direct effects include a grand mal epileptic seizure, convulsion, confusion, disorientation, and memory loss; long-term effects include permanent memory loss, brain damage, loss of intellectual or creative skills, and trauma. Electroshock is mainly prescribed to women and elderly people labelled "depressed"; 2 to 3 times more women than men are prescribed electroshock.

Epistemic violence: Refers to the violence done to people via particular worldviews or knowledge claims. Imposing biomedical explanations of mental distress and pharmaceutical treatments (by the use of force, including in the form of Community Treatment Orders) on a patient who believes that the cause and the solution for their distressing symptoms is a social one is an example of epistemic violence. In other words, epistemic violence involves ignoring someone's reality from their perspective, while informing them that they are too sick to be able to have insight into their condition when they disagree with psychiatric opinions.

Essentialize: To claim that particular attributes are a necessary part of a specific entity; to consider particular attributes to be a natural or inborn part of a specific entity; to reduce complex phenomena associated with particular groups or identities to simplistic biological or cultural explanations.

Extrapyramidal symptoms: Refers the damage caused by psychiatric drugs to the extrapyramidal system—the neural network that governs involuntary movements, reflexes, and physical coordination.

Healthification: The conversion of social problems into health problems. As with the medicalization of human distress at the level of the individual, healthification functions to divert attention from the systemic and hegemonic conditions that undermine human well-being. In the process, healthification privileges (bio)medicine as the primary instrument of individual recovery and social betterment, to the exclusion of political engagement, institutional reform, structural change, and the pursuit of human justice.

Hegemony: Refers to systemic dominance generally, although it is most commonly employed in reference to dominant ideological beliefs and the words that accompany them. When beliefs are hegemonic, they are so widely accepted that the average person takes them as common sense—in other words, is not aware that they are part of an ideology at all, never mind part of a regime of ruling.

Heteropatriarchy: A term used to refer to the intersection between the structures of heteronormativity and patriarchy. Heteronormativity designates fixed and binary categories of sex (male/female), gender (masculine/feminine), and sexuality (heterosexuality/homosexuality), and assumes a relationship of coherence between sex, gender, and sexuality whereby sex =

gender = sexuality (male = masculine = heterosexual). Patriarchy assumes that masculine attributes and ways of knowing are superior to feminine ones. The intersection between heteronormativity and patriarchy produces the naturalization of heterosexuality and the privileging of masculinity within social institutions. Importantly, heteropatriarchy is racialized and classed, and therefore, largely reflects the norms and values associated with the dominant white, middle-class, and heterosexual group.

Iatrogenesis: Damage caused by medical treatment.

Identity politics: Political engagement organized around group identification, common interest, and shared experience of oppression (as in the politics of gender, class, race, disability, sexual identity, and Mad identity).

Mad nationalism: The articulation of the Mad movement through an appeal to identity politics; analogous to "homonationalism," a term coined by anti-racist queer theorists to describe the process by which some queer people gain normative status through making rights claims on the state, thereby leveraging white privilege and liberal-nationalist ideas of progress.

Mad ontology: The idea that Mad people have trans-historical characteristics that make us distinct from non-Mad people; this idea may be discerned both in medical model approaches to madness, and in the Mad identity politics claim that we have existed, and have been persecuted, throughout history.

Mad pride: An international movement of psychiatric consumers/survivors/ex-patients/mental health service users who self-identify as proud of their Mad identity. The movement originated as Psychiatric Survivor Pride in Toronto, Canada, in 1993.

Mad Studies: An umbrella term that is used to embrace the body of knowledge that has emerged from psychiatric survivors, Mad-identified people, antipsychiatry academics and activists, critical psychiatrists, and radical therapists. This body of knowledge is wide-ranging and includes scholarship that is critical of the mental health system as well as radical and Mad activist scholarship. This field of study is informed by and generated by the perspectives of psychiatric survivors and Mad-identified researchers and academics.

Madness: A ubiquitous term for a range of phenomena (e.g., violence, extremity, creativity, excellence, chaos) historically used in the West to indicate irrationality, confusion, or distress in a situation or an individual (e.g., mania, melancholy, lunacy). Madness discourse was formulated into psycho-medical terms (e.g., psychosis, depression, asociality) and psycho-legal terms (e.g., insanity, incapacity), but has recently been reclaimed for broader social, cultural, even liberatory approaches to medicalized experience, especially by people treated involuntarily. Mad people (not the trope of madness per se) provide the grounds for these new discourses, often in tension with dominant explanations of experience.

Matrix of domination: Black feminist sociologist Patricia Hill Collins introduced this concept as a cornerstone of intersectionality theory to capture the overlapping, relational experiences and effects of multiple oppressions based on gender, race, class, culture, sexual orientation, youth, seniority, disability, and corresponding axes of domination and subjugation. In this book we argue that mentalities, and oppressions grounded in sanist and biopsychiatric ideologies, represent a key dimension of the matrix of domination.

MDI theory: Pioneered by Australian feminist psychologist and author Jane Ussher, MDI theory adopts a material-discursive-intrapsychic approach to understanding and addressing women's misery. Ussher argues that these three realms of experience operate interdependently and dialectically. Accordingly, it is incumbent on feminist theorists, activists, and clinical practitioners to simultaneously engage the material conditions that impinge on women's lives, the discursive fields that structure their thoughts and social relations, and the pains that they endure at the levels of consciousness, identity, and experience.

Minimum separation distance (MSD) requirements: Municipal bylaws that require particular types of land uses to be a specific distance away from one another.

Neoliberalism: A political philosophy and an economic system that gives expression to Margaret Thatcher's infamous maxim that "there is no such thing as society." Since the 1980s, neoliberals have dominated geopolitics and domestic governments in the "developed" world, promoting policies of "free" market economy, globalization, state minimalism, the expansion and deregulation of "private enterprise," lower taxation for corporations and the rich, the hollowing out of systems of social provision (including health, welfare, and education), and the celebration of the autonomous, self-governing, "responsibilized" citizen.

Neuroleptic: Literally "nerve-seizing," refers to the class of psychiatric drugs also known as phenothiazines or antipsychotics. These drugs are often often given to patients who are assessed as having unusual or bizarre thoughts, or who have been deemed to engage in violent or destructive behaviour. These drugs inhibit the activity of brain cells, and therefore have a powerful sedative effect. These drugs also have serious side effects.

Neuroleptic malignant syndrome: A fatal condition of the nervous system caused by an adverse reaction to neuroleptic drugs (see above).

Normalization: The social processes that allow for particular ideas, behaviours, attributes, and so on to be understood as normal/valuable within a given society. Those who deviate from a society's norms are required, if deemed possible, to go through rehabilitative procedures in order to attempt to achieve normalcy.

Participatory democracy: An organizational philosophy that prioritizes the collective over the individual and seeks to democratize social or political groups by enabling broad-based decision-making and equal participation, thus rendering traditional hierarchical power relationships null. An organizing principle of anarchist republicans in the Spanish Civil War, of the leftist groups of the 1960s and 1970s, and of the Occupy movement of 2011, participatory democracy is connected to the notion of small world networks, but is inherently political in nature.

Pathologization: The practice of construing thought and behaviour as symptoms of disease; a pretext for drugging/electroshocking people whose thoughts/behaviours others dislike (or who dislike their own thoughts/behaviours) and indeed for the existence of biomedical psychiatry.

Performativity: A term used to refer to how the compulsory repetition of speech and language, acts, expressions, and behaviours brings into existence that which it names. Judith Butler (1999) has used the concept of performativity to reveal the illusion of gender as naturally and logically arising from some *real* substance of the self. It is through the repetition of gendered acts, expressions, and behaviours that gender gets produced on the surface of bodies.

Gender is conceptualized as a performative speech act through which bodies are materialized and "naturalized" as man and woman.

Psychiatric knowledge: The discourses that the profession of psychiatry put forth as explanatory truths about the origins, causes, and treatments of madness. Psychiatric knowledge attempts to be the dominant way in which we construct and act upon madness, as well as influence the organizational strategies that are put in place to deal with difference.

Psychiatric survivor: Someone who considers herself/himself to have survived psychiatric treatment—often someone who has been treated by force.

Radicalism: Meaning "of the root(s)," radical refers to political policies, attitudes, or practices that advocate more sweeping political, economic, or social change than that traditionally supported by the mainstream political parties or mainstream society. In the context of mental health history, Mad liberation or survivor movements have embodied a radical approach by advocating the redistribution of power away from the psychiatric and medical professions and institutions to people who have received a psychiatric diagnosis or mental health services.

Refusal terms: Terms that people—oppressed communities in particular—use when combatting the hegemonic words of those in power. In various ways and to different degrees, just by being uttered or written, "refusal" terms call the hegemonic terms into question (see "hegemony" above).

Sanism: Originally coined by Morton Birnbaum but popularized by Michael Perlin, director of the Mental Disability Law Studies Program at New York Law School, sanism describes the systematic subjugation of people who have received mental health diagnoses or treatment. Also known as mentalism (see Judi Chamberlin's work for more information), sanism may result in various forms of stigma, blatant discrimination, and a host of microaggressions. These may include low expectations and professional judgments that individuals with mental health issues are "incompetent, not able to do things for themselves, constantly in need of supervision and assistance, unpredictable, violent and irrational" (Chamberlin, 1990, p. 2).

Social constructionism: Also known as social constructivism, this tradition of sociological theory advances the view that social facts are not inherent to people and things, but are rather the contingent product of historical processes, institutional contexts, discursive practices, and social relations. The "labelling" theory of mental "illness," pioneered by Thomas Scheff in the 1960s, is an example of social constructionism applied to Mad Studies.

Social death: To experience social death is to find oneself reduced to a less-than-fully-human status by governments, institutions, professions, and the wider culture. Many people who bear psychiatric labels are consigned to a state of social death by virtue of being objectified, pathologized, infantilized, rendered invisible, and otherwise relegated to society's margins.

Social mix: A government policy response that attempts to address social problems associated with concentrations of poor tenants in public housing. Social mix involves dispersing and/or "integrating" tenants on social assistance into areas with a large number of homeowners and private renters.

Spatial justice: An arrangement of space that encourages and/or enhances a just distribution of resources, e.g., the elimination of minimum separation distances by municipalities would enhance opportunities for psychiatric survivors to live in residential areas.

Structural violence: Understood as an institutionalized form of violence that is ingrained in everyday practices of institutions or social policies that disenfranchise some people but not others. Structural violence is hard to recognize because there is usually no individual perpetuator of violence and it receives no objection from society. Schools, hospitals, organized religions, and psychiatry can all engage in structural violence, while those who work within them can be unaware of the full implications of their taken-for-granted practices.

Survivor researchers: Former subjects of mental health research who have become health and social science researchers, creating new knowledge and advancing new researching methodologies and approaches that challenge traditional research agendas and products by inserting a user perspective. Closely connected in perspective and politics to the psychiatric survivor movement and hence generally critical of biomedical responses to madness, survivor research has developed as a field since the 1990s, and is particularly strong in the UK and continental Europe.

Systemic racism: The social and institutionalized processes that support and solidify racial discrimination and inequality as they are embedded in institutional, legal, organizational, economic, and everyday policies and procedures.

Tardive dyskinesia (TD): A disfiguring and sometimes incapacitating movement disorder resulting from a neurological syndrome commonly caused by psychiatric drugs (especially neuroleptics—see above). TD can cause tremors, tics, spasms, twitches, and other involuntary movements, especially of the face, tongue, and limbs. TD makes people look much crazier than they are. Due to increased use of neuroleptics, its incidence has reached epidemic proportions.

White liberal discourse: A (neo)colonialist tradition of narratives and truth claims that presents itself as upholding progressive, "tolerant" perspectives on "race relations," while implicitly marginalizing the histories and experiences of racialized peoples, and centring whiteness as the racial category against which all others are judged and found wanting.

White settler supremacy: White settlers in Canada are those who have settled within this nation-state and by doing so continue to partake in the displacement, forced assimilation, attempted genocide, and spatial containment of Indigenous peoples. White settler supremacy embodies the ongoing social, political, economic, and legal narratives that allow white settlers and their frameworks to be understood as central in origin to this land. By enacting white settler frameworks as dominant, all other people and their frameworks are understood as minority and marginalized.

The following *Mad Matters* authors and editors contributed terms to this glossary: Bonnie Burstow, Andrea Daley, Megan Davies, Shaindl Diamond, Lilith "Chava" Finkler, Rachel Gorman, Ji-Eun Lee, Brenda LeFrançois, Robert Menzies, Jennifer M. Poole, Geoffrey Reaume, Irit Shimrat, and Jijian Voronka.

References

Abdallah, C., Cohen, C.I., Sanchez-Almira, M., Reyes, P., & Ramirez, P. (2009). Community integration and associated factors among older adults with schizophrenia. *Psychiatric Services, 60*, 1642–1648.

Abraham, C. (2008, November 24). Psychiatry: A specialty relegated to the basement. *Globe and Mail*. Retrieved January 9, 2012, from http://v1.theglobeandmail.com/servlet/story/RTGAM.20081124.wmhstigma1125/BNStory/mentalhealth/.

ActiveHistory.ca. (n.d.). Retrieved from http://activehistory.ca/.

Adams, N., Daniels, A., & Compagni, A. (2009). International pathways to mental health transformation. *International Journal of Mental Health, 28*(1), 30–45.

Adamson, N., Briskin, L., & McPhail, M. (1988). *Feminists organizing for change: The contemporary women's movement in Canada*. Don Mills: Oxford University Press.

Ahmed, S. (2007). A phenomenology of whiteness. *Feminist Theory, 8*(2), 149–168.

Alarie, B., & Green, A. (2010). Interventions at the Supreme Court of Canada: Accuracy, affiliation, and acceptance. *Osgoode Hall Law Journal, 48*(3), 381–410.

American Civil Liberties Union. (n.d.). Retrieved November 6, 2011, from www.aclu.org/key-issues.

American Psychiatric Association. (2000). *Diagnostic and statistical manual of mental disorders* (4th ed.). Washington: American Psychiatric Association.

American Psychological Association. (2001). *Publication manual of the American Psychological Association* (5th ed.). Washington: American Psychological Association.

Anastakis, D., & Martel, M. (Eds.). (2008). *The sixties: Passion, politics and style*. Montreal: McGill-Queen's University Press.

Andre, L. (2009). *Doctors of deception: What they don't want you to know about shock treatment*. New Brunswick: Rutgers University Press.

Andreasen, N.C. (2008, September 16). A conversation with Nancy C. Andreasen: Using imaging to look at changes in the brain. *New York Times*.

Anglicare Tasmania. (2009). *Experts by experience: Strengthening the mental health consumer voice in Tasmania*. Anglicare Tasmania in association with the Tasmanian Mental Health Consumer Network.

Angus, W.A. (1966). The Mental Health Act of Alberta. *University of Toronto Law Journal, 16*(2), 423–430.

Anthony, W.A. (1993). Recovery from mental illness: The guiding vision of the mental health service system in the 1990s. *Psychosocial Rehabilitation Journal, 16*(4), 11–23.

Anthony, W.A., & Liberman, P.R. (1986). The practice of psychiatric rehabilitation: Historical, conceptual, and research base. *Schizophrenia Bulletin, 12*(4), 521–559.

Appignanesi, L. (2008). *Sad, mad and bad: Women and the mind-doctors from 1800–2007*. London: Virago.

Aronsen, L. (2011). *City of love and revolution: Vancouver in the sixties*. Vancouver: New Star Press.

Arthurson, K. (2002). Creating inclusive communities through balancing social mix: A critical relationship or tenuous link? *Urban Policy and Research, 20*(3), 245–261.

Arthurson, K. (2012). *Social mix and the city: Challenging the mixed communities consensus in housing and urban planning policies*. Victoria, AU: CSIRO Publishing.

Atkinson, R. (2005). *Neighbourhoods and impacts of social mix: Crime, tenure diversification and assisted mobility*. Hobart, TAS: Centre for Neighbourhood Research, University of Tasmania.

Attig, T. (2004). Meanings of death seen through the lens of grieving. *Death Studies, 28*(4), 341–360.

Aubry, T., & Myner, J. (1996). Community integration and quality of life: A comparison of persons with psychiatric disabilities in housing programs and community residents who are neighbours. *Canadian Journal of Community Mental Health, 15*(1), 5–20.

Aubry, T., Tefft, B., & Currie, R. (1995). Public attitudes and intentions regarding tenants of community mental health residences who are neighbours. *Community Mental Health Journal, 31*(1), 39–52.

August, M. (2008). Social mix and Canadian public housing redevelopment: Experiences in Toronto. *Canadian Journal of Urban Research, 17*(1), 82–100.

Austin, J.L. (1961). Performative utterances. In J.O. Urmsom & G.L. Warnock (Eds.), *Austin, philosophical papers* (pp. 239–251). Oxford: Oxford University Press.

Bagley, C., & Tremblay, P. (2000). Elevated rates of suicidal behaviour in gay, lesbian and bisexual youth. *Crisis, 21*(3), 111–117.

Baistow, K. (2000). Problems of powerlessness: Psychological explanations of social inequality and civil unrest in post-war America. *History of the Human Sciences, 13*(3), 95–116.

Baker, F.M., & Bell, C.C. (1999). Issues in the psychiatric treatment of African Americans. *Psychiatric Services, 50*(3), 362–368.

Balachandra, K., Swaminath, S., & Litman, L.C. (2004). Impact of Winko on absolute discharges. *Journal of the American Academy of Psychiatry and the Law, 32*(2), 173–177.

Baldwin, C. (2005). Narrative, ethics and people with severe mental illness. *Australian and New Zealand Journal of Psychiatry, 39*(6), 1022–1029.

Bannerji, H. (2000). *The dark side of the nation: Essays on multiculturalism, nationalism and gender*. Toronto: Canadian Scholars' Press.

Bannerji, H. (1995). *Thinking through: Essays on feminism, Marxism and anti-racism*. Toronto: Women's Press.

Barmak, S. (2008, January 19). Regent Park: Another attempt at "heaven." *Toronto Star*. Retrieved January 9, 2012, from www.thestar.com/living/article/294491.

Barnes, J. (2004). *Making policy, making law: An interbranch perspective*. Washington: Georgetown University Press.

Barnes, J. (2007). The mobilisation and diffusion of rights: Organizational responses to accessibility laws at the community level. Retrieved December 30, 2011, from http://escholarship.org/uc/item/39v186v186kh.

Barnes, M., & Berke, J. (1971). *Mary Barnes: Two accounts of a journey through madness*. New York: Harcourt Brace Jovanovich.

Barron, C., & Lacombe, D. (2005). Moral panic and the nasty girl. *Canadian Review of Sociology, 42*(1), 51–69.

Bartlett, A., King, M., & Smith, G. (2004). Treatments of homosexuality in Britain since the 1950s—an oral history: The experiences of professionals. *British Medical Journal, 328*(7437), 429–431.

Bartlett, P. (2001). English mental health reform: Lessons from Ontario. *Journal of Mental Health Law, 27,* 27–43.

Bartz, N., Joseph, M.L., & Chaskin, R.J. (2011, July 5). The new stigma of relocated public housing residents: Challenges to social identity in mixed-income communities. Presented at the European Network for Housing Research (ENHR) Conference, Toulouse, France.

Bay, M. (2003). The evolution of mental health law in Ontario. In Psychiatric Patient Advocate Office, *Mental health and patients' rights in Ontario: Yesterday, today and tomorrow* (p. 14). Psychiatric Patient Advocate Office 20th Anniversary. Toronto: Queen's Printer.

BC ECT Statistics, Health System Planning Division. (2008). Distinct patients count and number of services for electroconvulsive therapy, by client age group and gender, calendar years 2002 to 2007. Victoria: Ministry of Health.

Beal, G., Chan, A., Chapman, S., Edgar, J., McInnis-Perry, G., Osborne, M., & Mina, S. (2007). Consumer input into standards revision: Changing practice. *Journal of Psychiatric and Mental Health Nursing, 14,* 13–20.

Bentall, R. (2009). *Doctoring the mind: Why psychiatric treatments fail.* London: Penguin.

Beresford, P. (2002). User involvement in research and evaluation: Liberation or regulation? *Social Policy and Society, 1,* 95–105.

Beresford, P. (2005). Social approaches to madness and distress: User perspectives and user knowledges. In J. Tew (Ed.), *Social perspectives in mental health* (pp. 32–52). London: Jessica Kingsley.

Beresford, P., Branfield, F., Taylor, J., Brennan, M., Sartori, A., Lalani, M., & Wise, G. (2006). Working together for better social work education. *Social Work Education, 25*(4), 326–331.

Bielavitz, S., Wisdom, J., & Pollack, D. (2011). Effective mental health consumer education: A preliminary exploration. *The Journal of Behavioral Health Services and Research, 38*(1), 105–113.

Birnbaum, R. (2010). My father's advocacy for a right to treatment. *Journal of the American Academy of Psychiatry and the Law, 38*(1), 115–123.

Bishop, A. (1994). *Becoming an ally: Breaking the cycle of oppression.* Halifax: Fernwood.

Blackbridge, P. (1997). *Prozac highway.* Vancouver: Press Gang.

Blackbridge, P., & Gilhooly, S. (1985). *Still sane.* Vancouver: Press Gang.

Bonanno, G.A. (2009). *The other side of sadness: What the new science of bereavement tells us about life after loss.* Philadelphia: Basic Books.

Bordo, S. (1998). Bringing body into theory. In D. Welton (Ed.), *Body and flesh: A philosophical reader* (pp. 84–97). Oxford: Blackwell Publishers Ltd.

Bordone, S. (2003). Siting supportive housing facilities: An analysis of lessons learned. Master's thesis, University of Toronto.

Borland, K. (1991). "That's not what I said": Interpretive conflict in oral narrative research. In S.B. Gluck & D. Patai (Eds.), *Women's words: The feminist practice of oral history* (pp. 63–76). New York: Routledge.

Bourget, B., & Chenier, R. (2007). *Mental health literacy in Canada: Phase one report, mental health literacy project.* Retrieved September 20, 2011, from www.camimh.ca/files/literacy/MHL_REPORT_Phase_One.pdf.

Boyce, W. (2001). The Ontario Advocacy Act: Representing persons with intellectual disabilities. In W. Boyce, M.A. McColl, M. Tremblay, J. Bickenbach, A. Crichton, S. Andrews & N. Gerein (Eds.), *A seat at the table: Persons with disabilities and policy making* (pp. 85–108). Montreal & Kingston: McGill-Queen's University Press.

Boydell, K., Gladstone, B., & Crawford, E. (2002). The dialectic of friendship for people with psychiatric disabilities. *Psychiatric Rehabilitation Journal*, 26(2), 123–132.

Boydell, K., Gladstone, B., Crawford, E., & Trainor, J. (1999). Making do on the outside: Everyday life in the neighbourhoods of people with psychiatric disabilities. *Psychiatric Rehabilitation Journal*, 23(1), 11–19.

Boyer, M., Ku, J., & Shakir, U. (1997). *The healing journey: Phase II report—women and mental health: Documenting the voices of ethnoracial women within an anti-racist framework*. Toronto: Across Boundaries Mental Health Centre.

Boyle, M. (2006). Developing real alternatives to medical models. *Ethical Human Psychology and Psychiatry*, 8(3), 191–200.

Bracken, P., & Thomas, P. (2005). *Postpsychiatry: Mental health in a postmodern world*. Oxford: Oxford University Press.

Brandon, D. (1991). *Innovation without change? Consumer power in psychiatric services*. Basingstoke: Macmillan.

Brandon, D. (1998). *Speaking truth to power: Care planning with disabled people*. London: British Association of Social Workers.

Brean, J. (2010a, May 7). Mad pride: Movement to depose psychiatry emerges from the shadows. *National Post*. Retrieved January 25, 2011, from www.nationalpost.com/Mental+block+Opposers+Pride+protest+anti+psychiatrist/3996581/story.html.

Brean, J. (2010b, May 8). Mind control: Activists gather in Toronto for rare global event promoting the overthrow of psychiatry. *National Post*, A8.

Brean, J. (2010c, December 18). Mental block: Opposers of Mad Pride protest antipsychiatry. *National Post*. Retrieved January 25, 2011, from www.nationalpost.com/Mental+block+Opposers+Pride+protest+anti+psychiatrist/3996581/story.html.

Brean, J. (2011a, October 8). A rocky road to "recovery." *National Post*. Retrieved from www.nationalpost.com/scripts/rocky+road+recovery/5521554/story.html.

Brean, J. (2011b, October 8). Mental Health Commission struggles to find balance in developing strategy. *National Post*. Retrieved October 8, 2011, from http://news.nationalpost.com/2011/10/08/mental-health-commission-struggles-to-find-balance-in-developing-strategy/.

Breeding, J. (2000). Electroshock and informed consent. *Journal of Humanistic Psychology*, 40(1), 65–79.

Breeding, J. (2001). Testimony to New York assembly public hearing on forced electroshock, May 18, 2001. Retrieved from www.ect.org/effects/breeding_NYtestimony.html.

Breeding, J. (2011). A battle in Gaithersburg: Testimony presented at FDA hearings on reclassification of electroshock machines, January 27–28, Gaithersburg, MD.

Breen, L.J., & O'Connor, M. (2007). The fundamental paradox in the grief literature: A critical reflection. *Omega Journal of Death and Dying*, 53(3), 199–218.

Breggin, P. (1991). *Toxic psychiatry: Why therapy, empathy, and love must replace the drugs, electroshock, and biochemical theories of the new psychiatry*. New York: St. Martin's Press.

Breggin, P. (1997). *Brain-disabling treatments in psychiatry*. New York: Springer Publishing Company.

Breggin, P. (1998a). *Reclaiming our children: A healing plan for a nation in crisis.* New York: Perseus Books.

Breggin, P. (1998b). Electroshock: Scientific, ethical, and political issues. *International Journal of Risk and Safety in Medicine, 11,* 5–40.

Breggin, P. (1998c). *Talking back to Ritalin: What doctors aren't telling you about stimulants for children.* Monroe: Common Courage Press.

Breggin, P. (2001). *Talking back to Ritalin, revised: What doctors aren't telling you about stimulants and ADHD.* New York: Perseus Books.

Breggin, P. (2002). *The Ritalin fact book: What your doctor won't tell you about ADHD and stimulant drugs.* New York: Perseus Books.

Breggin, P. (2008a). Electroshock for depression. In P. Breggin, *Brain-disabling treatments in psychiatry* (2nd ed., pp. 129–156). New York: Springer Publishing Company.

Breggin, P. (2008b). *Medication madness: The role of psychiatric drugs in cases of violence, suicide and murder.* New York: St. Martin's Press.

Breggin, P., & Breggin, G.R. (1998). *The war against children of color: How the drugs, programs, and theories of the psychiatric establishment are threatening America's children with a medical "cure" for violence.* New York: Perseus Books.

Breggin, P., & Cohen, D. (1999). *Your drug may be your problem.* Reading: Perseus Books.

British Broadcasting Corporation. (2008). Capture Wales digital history website. Retrieved from www.bbc.co.uk/wales/arts/yourvideo/queries/capturewales.shtml.

British Columbia Schizophrenia Society. (n.d.). Retrieved from www.bcss.org/category/aboutbcss/.

Brown, J., & Isaacs, D. (2005). *The World Café: Shaping our futures through conversations that matter.* San Francisco: Berrett-Koehler Publishers.

Brown, M. (2011, August 15). Son who stabbed father to death was schizophrenic, court hears. *Sydney Morning Herald.* Retrieved January 21, 2012, from www.smh.com.au/nsw/son-who-stabbed-father-to-death-was-schizophrenic-court-hears-20110815-1ityg.html.

Brown, M.P. (2000). *Closet space: Geographies of metaphor from the body to the globe.* New York: Routledge.

Brown, P. (1990). The name game: Toward a sociology of diagnosis. *Journal of Mind and Behavior, 11,* 385–406.

Browne, A., Varcoe, C., & Fridkin, A. (2011). Addressing trauma, violence, and pain: Research on health services for women at the intersections of history and economics. In O. Hankivsky (Ed.), *Health inequities in Canada: Intersectional frameworks and practices* (pp. 295–311). Vancouver: UBC Press.

Budd, D. (1981, August 29). Presentation to workshop on movement history. Ninth Annual Conference on Human Rights and Psychiatric Oppression, Cleveland, OH.

Burbridge, K. (1986, March 12). Social agencies welcome easier group home bylaw. *Toronto Star.*

Burstow, B. (2003). Toward a radical understanding of trauma and trauma work. *Violence Against Women, 9*(11), 1293–1317.

Burstow, B. (2005). A critique of posttraumatic stress disorder and the DSM. *Journal of Humanistic Psychology, 45*(4), 429–445.

Burstow, B. (2006a). Electroshock as a form of violence against women. *Women Against Violence, 12*(4), 372–392.

Burstow, B. (2006b). Understanding and ending ECT: A feminist imperative. *Canadian Woman Studies, 25*(1,2), 115–122.

Burstow, B. (2010). The withering away of psychiatry. *Conference proceedings for PsychOUT*, Toronto. Retrieved from http://aecp.oise.utoronto.ca/psychout/.

Burstow, B., & Weitz, D. (1988). *Shrink resistant: The struggle against psychiatry in Canada*. Toronto: New Star Books.

Burstow, B., Gower, K., & Weitz, D. (1988, February 7). Abolish psychiatric institutions. *Toronto Star*, B2, SU2 Edition.

Butler, J. (1999). *Gender trouble: Feminism and the subversion of identity* (10th anniversary ed.). New York: Routledge.

Butler, R., & Parr, H. (1999). New geographies of illness, impairment and disability. In R. Butler & H. Parr, *Mind and body spaces: Geographies of illness, impairment and disability* (pp. 1–24). London: Routledge.

Cairney, R. (1996). "Democracy was never intended for degenerates": Alberta's flirtation with eugenics comes back to haunt it. *Canadian Medical Association Journal*, 155(6), 789–792.

Calloway, S.P., Dolan, R.J., Jacoby, R.J., & Levy, R. (1981). ECT and cerebral atrophy. *Acta Psychiatrica Scandinavica*, 64, 442–445.

Cameron, D.G. (1994). ECT: Sham statistics, the myth of convulsive therapy, and the case for consumer misinformation. *The Journal of Mind and Behavior*, 15(1,2), 177–198.

Caminero-Santangelo, M. (1998). *The madwoman can't speak: Or why insanity is not subversive*. Ithaca: Cornell University Press.

Camp, D. (1976, October 9). Saint John: A "dungeon." Campbellton outdated. *Telegraph Journal*, 15.

Campbell, P. (1996). The history of the user movement in the United Kingdom. In T. Heller, J. Reynolds, R. Gomm, R. Muston & S. Pattison (Eds.), *Mental health matters: A reader*. Buckingham: Open University Press.

Campbell, P. (1999). The service user/survivor movement. In C. Newnes, G. Holmes & C. Dunn (Eds.), *This is madness: A critical look at the future of mental health services*. Ross-on-Wye: PCCS Books.

Campbell, P. (2005). From little acorns—The mental health service user movement. In A. Bell & P. Lindley (Eds.), *Beyond the water towers: The unfinished revolution in mental health services 1985–2005*. London: Sainsbury Centre for Mental Health.

Campsie, P. (1994). A brief history of rooming houses in Toronto, 1972–94. Retrieved from www.ontariotenants.ca/research/rooming-houses.phtml.

Canadian Alliance on Mental Illness and Mental Health. (2011). About CAMIMH. Retrieved September 20, 2011, from http://camimh.ca/about-camimh/.

Canadian Civil Liberties Association. (n.d.). Retrieved November 6, 2011, from http://ccla.org/.

Canadian Medical Association. (2008). *8th annual national report card on health care*. Retrieved from www.cma.ca/multimedia/.../National_Report_Card_EN.pdf.

Canadian Psychiatric Association. (1979). Consent in psychiatry: The position of the Canadian Psychiatric Association, approved September 1979. *Canadian Journal of Psychiatry*, 25(1).

Canadian Task Force on Mental Health Issues Affecting Immigrants and Refugees. (1988). *After the door has been opened: Mental health issues affecting immigrants and refugees in Canada*. Ottawa: Health and Welfare Canada.

Caplan, P. (1996). *They say you're crazy: How the world's most powerful psychiatrists decide who's normal*. New York: Perseus.

Capponi, P. (1992). *Upstairs in the crazy house: The life of a psychiatric survivor*. Toronto: Viking.

Capponi, P. (1997). *Dispatches from the poverty line.* Toronto: Penguin.

Capponi, P. (2003). *Beyond the crazy house: Changing the future of madness.* Toronto: Penguin.

Carlson, K.T. (2009). *Mountains that see, and that need to be seen: Aboriginal perspectives on degraded visibility associated with air pollution in the BC Lower Mainland and Fraser Valley (A traditional knowledge study prepared for Environment Canada).* Retrieved from www.airhealthbc.ca/docs/aboriginal%20perspectives%20on%20visibility%20in%20lfv_carlson_2009.pdf .

Carver, P., & Langlois-Klassen, C. (2006). The role and powers of Forensic Psychiatric Review Boards in Canada: Recent developments. *Health Law Journal, 14,* 1–19.

Castel, R., Castel, F., & Lovell, A. (1982). *The psychiatric society.* New York: Columbia University Press.

Cellard, A, & Thifault, M-C. (2007). *Une toupie sur la tête. Visages de la folie à Saint-Jean-de-Dieu.* Montreal: Éditions du Boréal.

Centre for the Study of Gender, Social Inequities and Mental Health (CGSM). (2010). *A critical exploration of social inequities in mental health recovery: Summary of research.* Vancouver: CGSM.

Chadha, E. (2008). "Mentally defectives" not welcome: Mental disability in Canadian immigration law, 1859–1927. *Disability Studies Quarterly, 28*(1). Retrieved from www.dsq-sds.org/article/view/67/67.

Chamberlin, J. (1978). *On our own: Patient-controlled alternatives to the mental health system.* New York: McGraw-Hill.

Chamberlin, J. (1990). The ex-patients' movement: Where we've been and where we're going. *Journal of Mind and Behaviour, 11*(3), 323–336.

Chamberlin, J. (1995). Struggling to be born. In J. Grobe (Ed.), *Beyond bedlam: Contemporary women psychiatric survivors speak out* (pp. 59–64). Chicago: Third Side Press.

Chan, W., Chunn, D.E., & Menzies, R. (Eds.). (2005). *Women, madness and the law: A feminist reader.* London: GlassHouse, Cavendish.

Chesler, P. (1972). *Women and madness.* Garden City: Doubleday.

Chrisjohn, R.D., Young, S., & Maraun, M. (2006). *The circle game: Shadows and substance in the Indian residential school experience in Canada* (2nd ed.). Penticton: Theytus Books.

Church, K. (1993). Breaking down/breaking through: Multi-voiced narratives of psychiatric survivor participation in Ontario's mental health system. PhD diss., University of Toronto.

Church, K. (1995). *Forbidden narratives: Critical autobiography as social science.* Amsterdam: International Publishers Distributors. Reprinted by Routledge, London.

Church, K. (1997). *Because of where we've been: The business behind the business of psychiatric survivor economic development.* Toronto: Ontario Council of Alternative Businesses.

Church, K. (2006). Working like crazy on *Working Like Crazy*: Imag(in)ing CED practice through documentary film. In E. Shragge (Ed.), *Community economic development: Building for social change* (pp. 169–182). Sydney: University College of Cape Breton.

Church, K. (2011, April). Still "unsettled" after all these years? Exploring the contradictions of "mad" knowledge for professional practice in the academy. Presented at Unsettling Relations: Mad Activism and Academia, University of Central Lancashire, UK.

Church, K., & Reville, D. (1989). User involvement in the mental health field in Canada. *Canada's Mental Health, 37*(2), 22–25.

Church, K., & Reville, D. (2001). *"First we take Manhattan": Evaluation report on a community connections grant OCAB Regional Council Development*. Toronto, Ontario Council of Alternative Businesses.

Church, K., with Reville, D. (2010). Forward: Strike up the band! In M. McKoewn, L. Malihi-Shoja & S. Downe supporting the Comensus Writing Collective, *Service user and carer involvement in education for health and social care* (pp. ix–xiv). Oxford: Wiley-Blackwell.

Citizen's Commission on Human Rights. (2006). *Psychiatry: An industry of death*. Los Angeles: CCHR.

Clare, E. (2011, June 28). In whose interest? How psychiatric survivors can use our stories to change the world. Lecture presented by Recovering our Stories at Ryerson University, Toronto.

Claxton, T. (2008). From oppression to hope: Advocacy for voice and choice. The history of patient councils in Ontario—yesterday, today and tomorrow. In Psychiatric Patient Advocate Office, *Honouring the past, shaping the future: 25 years of progress in mental health advocacy and rights protection* (25th anniversary report, p. 83). Toronto: Queen's Printer for Ontario.

Clay, S. (2005). (Ed.). *On our own, together: Peer programs for people with mental illness*. Nashville: Vanderbilt University Press.

Cleary, A., & Dowling, M. (2009). The road to recovery. *Mental Health Practice, 12*(5), 28–31.

Coalition Against Psychiatric Assault. (2007, May 5). CAPA press statement: New study proves ECT damage conclusively: CAPA calls for action.

Coalition Against Psychiatric Assault. (2009, March 1). Letter to Ontario Health Minister David Caplan.

Coalition Against Psychiatric Assault. (2011a). CAPA statement to the FDA re shock machines. Docket No. FDA-2010-N-0585.

Coalition Against Psychiatric Assault. (2011b). Stop shocking our mothers and grandmothers. Retrieved from http://coalitionagainstpsychiatricassault.wordpress.com/?s=stop+shocking.

Cohen, C.I., & Timimi, S. (Eds.). (2008). *Liberatory psychiatry: Philosophy, politics and mental health*. New York: Cambridge University Press.

Cohen, D. (Ed.). (1990). *Challenging the therapeutic state: Critical perspectives on psychiatry and the mental health system*. New York: Institute of Mind and Behavior.

Cohen, M., Goldberg, M., Istvanffy, N., Stainton, T., Wasik, A., & Woods, K. (2008). *Removing barriers to work: Flexible employment options for people with disabilities in BC*. Vancouver: Canadian Centre for Policy Alternatives.

Cohn, T.A., Newcomer, J.W., Haupt, D.W., Sernyak, M.J., & Faulkner, G. (2006). Guest editorial and three review articles. *Canadian Journal of Psychiatry, 51*(8), 478–511.

Colbert, T. (2001). *Rape of the soul*. Tiscam: Kevco.

Coleman, E.G. (2008). The politics of rationality: Psychiatric survivors' challenge to psychiatry. In B. da Costa & K. Philip (Eds.), *Tactical biopolitics: Art, activism, and technoscience* (pp. 342–362). London: AK Press.

Collier, E. (2010). Confusion of recovery: One solution. *International Journal of Mental Health Nursing, 19*, 16–21.

Collins, A. (1988). *In the sleep room*. Toronto: Lester & Orpen Dennys.

Conle, C. (1999). Why narrative? Which narrative? Our struggle with time and place in teacher education. *Curriculum Inquiry, 29*(1), 7–33.

Conway, S. (2007). The changing face of death: Implications for public health. *Critical Public Health, 17*(3), 195–202.

Cooper, D. (Ed.). (1967). *Psychiatry and anti-psychiatry*. London: Paladin.

Coppock, V. (1997). "Mad," "bad" or misunderstood? In P. Scranton (Ed.), *"Childhood" in "crisis"?* (pp. 146–161). London: UCL Press.

Coppock, V. (2002). Medicalising children's behaviour. In B. Franklin (Ed.), *The new handbook of children's rights: Comparative policy and practice* (pp. 139–154). London: Routledge.

Corrigan, P. (2007). How clinical diagnosis may exacerbate the stigma of mental illness. *Social Work, 52*(1), 31–39.

Corrigan, P., Kerr, A., & Knudsen, L. (2005). The stigma of mental illness: Explanatory models and methods for change. *Applied and Preventive Psychology, 11*, 179–190.

Corrigan, P., Thompson, V., Lambert, D., Sangster, Y., Noel, J., & Campbell, J. (2003). Perceptions of discrimination among persons with serious mental illness. *Psychiatric Services, 54*(8), 1105–1110.

Corrigan, P., & Watson, A. (2002). The paradox of self-stigma and mental illness. *Clinical Psychology: Science and Practice, 9*(1), 35–53.

Corrigan, P., Watson, A., Gracia, G., Slopen, N., Rasinski, K., & Hall, L. (2005). Newspaper stories as measures of structural stigma. *Psychiatric Services, 56*, 551–556.

Corring, D.J., & Cook, J.V. (2007). Use of qualitative methods to explore the quality of life construct from a consumer perspective. *Psychiatric Services, 58*, 240–244.

Corry, M. (2008). *The final solution: Why ECT must be banned*. Dublin: The Wellbeing Foundation.

Costa, L. (2012, May 30–June 1). Consuming madness narratives: Uses and abuses in research. Paper presented at the annual meeting of the Canadian Disability Studies Association, Wilfrid Laurier University, Waterloo, ON.

Courvant, D., & Cook-Daniels, L. (1998). Transgender and intersex survivors of domestic violence: Defining terms, barriers and responsibilities. In National Coalition Against Domestic Violence, Conference manual, Denver, CO.

Crenshaw, K. (1991). Mapping the margins: Intersectionality, identity politics, and violence against women of color. *Stanford Law Review, 43*(6), 1241–1299.

Cresswell, M., & Spandler, H. (2012). The engaged academic: Academic intellectuals and the psychiatric survivor movement. *Social Movement Studies*.

Cribb, R. (2007, September 28). $5,800 bill for stats shocks researcher. *Toronto Star*.

Crossley, N. (2004). Not being mentally ill: Social movements, system survivors and the oppositional habitus. *Anthropology & Medicine, 11*(2), 161–180.

Crossley, N. (2006). *Contesting psychiatry: Social movements in mental health*. London: Routledge.

Crowe, M., & Alavi, C. (1999). Mad talk: Attending to the language of distress. *Nursing Inquiry, 6*, 26–33.

Crump, J. (2002). Deconcentration by demolition: Public housing, poverty and urban policy. *Environment and Planning, 20*, 581–596.

Culhane, D. (2009). Narratives of hope and despair in Downtown Eastside Vancouver. In L.J. Kirmayer & G.G. Valaskakis (Eds.), *Healing traditions: The mental health of Aboriginal Peoples in Canada* (pp. 160–177). Vancouver: UBC Press.

Culhane, D., Metraux, S., & Hadley, T. (2002). Public service reductions associated with placement of homeless persons with severe mental illness in supportive housing. *Housing Policy Debate, 13*, 107–163.

Curran, M.E. (2005). Geographic theorizations of sexuality: A review of recent works. *Feminist Studies, 31*(2), 380–398.

Currier, J.M., Neimeyer, R.A., & Berman, J.S. (2008). The effectiveness of psychothera-peutic interventions for the bereaved: A comprehensive quantitative review. *Psychological Bulletin, 134*, 648–661.

Cusack, R. (2006). Who was Mary Huestis Pengilly? *Our Voice/Notre Voix, 46*, 4.

Dain, N. (1980). *Clifford W. Beers: Advocate for the insane*. Pittsburgh: University of Pittsburgh Press.

Daley, A. (2010). Being recognized, accepted and affirmed: Self-disclosure of lesbian/queer sexuality within psychiatric and mental health service settings. *Social Work in Mental Health, 8*(4), 336–355.

Daley, A. (2011). The reconfiguration of lesbian/queer sexuality by service provider responses to self-disclosures. In G. Gonzalo Araoz (Ed.), *Proceedings of the Second Global Conference on Making Sense of Madness*. Oxford: Inter-Disciplinary Press.

Daley, A. (unpublished). A bodily presence of mind: Theorizing the invisibility of lesbian women with SMI in psychiatric and mental health services. Doctoral comprehensive paper, Faculty of Social Work, University of Toronto.

Daniels, A., Grant, E., Filson, B., Powell, I., Fricks, L., & Goodale, L. (Eds.). (2010). *Pillars of peer support: Transforming mental health systems of care through peer support services*. Atlanta: The Carter Center. Retrieved January 6, 2012, from www.iarecovery.org/docu-ments/PillarsofPS.pdf.

Danquah, M. (1999). *Willow weep for me: A Black woman's journey through depression*. New York: One World/Ballantine.

D'Augelli, A.R., Hershberger, S.L., & Pilkington, N.W. (2001). Suicidality patterns and sex-ual orientation-related factors among lesbian, gay, and bisexual youths. *Suicide and Life Threatening Behaviour, 31*(2), 250–254.

Davidson, L., Chinman, M., Sells, D., & Rowe, M. (2006). Peer support among adults with serious mental illness: A report from the field. *Schizophrenia Bulletin, 32*(3), 443–450.

Davidson, L., Rakfeldt, J., & Strauss, J. (2010). *The roots of the recovery movement in psy-chiatry: Lessons learned*. West Sussex: Wiley-Blackwell.

Davidson, L., & Roe, D. (2007). Recovery from versus recovery in serious mental illness: One strategy for lessening confusion plaguing recovery. *Journal of Mental Health, 16*(4), 459–470.

Davies, M.J. (1989). The patients' world: British Columbia's mental health facilities, 1910–1935. Master's thesis, University of Waterloo.

Davies, M.J. (2011). Mother's medicine: Women, home and health in BC's Peace River region, 1920–1940. In J.T.H. Conner & S. Curtis (Eds.), *Social medicine and rural health in the north in the 19th and 20th centuries* (pp. 199–214). London: Pickering and Chatto.

Davies, M.J. (forthcoming). La renaissance des sages-femmes dans la région de Kootenay en Colombie-Britannique, 1970–1990. In M-C. Thifault (Ed.), *L'incontournable caste des femmes. Histoire des services de soins de santé au Québec et au Canada*. Ottawa: University of Ottawa Press.

Davies, M.J., & Marshall, A. (2010). *Caring minds: Youth, mental health & community*. Retrieved from http://historyofmadness.ca/.

Davies, M.J., & Purvey, D. (2010). *More for the mind: Histories of mental health for the classroom*. Retrieved from http://historyofmadness.ca/.

Davis, L. (1995). *Enforcing normalcy: Disability, deafness and the body*. London: Verso.

Dear, M. (1992). Understanding and overcoming the NIMBY syndrome. *Journal of the American Planning Association, 58*(3), 288–300.

Dear, M., & Laws, G. (1986). Anatomy of a decision: Recent land use zoning appeals and their effect on group home locations in Ontario. *Canadian Journal of Community Mental Health, 5*(1), 5–17.

Dear, M., & Taylor, S.M. (1982). *Not on our street: Community attitudes to mental health care.* London: Pion Limited.

Dear, M., & Wolch, J. (1987). *Landscapes of despair: From deinstitutionalization to homelessness.* Oxford: Polity Press.

Deegan, P.E. (1988). Recovery: The lived experience of rehabilitation. *Psychosocial Rehabilitation Journal, 9*(4), 11–19.

Deegan, P.E. (2000). Spirit breaking: When the helping professions hurt. *The Humanistic Psychologist, 28,* 194–209.

Delahanty, J. (2001). Differences in rates of depression in schizophrenia by race. *Schizophrenia Bulletin, 152*(1), 29–38.

Dellar, R., Leslie, E., & Watson, B. (2001). *Mad pride: A celebration of mad culture.* London: Spare Change Books.

Dennis Jr., S.F., Gaulocher, S., Carpiano, R.M., & Brown, D. (2009). Participatory photo mapping (PPM): Exploring an integrated method for health and place research with young people. *Health & Place, 15,* 466–473.

Depla, M., De Graaf, R., & Heeren, T.J. (2006). The relationship between characteristics of supported housing and the quality of life of older adults with severe mental illness. *Aging & Mental Health, 10,* 592–598.

Desjarlait, R. (2011, October 11). Decolonization and Occupy Wall Street. Racialicious. Retrieved November 8, 2011, from www.racialicious.com/2011/10/11/decolonization-and-occupy-wall-street.

Deutsch, A. (1948). *The shame of the states (Mental illness and social policy: The American experience).* New York: Harcourt Brace.

De Wolff, A. (2008). *We are neighbours. The impact of supportive housing on community, social, economic and attitude changes.* Toronto: Wellesley Institute.

Dhand, R. (2009). Challenging exclusion: A critique of the legal barriers faced by ethno-racial psychiatric consumer/survivors in Ontario. LLM thesis, University of Toronto.

Diamond, S. (2012). Imagining possibilities outside the medicalization of humanity: A critical ethnography of a community trying to build a world free of sanism and psychiatric oppression. PhD diss., University of Toronto.

Dolan, M. (October 2009). Testimony of Moira Dolan, MD. Medical devices: Neurological devices: Electroconvulsive therapy device; Establishing a public docket. Re: Docket No. FDA-2009-N-0392.

Dominelli, L. (2002). *Anti-oppressive social work: Theory and practice.* London: Palgrave Macmillan.

Donnelly, M. (1992). *The politics of mental health in Italy.* London: Routledge.

Dorsey, K. (2008). The prosumer: An essay by Kevin Dorsey. *Open Minds Quarterly Writers Circle Online.* Retrieved January 11, 2012, from http://nisa.on.ca/index.php?option=com_content&task=view&id=327&Itemid=104.

Dorvil, H., Morin, P., Beaulieu, A., & Dominique, R. (2005). Housing as a social integration factor for people classified as mentally ill. *Housing Studies, 20,* 497–519.

Dossa, P. (2006). Disability, marginality and the nation-state: Negotiating social markers of difference: Fahimeh's story. *Disability and Society, 21*(4), 345–358.

Dotson, K. (2011). Tracking epistemic violence, tracking practices of silencing. *Hypatia*, 26(2), 236–257.

Dowbiggin, I. (2011). *The quest for mental health: A tale of science, medicine, scandal, sorrow, and mass society*. Cambridge: Cambridge University Press.

Drazen, J.M., & Curfman, G.D. (2002). Financial associations of authors. *New England Journal of Medicine*, 346(24), 1901–1902.

Dreezer, S., Bay, M., & Hoff, D. (2005). *Report on the legislated review of Community Treatment Orders, required under section 33.9 of the Mental Health Act for the Ontario Ministry of Health and Long-Term Care*. Toronto: Ontario Ministry of Health and Long-Term Care.

Drinkwater, C. (2005). Supported living and the production of individuals. In S. Tremain (Ed.), *Foucault and the government of disability*. Ann Arbor: University of Michigan Press.

Dyck, I. (1995). Hidden geographies: The changing lifeworlds of women with multiple sclerosis. *Social Science and Medicine*, 40(3), 307–320.

Ejiogu, N., & Ware, S.M. (2008, June). How disability studies stays white, and what kind of white it stays. Paper presented at the annual meeting of the Society for Disability Studies, CUNY, New York.

Enns, M.W., Reiss, J.P., & Chan. P. (2009). Electroconvulsive therapy: Position paper. *Canadian Psychiatric Association*.

Erevelles, N., & Minear, A. (2010). Unspeakable offenses: Untangling race and disability in discourses of intersectionality. *Journal of Literary and Critical Disability* Studies, 4(2), 127–145.

Erlich, S. (2011). Centering disability and accessibility. *Shameless: Your Regular Dose of Fresh Feminism for Girls and Trans Youth*. Retrieved September 10, 2011, from www.shamelessmag.com/blog/2011/08/centering-disability-and-accessibility/.

Everett, B. (2000). *A fragile revolution: Consumers and psychiatric survivors confront the power of the mental health system*. Waterloo: Wilfrid Laurier Press.

Eyler, A.E., & Witten, T.M. (1999). *Violence within and against the transgender community: Preliminary survey results*. Technical Report. San Antonio: International Longitudinal Transsexual and Transgender Aging Research Project.

Fabris, E. (2011). *Tranquil prisons: Chemical incarceration under Community Treatment Orders*. Toronto: University of Toronto Press.

Factum of the Intervenor, QSPC (Queen Street Patients Council). (n.d.)

Fakhoury, W.K.H., Murray, A., Shepherd, G., & Priebe, S. (2002). Research in supported housing. *Social Psychiatry and Psychiatric Epidemiology*, 37, 301–315.

Fanon, F. (1963). *The wretched of the earth*. New York: Grove Press.

Fanon, F. (1965). *A dying colonialism*. New York: Grove Press.

Farley, C. (2011, April 14). What your home is really worth. *Toronto Star*. Retrieved January 9, 2012, from www.thestar.com/news/article/974790.

Farnfield, S. (1995). *Research into the views of children, young people and their carers, of mental health services. A report to the Southampton and South West Hampshire Health Commission*.

Findlay, B. (1975). Shrink! Shrank! Shriek! In D.E. Smith & S.J. David (Eds.), *Women look at psychiatry* (pp. 59–71). Vancouver: Press Gang Publishers.

Finkler, L. (1997). Psychiatric Survivor Pride Day: Community organizing with psychiatric survivors. *Osgoode Hall Law Journal*, 35(3/4), 763–772.

Finkler, L. (2006). Re-placing (in)justice: Disability-related facilities at the Ontario Municipal Board. In Law Commission of Canada (Ed.), *The place of justice*. Halifax: Fernwood.

Finkler, L., & Grant, J. (2011). Minimum separation distance bylaws for group homes: The negative side of planning regulation. *Canadian Journal of Urban Research, 20*(1), 33–56.

Flaccus, G. (2011, August 4). Outrage on schizophrenic's beating death by cops. *Associated Press*. Retrieved November 5, 2011, from http://articles.sfgate.com/2011-08-04/bay-area/29849178_1_stun-gun-schizophrenic-man-confrontation.

Fletcher, C., & Cambre, C. (2009). Digital storytelling and implicated scholarship in the classroom. *Journal of Canadian Studies, 43*(1), 109–130.

Fong, P., & Mulgrew, I. (2001, December 3). Doctor loses job after electroshock controversy. *Vancouver Sun*. Retrieved from www.ect.org/doctor-loses-job-after-electroshock-controversy/.

Foote, C., & Frank, A. (1999). Foucault and therapy: The disciplining of grief. In A. Chambon, A. Irving & L. Epstein (Eds.), *Reading Foucault for social work* (pp. 156–187). New York: Columbia University Press.

Forchuk, C., Nelson, G., & Hall, B. (2006a). From psychiatric ward to the streets and shelters. *Journal of Psychiatric and Mental Health Nursing, 13*, 301–308.

Forchuk, C., Nelson, G., & Hall, B. (2006b). Surviving the tornado of mental illness: Psychiatric survivors' experiences of getting, losing and keeping housing. *Psychiatric Services, 57*(4), 558–562.

Forchuk, C., Nelson, G., & Hall, B. (2006c). "It's important to be proud of the place you live in": Housing problems and preferences of psychiatric survivors. *Perspectives in Psychiatric Care, 42*, 42–52.

Fortney, V. (2010, August 13). Former senator Michael Kirby saluted for mental health work. *Calgary Herald*. Retrieved December 10, 2010, from http://spon.ca/formersenator-michael-kirby-saluted-for-mental-health-work/2010/08/14/.

Foucault, M. (1962). *Madness and civilization: A history of insanity in the age of reason*. New York: Vintage.

Foucault, M. (1979). *Discipline and punish: The birth of the prison*. London: Penguin.

Foucault, M. (1980). *Power/Knowledge: Selected interviews and other writings, 1972–1977*. New York: Pantheon.

Foucault, M. (1991). Governmentality. In G. Burchell, C. Gordon & P. Miller (Eds.), *The Foucault effect: Studies in governmentality* (pp. 87–104). Chicago: University of Chicago Press.

Foucault, M. (1997). *"Society must be defended": Lectures at the Collège de France 1975–1976*. New York: Picador.

Foucault, M. (2006). *History of madness*. Ed. J. Khalfa, Trans. J. Murphy & J. Khalfa. London: Routledge.

Foucault, M. (2007). *Birth of the Clinic*. London: Tavistock.

Foucault, M. (2010). *The government of self and others: Lectures at the Collège de France 1982–1983*. Ed. A.I. Davidson, Trans. G. Burchell. New York: Palgrave Macmillan.

Fox, N.J. (1994). *Postmodernism, sociology, and health*. Toronto: University of Toronto Press.

Frances, A. (2009). A warning sign on the road to DSM-V: Beware of its unintended consequences. *Psychiatric Times, 26*(8).

Frank, L.R. (1983). Reflections on the campaign. *Madness Network News, 7*(1), 5.

Frank, L.R. (1990). Electroshock, death, brain damage, memory loss, and brainwashing. *Journal of Mind and Behavior, 11*, 489–512.

Frank, L.R. (2006a). A petition to enact an ordinance. The electroshock quotationary. Retrieved from http://endofshock.com.

Frank, L.R. (2006b). The electroshock quotationary. Retrieved from http://endofshock.com.

Frankenburg, F. (1982). The 1978 Ontario Mental Health Act in historical context. *HSTC Bulletin: Journal of the History of Canadian Science, Technology and Medicine*, 6(3), 172–177.

Freeman, S.J. (1994). An overview of Canada's mental health system. *New Directions for Mental Health Services*, 61, 11–20.

Freire, P. (1970). *Pedagogy of the oppressed*. New York: Seabury Press.

Friedberg, J. (1977). Shock treatment, memory loss and brain damage: A neurological perspective. *American Journal of Psychiatry*, 134, 1010–1014.

Friedli, L. (2009). *Mental health, resilience and inequalities*. Geneva: WHO.

Frisch, M. (1990). *A shared authority: Essays on the craft and meaning of oral and public history*. Albany: State University of New York Press.

Frisch, M. (2003). Sharing authority: Oral history and the collaborative process. *Oral History Review*, 30(1), 111–113.

Frost, L., Heinz, T., & Bach, D.H. (2011). Promoting recovery-oriented mental health services through a peer specialist employer learning community. *Journal of Participatory Medicine*, 3. Retrieved January 6, 2012, from www.jopm.org/evidence/case-studies/2011/05/09/promoting-recovery-oriented-mental-health-services-through-a-peer-specialist-employer-learning-community/.

Funk, W. (1998). *"What difference does it make?": The journey of a soul survivor*. Cranbrook: Wildflower Publishing.

Galster, G.C., Tatian, P.A., Santiago, A.M., Pettit, K.L.S., & Smith, R.E. (2003). *Why not in my backyard? Neighborhood impacts of deconcentrating assisted housing*. New Brunswick: Centre for Urban Policy Research.

Gary, F. (2005). Stigma: Barrier to mental health care among ethnic minorities. *Issues in Mental Health Nursing*, 26, 979–999.

Gash, A. (2011). To tell or not to tell: Adversarialism v. collaboration in group home location. Paper presented at the American Political Science Association, Seattle, WA. Retrieved from http://ssrn.com/abstract=1901096.

Giannakali. (2007). Beyond meds: Alternatives to psychiatry. Retrieved March 19, 2008, from https://bipolarblast.wordpress.com/.

Gilman, C. Perkins (1892). The yellow wallpaper. *New England Magazine*, 11(5).

Gilman, S.L. (1988). *Disease and representation: Images of illness from madness to AIDS*. New York: Cornell University Press.

Gilmore, R. (2007). *Golden Gulag: Prisons, surplus, crisis, and opposition in globalizing California*. Berkeley: University of California Press.

Glaser, B., & Strauss, A. (1968). *The discovery of grounded theory*. Hawthorne: Aldine de Gruyter.

Glenmullen, J. (2000). *Prozac backlash*. New York: Simon & Schuster.

Globe and Mail. (2008). Breakdown: Canada's mental health crisis. *Globe and Mail*. Retrieved December 5, 2010, from http://v1.theglobeandmail.com/breakdown/.

Goetz, E.G. (2003). *Clearing the way: Deconcentrating the poor in urban America*. Washington: Urban Institute Press.

Goffman, E. (1961). *Asylums: Essays on the social situation of mental patients and other inmates*. Chicago: Aldine.

Goffman, E. (1963). *Stigma: Notes on the management of a spoiled identity*. Englewood Cliffs: Prentice-Hall.

Goldenberg, M. (2007). The problem of exclusion in feminist theory and politics: A metaphysical investigation into constructing a category of "woman." *Journal of Gender Studies*, 16(2), 139–153.

Gondry, M. (2008). *You'll like this film because you're in it: The be kind rewind protocol.* Brooklyn: PictureBox.

Goodkin, K., Lee, D., Frasca, A., Molina, R., Zheng, W., O'Mellan, S., et al. (2005). Complicated bereavement: A commentary on its state and evolution. *Omega Journal of Death and Dying, 52*(1), 99–105.

Goodley, D. (2010). *Disability studies: An interdisciplinary introduction.* Thousand Oaks: Sage.

Gorman, R. (2005). Class consciousness, disability, and social exclusion: A relational/reflexive analysis of disability culture. PhD diss., University of Toronto.

Gorman, R. (2009a, June). Time out: A life narrative approach to ADHD, racialization, and gender non-conformity. Paper presented at the annual meeting of the Society for Disability Studies, University of Arizona, Tucson.

Gorman, R. (2009b, May). Good mothering and medical compliance: Mothers' agency in child quasi-psychiatric diagnoses. Paper presented at the meeting of the Association for Research on Mothering, Nola Studios, New York.

Gorman, R., & Udegbe, O. (2010). Disabled woman/nation: Re-narrating the erasure of (neo)colonial violence in Ondjaki's *Good Morning Comrades* and Tsitsi Dangarembga's *Nervous Conditions. Journal of Literary and Cultural Disability Studies, 4*(3), 309–325.

Government of Ontario. (2011). *Open minds, healthy minds. Ontario's comprehensive mental health and addictions strategy.* Toronto: Queen's Printer.

Graham, R. (1988). The Graham report. Toronto: Provincial Mental Health Committee.

Greaves, L., Varcoe, C., Poole, N., Morrow, M., Johnson, J., Pederson, A., & Irwin, L. (2002). *A motherhood issue: Mothering under duress.* Ottawa: Status of Women Canada.

Greenberg, G. (2010). *Manufacturing depression: The secret history of a modern disease.* New York: Simon & Schuster.

Greene, B. (2000). *The elegant universe: Superstrings, hidden dimensions, and the quest for the ultimate theory.* New York: Random House.

Grekul, J., Krahn, A., & Odynak, D. (2004). Sterilizing the "feeble-minded": Eugenics in Alberta, Canada, 1929–1972. *Journal of Historical Sociology, 17*(4), 358–384.

Grenier, G. (1999). *Les monstres, les fous et les autres: La folie criminelle au Québec.* Montreal: Éditions Trait d'union.

Grief-Healing-Support.com. (2011, November 1). Complicated grief—prolonged grief disorder. Retrieved from www.grief-healing-support.com/index.html.

Griffin, J.D. (1963). *More for the mind.* Toronto: Canadian Mental Health Association.

Gudmundsdottir, M. (2009). Embodied grief: Bereaved parents' narratives of their suffering body. *Omega Journal of Death and Dying, 59*(3), 253–269.

Habermas, J. (1971). *Knowledge and human interest.* Boston: Beacon Press.

Habitat Services & Ontario Coalition of Alternative Businesses (OCAB). (2010). *Breaking ground: Peer support for congregate living settings.* Toronto: Wellesley Institute.

Hacking, I. (2002). *Mad travelers: Reflections on the reality of transient mental illnesses.* Boston: Harvard University Press.

Hadad, M. (2009). *The ultimate challenge: Coping with death, dying and bereavement.* Toronto: Nelson Education.

Hall, W. (2007). The freedom to sit: Welcoming people with psychiatric disabilities at Buddhist retreats. *Turning Wheel: The Journal of Socially Educated Buddhism*, Summer, 34–36.

Hanafi, S. (2009a). Spacio-cide and bio-politics: The Israeli colonial project from 1947 to the wall. In M. Sorkin (Ed.), *Against the wall* (pp. 158–173). New York: The New Press.

Hanafi, S. (2009b). Palestinian refugee camps in Lebanon: Laboratory of indocile identity formation. In M.A. Khalidi (Ed.), *Citizenships and identities: Palestinian refugees in Lebanon*. Washington: Institute of Palestinian Studies.

Harding, S. (1987). Conclusion: Epistemological questions. In S. Harding (Ed.), *Feminism and methodology* (pp. 181–189). Bloomington: Indiana University Press.

Harding, S. (2006). *Science and social inequality*. Chicago: University of Illinois Press.

Harris, A.P. (2000). Gender, violence, race and criminal justice. *Stanford Law Review, 52*(4), 777–807.

Harris, G. (2009, October 21). Drug makers are advocacy group's biggest donors. *New York Times*. Retrieved from www.nytimes.com/2009/10/22/health/22nami.html#.

Hartford, K., Schrecker, T., Wiktorowicz, M., Hoch, J.S., & Sharp, C. (2003). Four decades of mental health policy in Ontario, Canada. *Administration and Policy in Mental Health, 31*(1), 1–11.

Hawker, S. (2003). *Little Oxford dictionary, thesaurus and wordpower guide*. Oxford: Oxford University Press.

Health Canada. (2000). *A statistical profile on the health of First Nations in Canada for the year 2000*. Ottawa: Health Canada.

Healy, D. (2004). *Let them eat Prozac: The unhealthy relationship between the pharmaceutical industry and depression*. New York: NYU Press.

Healy, D. (2008). *Mania: A short history of bipolar disorder*. Baltimore: The Johns Hopkins University Press.

Healy, K. (2005). Social work theories in context: Creating frameworks for practice. London: Palgrave MacMillan.

Hekman, S. (1998). Material bodies. In D. Welton (Ed.), *Body and flesh: A philosophical reader* (pp. 61–70). Oxford: Blackwell.

Henderson, H. (2010, April 16). Exploring madness and mental health. *Toronto Star*. Retrieved November 6, 2011, from www.thestar.com/living/disabilities/article/796516-exploring-madness-and-mental-health.

Hepburn, A.W., & Deman, A.F. (1980). Patient rights and the Dutch Clientenbond. *Canada's Mental Health, 28*, 17.

Herman, N.J., & Musolf, G.R. (1998). Resistance among ex-psychiatric patients: Expressive and instrumental rituals. *Journal of Contemporary Ethnography, 26*(4), 426–449.

High, S. (2009). Shared authority: An introduction. *Journal of Canadian Studies, 43*(1), 12–34.

Hill Collins, P. (2000). *Black feminist thought: Knowledge, consciousness, and the politics of empowerment*. New York: Routledge.

Hill Collins, P. (2003). Toward a new vision: Race, class, and gender as categories of analysis and connection. In M.S. Kimmel & A.L. Ferber (Eds.), *Privilege: A reader* (pp. 331–348). Colorado: Westview Press.

Hoekstra, T., Lendemeijer, H.H., & Jansen, M.G. (2004). Seclusion: The inside story. *Journal of Psychiatric and Mental Health Nursing, 11*, 276–283.

Hollander, E.M. (2004). Am I alright? *Journal of Loss and Trauma, 9*, 201–204.

Hook, D. (2007). *Foucault, psychology and the analytics of power.* New York: Palgrave Macmillan.

Hook, H., Goodwin, S., & Fabris, E. (2005). Psycho, patient, person: Perspectives on being labeled mentally ill. Retrieved July 11, 2011, from www.camh.net/Publications/Cross_Currents/Autumn_2005/psychopatient_crcuautumn05.html.

hooks, b. (1992). Dialectically down with the critical program. In M. Wallace & G. Dent (Eds.), *Black popular culture* (pp. 48–55). Seattle: Bay Press.

hooks, b. (2000). *Feminism is for everybody: Passionate politics.* Cambridge: South End.

Horwitz, A., & Wakefield, J. (2007). *The loss of sadness: How psychiatry transformed normal sorrow into depressive disorder.* New York: Oxford University Press.

Howell, A. (2007). Victims or madmen? The diagnostic competition over "terrorist" detainees at Guantánamo Bay. *International Political Sociology,* 1(1), 29–47.

Howell, A. (2011). *Madness in international relations: Psychology, security, and the global governance of mental health.* New York: Routledge.

Huxley, M. (2002). Governmentality, gender, planning: A Foucauldian perspective. In P. Allmendinger & M. Tewdwr-Jones (Eds.), *Planning futures: New directions for planning theory* (pp. 136–153). London: Routledge.

ICBE. (2009). International Campaign to Ban Electroshock. Retrieved from http://intcamp.wordpress.com/.

Illich, I. (1973). *Tools for conviviality.* New York: Harper & Row.

Illich, I. (1976). *Medical nemesis: The expropriation of health.* New York: Pantheon.

Illich, I., Zola, I.K., McKnight, J., Caplan, J., & Shaiken, H. (Eds.). (2005). *Disabling professions.* New York: M. Boyars.

Ingleby, D. (Ed.). (1980). *Critical psychiatry: The politics of mental health.* New York: Pantheon.

Ingram, R. (2005). Troubled being and being troubled: Subjectivity in the light of problems of the mind. PhD diss., University of British Columbia.

Ingram, R. (2008, May 3). Mapping "Mad Studies": The birth of an in/discipline. Disability Studies Student Conference, Syracuse University, Syracuse, NY.

Ingram, R. (2011a). Recovery from compulsory sanity. Presented at Society for Disabilities Studies Conference, San Jose, CA.

Ingram, R. (2011b, December). Personal communication.

Ingram, R. (2012, January). Personal communication.

Inman, S. (2011a, July 29). Susan Inman: The right to be sane. *National Post.* Retrieved from http://fullcomment.nationalpost.com/2011/07/29/susan-inman-the-right-to-be-sane/.

Inman, S. (2011b, August 29). Suppressing schizophrenia. Schizophrenia is invisible in Canada's new mental health strategy. *Tyee.* Retrieved from http://thetyee.ca/Opinion/2011/08/29/Review-Mental-Health-Strategy/.

International Committee of Medical Journal Editors. (2001, September). *Sponsorship, authorship, and accountability.* Retrieved from www.icmje.org/update_sponsor.html.

Jackson, D. (1990). *Unmasking masculinity: A critical autobiography.* London: Unwin Hyman.

Jacobson, N., Farah, D., & The Toronto Recovery and Cultural Diversity Community of Practice. (2010). *Recovery through the lens of cultural diversity.* Toronto: Community Resource Connections of Toronto; Centre for Addiction and Mental Health; Wellesley Institute.

Jamison, K.R. (2009). *Nothing was the same.* New York: Random House.

Janis, I. (1948). Memory loss following electroconvulsive treatments. *Journal of Personality, 17*, 29–32.

Janis, I. (1950). Psychological effects of electric convulsive treatments. *Journal of Nervous and Mental Disease, 111*, 359–397, 469–489.

Janis, I., & Astrachan, M. (1951). The effects of electroconvulsive treatments on memory efficiency. *Journal of Abnormal Psychology, 46*, 501–511.

Johnson, L.C. (2001). The community/privacy trade-off in supportive housing: Consumer/survivor preferences. *Canadian Journal of Community Mental Health, 20*(1), 123–133.

Johnstone, L. (2000). *Users and abusers of psychiatry: A critical look at psychiatric practice* (2nd ed.). London: Routledge.

Jones, C. (1992). Listening to hidden voices: Power, domination, resistance and pleasure within Huronia Regional Centre. *Disability, Handicap and Society, 7*(4), 339–348.

Jones, L., & Newman, L. (1998). *Our America. Life and death on the south side of Chicago.* New York: Washington Square Press.

Kaba, E., Thompson, D.R., Burnard, P., Edwards, D., & Theodosopoulou, E. (2005). Somebody else's heart inside me: A descriptive study of psychological problems after heart transplantation. *Issues in Mental Health Nursing, 26*, 611–625.

Kaiser, A. (2001). Restraint and seclusion in Canadian mental health facilities: Assessing the prospects for improved access to justice. *Windsor Yearbook of Access to Justice, 19*, 391–417.

Kalinowski, C., & Risser, P. (2005). Identifying and overcoming mentalism. InforMed Health Publishing & Training. Retrieved March 10, 2010, from www.newmediaexplorer.org/sepp/Mentalism.pdf.

Kallos, S. (2009). *Sing them home.* New York: Grove Press.

Kearns, R. (1997). Narrative and metaphor in health geographies. *Progress in Human Geography, 21*(2), 269–277.

Kendall, K. (2005). Beyond reason: Social constructions of mentally disordered female offenders. In W. Chan, D.E. Chunn & R. Menzies (Eds.), *Women, madness and the law: A feminist reader* (pp. 41–57). London: GlassHouse/Cavendish.

Kendall, K. (2009). Suffering and the double-edged sword of the psy-sciences. *Community Corrections Report, 16*(2), 1–29.

Kerr, D. (2003). "We know what the problem is": Using oral history to develop a collaborative analysis of homelessness from the bottom up. *Oral History Review, 30*(1), 27–45.

Kesey, K. (1962). *One flew over the cuckoo's nest.* New York: Viking.

Kibble, T. (2009, January 28). Domiciliary residence under fire by businesses. Petition asks for review of all such homes before more beds can be added. *Georgina Advocate.* Retrieved January 9, 2012, from www.yorkregion.com/yorkregion/article/555457.

Kickbusch, I.S. (2001). Health literacy: Addressing the health and education divide. *Health Promotion International, 16*(3), 289–297.

Kilty, J. (2008). Governance through psychiatrization: Seroquel and the new prison order. *Radical Psychology, 7*(2). Retrieved from http://radicalpsychology.org/vol7-2/kiltys.html.

Kinsman, G. (2006). Mapping social relations of struggle: Activism, ethnography, social organization. In C. Frampton, G. Kinsman, A. Thompson & K. Tilleczek (Eds.), *Sociology for changing the world: Social movements/social research* (pp. 135–158). Halifax: Fernwood.

Kipfer, S., & Petrunia, J. (2009). Recolonization and public housing: A Toronto case study. *Studies in Political Economy, 83*, 111–139.

Kirby, M. (2006). *Out of the shadows at last: Transforming mental health, mental illness and addiction services in Canada*. Final Report of the Standing Senate Committee on Social Affairs, Science and Technology.

Kirmayer, L., Brass, G.M., & Tait, C.L. (2001). The mental health of Aboriginal peoples: Transformations of identity and culture. *Canadian Journal of Psychiatry, 45*(7), 607–617.

Kisely, S., Smith, M., Lawrence, D., Cox, M., Campbell, L.A., & Maaten, S. (2007). Inequitable access for mentally ill patients to some medically necessary procedures. *Canadian Medical Association Journal, 176*(6), 779–788.

Klass, D. (1996). Grief in an Eastern culture: Japanese ancestor worship. In D. Klass, P.R. Silverman & S.L. Nickman (Eds.), *Continuing bonds: New understandings of grief* (pp. 59–70). Washington: Taylor and Francis.

Kleinman, A. (1988). *The illness narratives: Suffering, healing & the human condition*. New York: Basic Books.

Knowles, C. (2000). *Bedlam on the streets*. London: Routledge.

Kübler-Ross, E. (1969). *On death and dying*. London: Routledge.

Kübler-Ross, E., & Kessler, D. (2005). *On grief and grieving: Finding the meaning of grief through the five stages of loss*. New York: Scribner.

Kumar, S. (2000). Client empowerment in psychiatry and the professional abuse of clients: Where do we stand? *International Journal of Psychiatry in Medicine, 30*(1), 61–70.

Kupfer, D.J., First, M.B., & Regier, D.A. (2002). *A research agenda for DSM-V*. Washington: American Psychiatric Association.

Kutchins, H., & Kirk, S.A. (1997). *Making us crazy: DSM: The psychiatric bible and the creation of mental disorders*. New York: Free Press.

Kyle, T., & Dunn, J.R. (2008). Effects of housing circumstances on health, quality of life and healthcare use for people with severe mental illness: A review. *Health and Social Care in the Community, 16*, 1–15.

Laing, R.D. (1960). *The divided self: An existential study in sanity and madness*. Harmondsworth: Penguin.

Laing, R.D. (1967). *The politics of experience and the bird of paradise*. Harmondsworth: Penguin.

Laing, R.D. (1971). *The politics of the family, and other essays*. Harmondsworth: Pelican.

Laing, R.D., & Esterson, A. (1964). *Sanity, madness and the family: Families of schizophrenics*. London: Tavistock.

Lane, C. (2007). *Shyness: How normal behavior became a sickness*. New Haven: Yale University Press.

Lawn, S. (2005). Cigarette smoking in psychiatric settings: Occupational health, safety, welfare and legal concerns. *Australian and New Zealand Journal of Psychiatry, 39*(10), 886–891.

Lawrence, B., & Dua, E. (2005). Decolonizing antiracism. *Social Justice, 32*(4), 120–143.

Laws, S., Armitt, D., Metzendorf, W., Percival, P., & Reisel, J. (1999). *Time to listen: Young people's experiences of mental health services*. London: Save the Children.

LeBlanc, E. (2006). A diary that speaks to me. *Our Voice/Notre Voix, 46*, 1–3.

LeBlanc, E., & St-Amand, N. (2008). *Dare to imagine: From lunatics to citizens*. Moncton: Our Voice/Notre Voix.

LeClaire, J. (2011). Should nurses blow the whistle? Retrieved from http://allhealthcare.monster.com/benefits/articles/2824-should-nurses-blow-the-whistle.

LeFrançois, B.A. (2006). "They will find us and infect our bodies": The views of adolescent inpatients taking psychiatric medication. *Radical Psychology, 5*(1).

LeFrançois, B.A. (2007). Psychiatric childhood(s): Child-centred perspectives on mental health inpatient treatment and care. PhD diss., University of Kent.

LeFrançois, B.A. (2008). "It's like mental torture": Participation and mental health services. *International Journal of Children's Rights, 16,* 211–227.

LeFrançois, B.A. (2010). Organizing collective resistance through children's rights legislation and children's agency. *Conference proceedings for PsychOUT: A Conference for Organizing Resistance Against Psychiatry,* OISE, University of Toronto.

LeFrançois, B.A. (2012). And we are still being psychiatrised. *Asylum: The Magazine for Democratic Psychiatry, 19*(1), 7–9.

LeFrançois, B.A. (2013). Queering child and adolescent mental health services: The subversion of heteronormativity in practice. *Children & Society, 27*(1), 1–12.

Lewis, C.S. (1961). *A grief observed.* New York: Harper Collins.

Lieblich, A., Tuval-Mashiach, R., & Zilber, T. (1998). *Narrative research: Reading, analysis, and interpretation.* Thousand Oaks: Sage.

Lightman, E., & Aviram, U. (2000). Too much, too late: The Advocacy Act in Ontario. *Law & Policy, 22*(1), 25–48.

Link, B., Cullen, F., Frank, J., & Wozniak, J. (1987). The social rejection of former mental patients: Understanding why labels matter. *American Journal of Sociology, 92*(6), 1461–1500.

Linter, J. (1979). Reflections on the media and the mental patient. *Hospital and Community Psychiatry, 30*(6), 415–416.

Livingston, J. (2006). Insights from an African history of disability. *Radical History Review, 94,* 111–126.

Lorde, A. (1984, 2007). *Sister outsider: Essays and speeches by Audre Lorde.* Berkeley: Crossing.

Lupton, D. (1997). Consumerism, reflexivity and the medical encounter. *Social Science and Medicine, 45*(3), 373–381.

Lyons, T. (2002, September 29). Debate rages over safety of ECT, or shock therapy, used on elderly. *Canadian Press.*

MacLeod, C., & Durrheim, K. (2002). Foucauldian feminism: The implications of governmentality. *Journal for the Theory of Social Behaviour, 32*(1), 41–60.

Makin, K. (2010, November 17). Mentally ill offenders swamping prisons. *Globe and Mail.* Retrieved December 30, 2010, from www.theglobeandmail.com/news/national/ontario/mentally-ill-offenders-swamping-prisons/article1803550/.

Makin, K. (2011, January 22). To heal and protect. *Globe and Mail,* pp. F6, F7.

Mama, A. (1995). *Beyond the masks: Race, gender and subjectivity.* London: Routledge.

Marker, M. (2003). Indigenous voice, community, and epistemic violence: The ethnographer's "interests" and what "interests" the ethnographer. *Qualitative Studies in Education, 16*(3), 361–375.

Markman, A. (1981, August 29). Presentation to workshop on movement history. Ninth Annual Conference on Human Rights and Psychiatric Oppression, Cleveland, OH.

Marsh, D.T. (2000). Personal accounts of consumer/survivors: Insights and implications. *Journal of Clinical Psychology/In Session: Psychotherapy in Practice, 56*(11), 1447–1457.

Marshall, J. (1982). *Madness: An indictment of the mental health care system in Ontario.* Toronto: Ontario Public Service Employees Union.

Martens, C. (2008). Theorizing distress: Critical reflections on bipolar and borderline. *Radical*

Psychology, 7(2). Retrieved from http://radicalpsychology.org/vol7-2/Martens.html.

Martensson, L. (1998). *Deprived of our humanity: The case against neuroleptic drugs.* Geneva, SUI: The Voiceless Movement.

Martinot, S., & Sexton, J. (2003). The avant-garde of white supremacy. *Social Identities*, 9(2), 169–180.

Mason, G. (2001). Body maps: Envisaging homophobia, violence and safety. *Social & Legal Studies*, 10(1), 23–44.

Masterson, S., & Owen, S. (2006). Mental health service user's social and individual empowerment: Using theories of power to elucidate far-reaching strategies. *Journal of Mental Health*, 15(1), 19–34.

Masuda, J., & Crabtree, A. (2010). Environmental justice in the therapeutic inner city. *Health & Place*, 16, 656–665.

Mazer, K., & Rankin, K. (2011). The social space of gentrification: The politics of neighbourhood accessibility in Toronto's downtown west. *Environment and Planning D: Society and Space*, 29, 822–839.

Mbembé, A. (2002). African modes of self-writing. *Public Culture*, 14(1), 239–273.

McCubbin, M. (1998). The political economy of mental health: Power and interests within a complex system. PhD diss., Université de Montréal.

McCubbin, M. (2003). Biomedical cooptation of the psychological care and support continuum for severely distressed persons. *Ethical Human Sciences and Services*, 5(1), 57–62.

McCubbin, M., & Cohen, D. (1998). The rights of users of the mental health system: The tight knot of power, law and ethics. *Santé Mentale Québec*, 23(2), 212–224.

McIntosh, P. (1989). White privilege: Unpacking the invisible knapsack. *Peace and Freedom*, 49(4), 10–12.

McKague, C. (1979). Myths of mental illness: Publication for *Phoenix Rising.* Toronto.

McKay, I. (2005). *Rebels, reds, radicals: Rethinking Canada's left history.* Toronto: Between the Lines.

McKeown, M., Malihi-Shoja, L., Downe, S., supporting the Comensus Writing Collective. (2010). *Service user and carer involvement in education for health and social care.* Oxford: Wiley-Blackwell.

McKnight, J.L. (1984). John Deere and the bereavement counselor. E.F. Schumacher Society: Linking people, land and community by building local economies. Retrieved July 22, 2011, from www.smallisbeautiful.org/publications/mcknight_84.html.

McMurtry, R., & Curling, A. (2008a). *The review of the roots of youth violence: Volume 1, Findings, analysis and conclusions.* Toronto: Queen's Printer for Ontario. Available at www.rootsofyouthviolence.on.ca.

McMurtry, R., and Curling, A. (2008b). *The review of the roots of youth violence: Executive summary.* Toronto: Queen's Printer for Ontario. Available at www.rootsofyouthviolence.on.ca.

McNamara, A., & DuBrul, S. (Eds.). (2006). *Navigating the space between brilliance and madness: A reader and roadmap of bipolar worlds* (2nd ed.). Oakland: AK Press.

McRuer, R. (2010). Disability nationalism in crip times. *Journal of Literary and Cultural Disability Studies*, 4(2), 163–178.

MedPage Today (2011, January 28). FDA panel: Keep ECT devices as high risk. Retrieved from www.medpagetoday.com/Psychiatry/Depression/24590.

Meekosha, H. (2011). Decolonising disability: Thinking and acting globally. *Disability & Society*, 26(6), 667–682.

Meekosha, H., & Dowse, L. (2007). Integrating critical disability studies into social work. *Practice: Social Work in Action, 19*(3), 169–183.

Meekosha, H., & Soldatic, K. (2011). Special issue. *Third World Quarterly: Disability in the Global South, 32*(8).

Melinda, M. (2005, March-April). Can international law improve mental health? Some thoughts on the proposed convention on the rights of people with disabilities. *International Journal of Law and Psychiatry, 28*(2), 183–205.

Mental Health Commission of Canada. (2009a). Into the light. MHCC. Retrieved December 10, 2010, from www.mentalhealthcommission.ca/English/Pages/IntotheLight.aspx.

Mental Health Commission of Canada. (2009b). *Toward recovery and well-being: A framework for a mental health strategy for Canada.* Retrieved August 29, 2011, from www.mentalhealthcommission.ca/SiteCollectionDocuments/boarddocs/15507_MHCC_EN_final.pdf.

Mental Health Commission of Canada (n.d.). Vision and mission of the MHCC. MHCC. Retrieved January 20, 2011, from www.mentalhealthcommission.ca/English/Pages/TheMHCC.aspx.

Mental Health "Recovery" Study Working Group. (2009). *Mental health "recovery": Users and refusers.* Toronto: Wellesley Institute.

Menzies, R. (1989). *Survival of the sanest: Order and disorder in a pre-trial psychiatric clinic.* Toronto: University of Toronto Press.

Menzies, R. (2001). Contesting criminal lunacy: Narratives of law and madness in west coast Canada, 1874–1950. *History of Psychiatry, 7,* 123–156.

Menzies, R. (2002). Race, reason and regulation: British Columbia's mass exile of Chinese "lunatics" aboard the *Empress of Russia,* 9 February 1935. In J. McLaren, R. Menzies & D.E. Chunn (Eds.), *Regulating lives: Historical essays on the state, society, the individual, and the law* (pp. 196–230). Vancouver: University of British Columbia Press.

Metzl, J. (2009). *The protest psychosis: How schizophrenia became a black disease.* Boston: Beacon Press.

Meyer, I., & Schwartz, S. (2000). Social issues as public health: Promise and peril. *American Journal of Public Health, 90*(8), 1189–1191.

Michener, A.J. (1998). *Becoming Anna: The autobiography of a sixteen-year-old.* Chicago: University of Chicago Press.

Miettinen, R., Samra-Fredericks, D., & Yanow, D. (2009). Return to practice: An introductory essay. *Organization Studies, 30*(2), 1309–1327.

Mill, J.S. (1986 [1859]). *On liberty.* Buffalo: Prometheus Books.

Miller, R.B. (2004). *Facing human suffering: Psychology and psychotherapy as moral engagement.* Washington: American Psychological Association.

Millett, K. (1991). Untitled lecture. In B. Burstow, K. Millett, M. Pratt & H. Levine, *Feminist antipsychiatry perspectives. Resistance against psychiatry.* Public lecture sponsored by Resistance Against Psychiatry. Toronto: Ontario Institute for Studies in Education.

Milner, P., & Kelly, B. (2009). Community participation and inclusion: People with disabilities defining their place. *Disability and Society, 24*(1), 47–62.

MindFreedom Ghana. (2005). Report of psychiatric services in Ghana: Activities of MindFreedom Ghana. MindFreedom International. Retrieved December 28, 2011, from www.mindfreedom.org/as/act-archives/inter/mfghana/mfghana2005.

MindFreedom International. (2009). Retrieved from www.mindfreedom.org/electroshock/fda.

MindFreedom International. (2011). Occupy normal. MFI Portal. Retrieved November 8, 2011, from www.mindfreedom.org/campaign/boycott-normal/occupy.

MindFreedom International. (n.d.). Retrieved December 28, 2011, from www.mindfreedom. org/campaign/media.

MindFreedom International Global Campaign Committee. (2011). Global mental health empowerment handbook. MindFreedom International. Retrieved December 28, 2011, from www.mindfreedom.org/globalhandbook.

MindFreedom Media Campaign Committee. (n.d.). MindFreedom media action. MindFreedom International. Retrieved from www.mindfreedom.org/campaign/media.

Mirowski, J. (1990). Subjective boundaries and combinations in diagnoses. *Journal of Mind and Behavior, 11*, 407–423.

Mitchell, D., & Snyder, S. (2000). *Narrative prosthesis: Disability and the dependencies of discourse.* Ann Arbor: University of Michigan Press.

Mitchinson, W. (1991). *The nature of their bodies: Women and their doctors in Victorian Canada.* Toronto: University of Toronto Press.

Mohanty, C.T. (2003). *Feminism without borders: Decolonizing theory, practicing solidarity.* Durham: Duke University.

Moncrieff, J. (2008). *The myth of the chemical cure: A critique of psychiatric drug treatment.* London: Palgrave.

Mood Disorders Association of British Columbia (MDA). (n.d.). Retrieved from www.mdabc. net/.

Moore, T.J., Glenmullen, J., & Furberg, C.D. (2010). *Prescription drugs associated with reports of violence towards others. PLoS ONE, 5*(12). Retrieved from www.plosone.org/ article/info%3Adoi%2F10.1371%2Fjournal.pone.0015337.

Moran, J.E. (2000). *Committed to the state asylum: Insanity and society in nineteenth century Quebec and Ontario.* Montreal: McGill-Queen's University Press.

Morley, C. (2003). Towards a critical social work practice in mental health: A review. *Journal of Progressive Human Services, 14*(1), 61–84.

Morris, B. (2001). Policing racial fantasy in the far west of New South Wales. *Oceania, 71*(3), 242–262.

Morris, J., & Stone, G. (2011). Children and psychotropic medication: A cautionary note. *Journal of Marital and Family Therapy, 37*(3), 299–306.

Morris, K. (2010). *Unfinished revolution: Daniel Ortega and Nicaragua's struggle for liberation.* Chicago: Lawrence Hill Books.

Morrison, L.J. (2005). *Talking back to psychiatry: The psychiatric/consumer/ex-patient movement.* New York: Routledge.

Morrison, L.J. (2006). A matter of definition: Acknowledging consumer/survivor experiences through narrative. *Radical Psychology, 5.* Retrieved from www.radicalpsychology.org/ vol5/Morrison.html.

Morrow, M. (2003). *Demonstrating progress: Innovations in women's mental health.* Vancouver: BC Centre of Excellence for Women's Health.

Morrow, M. (2005). Mental health reform, economic globalization and the practice of citizenship. *Canadian Journal of Community Mental Health, 23*(2), 39–50.

Morrow, M., Frischmuth, S., & Johnson, A. (2006). *Community based mental health services in BC: Changes to income, employment and housing security.* Vancouver: Canadian Centre for Policy Alternatives.

Morrow, M., Jamer, B., & Weisser, J. (2011). *The recovery dialogues: A critical exploration of social inequities in mental health recovery.* Vancouver: Centre for the Study of Gender,

Social Inequities and Mental Health. Retrieved from www.socialinequities.ca/wordpress/wp-content/uploads/2011/02/The-Recovery-Dialogues-Team-Report.Final_.style_.pdf.

Morrow, M., Pederson, A., Smith, J., Josewski, V., Jamer, B., & Battersby, L. (2010). *Relocating mental health care in British Columbia: Riverview Hospital redevelopment, regionalization and gender in psychiatric and social care.* Vancouver: Centre for the Study of Gender, Social Inequities and Mental Health.

Morrow, M., Smith, J., Lai, Y., & Jaswal, S. (2008). Shifting landscapes: Immigrant women and postpartum depression. *Health Care for Women International, 29*(6), 593–617.

Morrow, M., Wasik, A., Cohen, M., & Perry, K. (2009). Removing barriers to work: Building economic security for people with mental illness. *Critical Social Policy, 29*(4), 655–676.

Mosher, L. (1995). The Soteria project: The first-generation American alternatives to psychiatric hospitalization. In R. Warner (Ed.), *Alternatives to the hospital for acute psychiatric treatment* (pp. 111–132). Washington: American Psychiatric Publishing.

Mosoff, J. (1997). "A jury dressed in medical white and judicial black": Mothers with mental health histories in child welfare and custody. In S. Boyd (Ed.), *Challenging the public/private divide: Feminism, law and public policy* (pp. 227–252). Toronto: University of Toronto Press.

Motivation, Power and Achievement Society (MPA). (2011). Retrieved from www.mpa-society.org/.

Myers, J., & Burstow, B. (2006). *ECT report,* DVD. Enquiry Into Psychiatry, Coalition Against Psychiatric Assault.

National Film Board. (1999). *Working like crazy.* Directed by Gwynne Basen and Laura Sky. Montreal: NFB.

National Institute of Mental Health. (n.d.(a)). *Depression.* Retrieved November 6, 2011, from www.nimh.nih.gov/health/publications/depression/complete-index.shtml.

National Institute of Mental Health. (n.d.(b)). *Schizophrenia.* Retrieved November 6, 2011, from www.nimh.nih.gov/health/publications/schizophrenia/complete-index.shtml.

National Network for Mental Health. (n.d.). About us. Retrieved from www.nnmh.ca/AboutUs/tabid/444/language/en-CA/Default.aspx.

Neimeyer, R.A. (2005). Complicated grief and the quest for meaning: A constructivist contribution. *Omega Journal of Death and Dying, 2*(1), 37–52.

Nelson, G., Ochocka, J., Janzen, R., & Trainor, J. (2006a). A longitudinal study of mental health consumer/survivor initiatives: Part 1—Literature review and overview of the study. *Journal of Community Psychology, 34*(3), 247–260.

Nelson, G., Ochocka, J., Janzen, R., & Trainor, J. (2006b). A longitudinal study of mental health consumer/survivor initiatives: Part 2—A quantitative study of impacts of participation on new members. *Journal of Community Psychology, 34*(3), 272–260.

Nelson, G., Ochocka, J., Janzen, R., & Trainor, J. (2006c). A longitudinal study of mental health consumer/survivor initiatives: Part 3—A qualitative study of impacts of participation on new members. *Journal of Community Psychology, 34*(3), 273–283.

Nelson, G., Ochocka, J., Janzen, R., & Trainor, J. (2006d). A longitudinal study of mental health consumer/survivor initiatives: Part 4—Benefits beyond the self? A quantitative and qualitative study of system-level activities and impacts. *Journal of Community Psychology, 34*(3), 285–303.

Nelson, G., & Saegert, S. (2009). Housing and quality of life: An ecological perspective. In V.R. Preedy & R.R. Watson (Eds.), *Handbook of disease burdens and quality of life measures* (pp. 3363–3382). Heidelberg: Springer-Verlag.

Nelson, G., Sylvestre, J., Aubry, T., George, L., & Trainor, J. (2007). Housing choice and control, housing quality, and control over professional support as contributors to the subjective quality of life and community adaptation of people with severe mental illness. *Administration and Policy in Mental Health and Mental Health Services Research, 34*, 89–100.

Neugeboren, J. (1997). *Imagining Robert: My brother, madness and survival.* New York: Henry Holt.

Ninth International Conference on Human Rights and Psychiatric Oppression. (1981, August 31). Press release. *Phoenix Rising, 2*(3).

NPR (National Public Radio). (2011). Exploring Occupy Wall Street's "Adbuster" origins. Retrieved January 28, 2012, from http://www.npr.org/2011/10/20/141526467/exploring-occupy-wall-streets-adbuster-origins.

Oaks, D.W. (2008). Prospects for a nonviolent revolution in the mental health system during a time of psychiatric globalization. Keynote address at Madness, Citizenship, and Social Justice: A Human Rights Conference, Simon Fraser University, Vancouver, BC.

Oaks, D.W., Imai, A., & Erickson, K. (2011, October 8). Web radio interview on MindFreedom Mad Pride live free web radio: Occupy Normal show. Retrieved November 8, 2011, from www.blogtalkradio.com/davidwoaks/2011/10/08/.mindfreedom-occupy-normal-show-guest-aki-imai.

O'Hagan, M. (2004a). Force in mental health services: International user and survivor perspectives. *Mental Health Practice, 7*(5), 12–17.

O'Hagan, M. (2004b). Guest editorial: Recovery in New Zealand: Lessons for Australia. *Australian e-Journal for the Advancement of Mental Health, 3*(1), 1–3.

O'Hagan, M., Cyr, C., McKee, H., & Priest, R. (2010). *Making the case for peer support: Report to the Mental Health Commission of Canada, Mental Health Peer Support Project Committee.* Retrieved January 7, 2012, from www.mentalhealthcommission.ca/English/Pages/servicesystemsinformation.aspx.

O'Hara, K. (2006). *A grief like no other: Surviving the violent death of someone you love.* New York: Marlowe and Company.

Oldenburg, R. (1989). *The great good place.* New York: Paragon House.

Oliver, M. (1992). Changing the social relations of research production. *Disability, Handicap and Society, 7*(2), 101–115.

Omi, M., & Winant, H. (1994). Toward a racial formation perspective. In M. Omi & H. Winant (Eds.), *Racial formation in the United States: From the 1960s to the 1990s* (2nd ed., pp. 48–76). New York: Routledge.

On Our Own. (1980–1990). *Phoenix Rising: The Voice of the Psychiatrized.* Toronto.

Ontario Ministry of Health. (1985). *Report of the Electro-Convulsive Therapy Review Committee.* Toronto: Government of Ontario.

Ontario Ministry of Health and Long-Term Care. (2000–2004). Services and payments for electroconvulsive therapy; PPH ECT statistics: 2002–2004.

Ontario Ministry of Health and Long-Term Care. (n.d.). *Community mental health careers.* Retrieved January 6, 2012, from www.mentalhealthcommission.ca/SiteCollectionDocuments/Peer%20Support/Service%20Systems%20AC%20-%20Peer%20support%20report%20EN.pdf.

Ontario Psychiatric Association. (2008). Medicine's blind spot. Mental health stigma: Are some patients worth less than others? *OPA Dialogue,* Summer, 11–13.

OPSA (Ontario Psychiatric Survivor Alliance). (1992). OPSA newsletter. Toronto.

Ontario Review Board. (2009–2010). *Annual reports*. Retrieved November 5, 2011, from www.orb.on.ca/scripts/en/resources.asp.

Ord, R. (2009). "It's like a tattoo": Dominant discourses on grief. *Canadian Social Work Review*, 26(2), 195–212.

Overton, S., & Medina, S. (2008). The stigma of mental illness. *Journal of Counselling & Development*, 86, 143–151.

Owram, D. (1996). *Born at the right time: A history of the baby boom generation*. Toronto: University of Toronto Press.

Packard, E.P.W. (1866). *Marital power exemplified: Three years' imprisonment for religious belief*. Hartford: Published by the author.

Packard, E.P.W. (1869). Mrs. Packard's address to the Illinois Legislature. February 12. Chicago: Clarke & Co.

Packard, E.P.W. (1882, June). Emancipation of married women! An argument of providential events in support of the Identity Act. *Colorado Antelope*.

Page, M. (2001). Radical public history in the city. *Radical History*, 79, 114–116.

Palmer, B.D. (2009). *Canada's 1960s: The ironies of identity in a rebellious era*. Toronto: University of Toronto Press.

Parkes, C. (1996). *Bereavement: Studies in grief in adult life*. Philadelphia: Taylor and Francis.

Pasternak, S. (2011, October 20). Occupy(ed) Canada: The political economy of Indigenous dispossession in Canada. Rabble.ca. Retrieved November 8, 2011, from rabble.ca/news/2011/10/occupyed-canada-political-economy-indigenous-dispossession-canada.

Patterson, M., Somers, J., McIntosh, K., Shiell, A., & Frankish, C.J. (2008). *Housing and support for adults with severe addictions and/or mental illness in British Columbia*. Vancouver: Centre for Applied Research in Mental Health and Addiction.

Peach, C. (1996). Good segregation, bad segregation. *Planning Perspectives*, 11, 379–398.

Pearson, G. (1975). *The deviant imagination: Psychiatry, social work and social change*. London: Macmillan.

Penfold, S., & Walker, G. (1983). *Women and the psychiatric paradox*. Montreal: Eden Press.

Pengilly, M.H. (1885). *Diary written in the Provincial Lunatic Asylum*. Lowell: Monitor Steam Job Print; also at Early Canadiana Online. Retrieved January 12, 2012, from www.canadiana.org/cgi-bin/ECO/mtq?id=c5fd0156b2&doc=11978.

Peris, T.S., Teachman, B.A., & Nosek, B.A. (2008). Implicit and explicit stigma of mental illness: Links to clinical care. *Journal of Nervous and Mental Disease*, 196, 752–760.

Perlin, M.L. (1991). Competency, deinstitutionalization and homelessness: A story of marginalization. *Houston Law Review*, 28, 63–142.

Perlin, M.L. (2000). *The hidden prejudice: Mental disability on trial*. Washington: American Psychological Association.

Perlin, M.L. (2003). "You have discussed lepers and crooks": Sanism in clinical teaching. *Clinical Law Review*, 9, 683–730.

Perlin, M.L. (2008). "I might need a good lawyer, could be your funeral, my trial": Global clinical legal education and the right to counsel in civil commitment cases. *Washington University Journal of Law and Policy*, 28, 241–272.

Perreault, I. (2009). Psychiatrie et ordre social: Analyse des causes d'internement et des diagnostics donnés à Saint-Jean-de-Dieu dans une perspective de genre, 1920–1950. PhD diss., University of Ottawa.

Pescosolido, B., Monahan, J., Link, B., Stueve, A., & Kikuzawa, S. (1999). The public's view of the competence, dangerousness, and need for legal coercion of persons with mental health problems. *American Journal of Public Health, 89*(9), 1339–1345.

Peters, Y. (2004). Twenty years of litigating for disability equality rights: Has it made a difference? Retrieved December 29, 2011, from www.ccdonline.ca/en/humanrights/promoting/20years.

Phelan, J.C. (2005). Geneticization of deviant behavior and consequences for stigma: The case of mental illness. *Journal of Health and Social Behavior, 46*, 307–322.

Phoenix Rising Collective. (1980). Being an inmate. *Phoenix Rising, 1*(2), 1–3.

Piat, M., & Sabetti, J. (2009). The development of a recovery-oriented mental health system in Canada: What the experience of commonwealth countries tells us. *Canadian Journal of Community Mental Health, 28*(2), 17–33.

Piat, M., Sabetti, J., & Couture, A. (2008). Do consumers use the word recovery? *Psychiatric Services, 59*(4), 446.

Picard, A. (2011, August 31). Mental health strategy draft doesn't go far enough. *Globe and Mail.* Retrieved from www.theglobeandmail.com/life/health/new-health/andre-picard/mental-health-strategy-draft-doesnt-go-far-enough/article2149012/.

Pilgrim, D., & Rogers, A. (2005). The troubled relationship between psychiatry and sociology. *International Journal of Social Psychiatry, 51*, 228–41.

Piner, K., & Kahle, L. (1984). Adapting to the stigmatizing label of mental illness: Forgone but not forgotten. *Journal of Personality and Social Psychology, 47*(4), 805–811.

Plath, S. (1966). *The bell jar.* London: Faber & Faber.

Polletta, F. (2002). *Freedom is an endless meeting: Democracy in American social movements.* Chicago: University of Chicago Press.

Pollock, S. (1974). Social policy for mental health in Ontario. PhD diss., University of Toronto.

Poole, J. (2011). *Behind the rhetoric: Mental health recovery in Ontario.* Halifax: Fernwood.

Poole, J., Jivraj, T., Arslanian, A., Bellows, K., Chiasson, S., Hakimy, H., Pasini, J., & Reid, J. (2012). Sanism, "mental health" and social work/education: A review and call to action. *Intersectionalities: A Global Journal of Social Work Analysis, Research, Polity and Practice, 1*(1), 20–36.

Porter, R. (2002). *Madness: A brief history.* Oxford: Oxford University Press.

PPAO (Psychiatric Patient Advocate). (1994). *Bringing balance to mental health care: Consumer/survivor empowerment in the psychiatric hospital system.* Psychiatric Patient Advocate Office 10th anniversary report. Toronto: Queen's Printer for Ontario.

Pratt, M. (1988). Just make it to tomorrow. In B. Burstow & D. Weitz (Eds.), *Shrink resistant: The struggle against psychiatry in Canada* (pp. 55–70). Vancouver: New Star Books.

Prendergast, C. (2008). The unexceptional schizophrenic: A post-postmodern introduction. *Journal of Literary and Cultural Disability Studies, 1*(1), 55–62.

Price, M. (2011). *Mad at school.* Ann Arbor: University of Michigan Press.

Probyn, E. (1995). Lesbians in space: Gender, sex and the structure of missing. *Gender, Place & Culture, 2*(1), 77–84.

Probyn, E. (2003). The spatial imperative of subjectivity. In K. Anderson, M. Domosh, S. Pile, and N. Thrift (Eds.), *Handbook of cultural geography* (pp. 290–299). London: Sage.

PsychOUT. (2010). Retrieved from http://ocs.library.utoronto.ca/index.php/psychout/PsychOUT.

Puar, J.K. (2005). Queer times, queer assemblages. *Social Text, 23*(3–4), 122–139.

Puar, J.K. (2009). Prognosis time: Toward a geopolitics of affect, debility and capacity. *Women & Performance: A Journal of Feminist Theory, 19*(2), 161–172.

Puar, J.K. (2010, November 16). In the wake of It Gets Better: The campaign prompted by recent gay youth suicides promotes a narrow version of gay identity that risks further marginalization. *Guardian.* Retrieved November 8, 2011, from www.guardian.co.uk/commentisfree/cifamerica/2010/nov/16/wake-it-gets-better-campaign.

Puar, J.K., Pitcher, B., & Gunkel, H. (2008). *Q&A with Jasbir Puar.* Interview transcript. Retrieved from www.darkmatter101.org/site/2008/05/02/qa-with-jasbir-puar.

Public Health Agency of Canada. (2011). *Schizophrenia: A handbook for families.* Retrieved from www.phac-aspc.gc.ca/mh-sm/pubs/schizophrenia-schizophrenie/chpt01-eng.php.

Putnam, R. (1995). Bowling alone: America's declining social capital. *Journal of Democracy, 6*(1), 65–78.

Qadeer, M. (2005). Ethnic segregation in a multicultural city. In D. Varady (Ed.), *Desegregating the city: Ghettos, enclaves and inequality.* Albany: State University of New York Press.

QSPC (Queen Street Patients Council) & Urban Alliance on Race Relations. (2002). Saving lives: Alternatives to the use of lethal force by police. Toronto.

Quayson, A. (2007). *Aesthetic nervousness: Disability and the crisis of representation.* New York: Columbia University Press.

Quigley, B. (1983). Berkeley electorate bans electroshock. *Madness Network News, 7*(1), 1,3,4.

Rabaia, Y., Giacaman, R., & Nguyen-Gillham, V. (2010). Violence and adolescent mental health in the occupied Palestinian territory: A contextual approach. *Asia Pacific Journal of Public Health, 22*(3), 216S–221S.

Race, D., Boxall, K., & Carson, I. (2005). Towards a dialogue for practice: Reconciling social role valorization and the social model of disability. *Disability & Society, 20*(5), 507–521.

Radley, A. (1999). The aesthetics of illness: Narrative, horror and the sublime. *Sociology of Health & Illness, 21*(6), 778–796.

Rakoff, V. (1979). Review of *Blue Jolts. Canadian Journal of Psychiatry, 24*(5), 494.

Ralph, D.S. (1983). *Work and madness: The rise of community psychiatry.* Montreal: Black Rose Books.

Ramon, S. (2008). Neoliberalism and its implications for mental health in the UK. *International Journal of Law and Psychiatry, 31*(2), 116–125.

Ramon, S., Healy, B., & Ranouf, N. (2007). Recovery from mental illness as an emergent concept and practice in Australia and the UK. *International Journal of Social Psychiatry, 53*(2), 108–122.

Rancière, J. (1994). *The politics of aesthetics.* Britain: Continuum.

Rando, T. (1993). *Treatment of complicated mourning.* Champaign: Research Press.

Razack, S. (1991). *Canadian feminism and the law: The Women's Legal Education and Action Fund and the pursuit of equality.* Toronto: Second Story Press.

Razack, S. (1998). *Looking white people in the eye: Gender, race, and culture in courtrooms and classrooms.* Toronto: University of Toronto Press.

Razack, S. (2002). Gendered racial violence and spatialized justice. In S. Razack (Ed.), *Race, space, and the law: Unmapping a white settler society* (pp. 121–156). Toronto: Between the Lines.

Razack, S. (2004). *Dark threats and white nights: The Somalia Affair, peacekeeping and the new imperialism.* Toronto: University of Toronto Press.

Read, J., & Bentall, R. (2010). The effectiveness of electroconvulsive therapy: A literature review. *Epidemiologia e Psichiatria Sociale, 19*(3), 333–347.

Read, J., Haslam, N., Sayce, L., & Davies, E. (2006). Prejudice and schizophrenia: A review of the "mental illness is an illness like any other" approach. *Acta Psychiatrica Scandinavica, 114*(5), 303–318.

Reaume, G. (2000). *Remembrance of patients past: Patient life at the Toronto Hospital for the Insane, 1870–1940*. Toronto: Oxford University Press.

Reaume, G. (2002). Lunatic to patient to person: Nomenclature in psychiatric history and the influence of patients' activism in North America. *International Journal of Law and Psychiatry, 25*(4), 405–426.

Reaume, G. (2004). No profits, just a pittance: Work, compensation and people defined as mentally disabled in Ontario, 1964–1990. In S. Noll & J.W. Trent (Eds.), *Mental retardation in America: A historical reader* (pp. 466–493). New York: New York University Press.

Reaume, G. (2006). Teaching radical history: Mad people's history. *Radical History Review, 94*, 170–182.

Reaume, G. (2011). Psychiatric patient built wall tours at the Centre for Addiction and Mental Health (CAMH), Toronto, 2000–2010. *Active History/History Matters*. Retrieved October 21, 2011, from http://activehistory.ca/papers/historypaper-10/.

Reid, J. (2008). Social work practice with the mad community: Presenting an alternative. Unpublished paper, Toronto.

Renke, W. (1995). No present danger: A comment on Lepage v. The Queen. *Health Law Review, 1*, 30–40.

Reoch, P. (2011, August 26). Paranoid schizophrenic cut woman's arm with screwdriver. *Courier*. Retrieved January 21, 2012, from www.thecourier.co.uk/News/Perthshire/article/16812/paranoid-schizophrenic-cut-woman-s-arm-with-screwdriver.html.

Report of the Panel on Electroshock. (2005). *Electroshock is not a healing option. Inquiry into psychiatry*. Retrieved from http://capacanada.wordpress.com, 9–10.

Reville, D. (2011, July 25). Personal communication with J. Ward.

Richard, A.L., Jongbloed, L.E., & MacFarlane, A. (2009). Integration of peer support workers into community mental health teams. *International Journal of Psychosocial Rehabilitation, 14*(1), 99–110.

Roberts, G.A. (2000). Narrative and severe mental illness: What place do stories have in an evidence-based world? *Advances in Psychiatric Treatment, 6*, 432–441.

Roberts, M. (2005). The production of the psychiatric subject: Power, knowledge and Michel Foucault. *Nursing Philosophy, 6*, 33–42.

Robertson, R. (2007). Taming space: Drug use, HIV, and homemaking in Downtown Eastside Vancouver. *Gender, Place and Culture, 14*(5), 527–549.

Robins, C.S., Sauvageot, J.A., Cusack, K.J., Suffoletta-Maierle, S., & Frueh, B.C. (2005). Consumers' perceptions of negative experiences and "sanctuary harm" in psychiatric settings. *Psychiatric Services, 56*(9), 1134–1138.

Roe, D., & Ronen, Y. (2003). Hospitalization as experienced by the psychiatric patient: A therapeutic jurisprudence perspective. *International Journal of Law and Psychiatry, 26*, 317–332.

Roman, L., Brown, S., Noble, S., Wainer, R., & Young, A.E. (Eds.). (2009). No time for nostalgia!: Asylum-making, medicalized colonialism in British Columbia (1859–97) and artistic praxis for social transformation. *International Journal of Qualitative Studies in Education, 22*(1), 17–63.

Rooming House Working Group. (2011, March 14). Rooming House Working Group meeting notes.

Rose, D. (2004). Discourses and experiences of social mix in gentrifying neighbourhoods: A Montreal case study. *Canadian Journal of Urban Research, 13*(2), 278–327.

Rose, N. (1990). *Governing the soul: The shaping of the private self.* New York: Routledge.

Rose, N. (1998). *Inventing our selves: Psychology, power, and personhood.* Cambridge: Cambridge University Press.

Rose, N. (1999). *Powers of freedom: Rethinking political thought.* Cambridge: Cambridge University Press.

Rose, N. (2006). *The politics of life itself: Biomedicine, power, and subjectivity in the twenty-first century.* Princeton: Princeton University Press.

Rosenhan, D.L. (1973). On being sane in insane places. *Science, 179*(4070), 250–258.

Ross, J. (2007). Balancing supportive housing with civic engagement. Toronto: Centre for Urban and Community Studies. Retrieved January 9, 2012, from www.new.homecoming-coalition.com/wp-content/uploads/2009/08/RossSupportiveHousingstudy.pdf.

Ross, R. (2009). Heartsong: Exploring emotional suppression and disconnection in Aboriginal Canada. A discussion paper. In author's possession.

Roth Edney, D. (2004). *Mass media and mental illness: A literature review.* Toronto: Canadian Mental Health Association, Ontario Division. Retrieved November 5, 2011, from www.ontario.cmha.ca/about_mental_health.asp?cID=7600.

Rough Times Staff. (1973). *Rough times.* New York: Ballantyne Books.

Ruming, K., Mee, K., & McGuirk, P. (2004). Questioning the rhetoric of social mix: Courteous community or hidden hostility? *Australian Geographical Studies, 42*(2), 224–248.

Rusch, N., Angermeyer, M., & Corrigan, P. (2005). Mental illness stigma: Concepts, consequences, and initiatives to reduce stigma. *European Psychiatry, 20,* 529–539.

Ryersonian. (2006, October 11). "Schizophrenic team" leads madness class. *Ryersonian.* Ryerson University.

Sackeim, H., Prudic, J., Fuller, R., et al. (2007). The cognitive effects of electroconvulsive therapy in community settings. *Neuropsychopharmacology, 32,* 244–254.

Saïd, E. (1983). Opponents, audiences, constituencies and community. In H. Foster (Ed.), *The anti-aesthetic: Essays on postmodern culture* (pp. 135–159). Seattle: Bay Press.

Salie, M. (2010). WNUSP co-chair Moosa Salie responds to draft report: Reforming Mental Health Law in Africa: Practical tips and suggestions. World Network of Users and Survivors of Psychiatry. Retrieved December 28, 2011, from www.wnusp.net/.

Samuel, R. (1994). *Theatres of memory: Volume I: Past and present in contemporary culture.* London: Verso.

Sandburg, C. (1914). *Poetry.* March.

Sangster, J. (1994). Telling our stories: Feminist debates and the use of oral history. *Women's History Review, 3*(1), 5–28.

Savage, D., & Miller, T. (Eds.). (2011). *It gets better: Coming out, overcoming bullying, and creating a life worth living.* New York: Dutton.

Savage, H., & McKague, C. (1987). *Mental health law in Canada.* Toronto: Butterworths.

Sayce, L. (2000). *From psychiatric patient to citizen: Overcoming discrimination and social exclusion.* London: Palgrave Macmillan.

Scheff, T. (1966). *Being mentally ill: A sociological theory.* Chigago: Aldine.

Scheff, T., Phillips, B., & Kincaid, H. (2006). *Goffman unbound!: A new paradigm for social science—The sociological imagination.* Boulder: Paradigm.

Scheper-Hughes, N. (1992). *Death without weeping: The violence of everyday life in Brazil.* Berkeley: University of California Press.

Scheper-Hughes, N., & Lovell, A.M. (Eds.). (1987). *Psychiatry inside out: Selected writings of Franco Basaglia.* New York: Columbia University Press.

Schively, C. (2007). Understanding the NIMBY and LULU phenomena: Reassessing our knowledge base and informing future research. *Journal of Planning Literature, 21*(3), 255–266.

Schizophrenia Society of Canada. (n.d.). *Annual report 2010–2011.* Retrieved from www.schizophrenia.ca/SSCAnnualReport2011.pdf.

Schrag, P. (1978). *Mind control.* New York: Pantheon.

Schubert, J.D. (2002). Defending multiculturalism: From hegemony to symbolic violence. *American Behavioral Scientist, 45*(7), 1088–1102.

Scull, A. (1977). *Decarceration: Community treatment and the deviant: A radical view.* Englewood Cliffs: Prentice-Hall.

Scull, A. (2010). A psychiatric revolution. *Lancet, 375*(9722), 1246–1247.

Scull, A. (2011). *Madness: An introduction.* Oxford: Oxford University Press.

Secretariat for Social Development. (1983). *Ontario group homes resource manual.* Toronto: Province of Ontario.

Sedgwick, P. (1982). *Psycho politics: Laing, Foucault, Goffman, Szasz, and the future of mass psychiatry.* New York: Harper & Row.

Shagan, E. (2003). *Popular politics and the English Reformation.* Cambridge: Cambridge University Press.

Sharfstein, S.S. (2005). Big Pharma and American psychiatry: The good, the bad, and the ugly. A letter from the president of the American Psychiatric Association. *Psychiatric News, 40,* 16.

Sharma, N., & Wright, C. (2008). Decolonizing resistance, challenging colonial states. *Social Justice, 35*(3), 120–138.

Shear, M.K. (2010). Complicated grief treatment: The theory, practice and outcomes. *Bereaved Care, 29*(3), 10–14.

Shera, W., Aviram, U., Healy, B., & Ramon, S. (2002). Mental health system reform: A multi country comparison. *Social Work in Health Care, 35*(1-2): 547–575.

Shimrat, I. (1990). Analyzing psychiatry. CBC *Ideas* transcript. Toronto: Canadian Broadcasting Corporation.

Shimrat, I. (1991). By reason of insanity. CBC *Ideas* transcript. Toronto: Canadian Broadcasting Corporation.

Shimrat, I. (1997). *Call me crazy: Stories from the mad movement.* Vancouver: Press Gang.

Shimrat, I. (2011). The Mental Patients Association and the Vancouver Emotional Emergency Centre. *Networker, 16*(3), 13.

Shone, G., & Gray, L. (2000). *Canadian mental health law and policy.* Cited in Standing Senate Committee on Social Affairs, Science and Technology. (2004). *Interim report 1— Mental health, mental illness and addiction: Overview of policies and programs in Canada* (p. 5). Retrieved from www.parl.gc.ca/38/1/parlbus/commbus/senate/com-e/soci-e/rep-e/repintnov04-e.htm.

Shopes, L. (2003). Sharing authority. *Oral History Review, 30*(1), 103–110.

Showalter, E. (1985). *The female malady: Women, madness and English culture, 1830–1980.* New York: Pantheon.

Shragge, E. (2003). *Activism and social change: Lessons for community and local organizing.* Peterborough: Broadview Press.

Simmons, H.G. (1990). *Unbalanced: Mental health policy in Ontario, 1930–1989.* Toronto: Wall & Thompson.

Singal, N. (2010). Doing disability research in a southern context. *Disability & Society, 25*(4), 415–426.

Sinson, J.C. (1993). *Group homes and community integration of developmentally disabled people: Micro-Institutionalization?* London: Jessica Kingsley.

Sjöström, S. (2006). Invocation of coercion context in compliance communication—power dynamics in psychiatric care. *International Journal of Law and Psychiatry, 29,* 36–47.

Slater, T. (2004). Municipally managed gentrification in South Parkdale, Toronto. *Canadian Geographer, 48*(3), 303–325.

Slave labor in California psychiatric institutions. (1976). *Madness Network News. 3*(6), 7.

Sleeter, C. (1987:2010). Why is there learning disabilities? A critical analysis of the birth of the field in its social context. Reprinted in *Disability Studies Quarterly, 30*(2). Retrieved from www.dsq-sds.org/issue/view/46.

Slovenko, R. (2009). *Psychiatry in law/law in psychiatry.* New York: Routledge.

Smith, A. (2005). *Conquest. Sexual violence and American Indian genocide.* Boston: South End Press.

Smith, A. (2006). Heteropatriarchy and the three pillars of white supremacy. In *Rethinking women of color organizing. Color of violence: The Incite! anthology* (pp. 66–73). Boston: South End Press.

Smith, B., & Sparkes, A. (2008). Narrative and its potential contribution to disability studies. *Disability & Society, 23*(1), 17–28.

Smith, D. (1978). "K is mentally ill": The anatomy of a factual account. *Sociology, 12*(23), 23–53.

Smith, D. (1987). *The everyday world as problematic: A feminist sociology.* Toronto: University of Toronto Press.

Smith, D. (1990). *The conceptual practices of power: A feminist sociology of knowledge.* Toronto: University of Toronto Press.

Smith, D. (2003). Resisting institutional capture as a research practice. In B. Glassner & R. Hertz (Eds.), *Our studies, ourselves: Sociologists' lives and work* (pp. 150–161). New York: Oxford University Press.

Smith, D. (2005). *Institutional ethnography: A sociology of the people.* Landham: Altamira Press.

Smith, D., & David, S.J. (Eds.). (1975). *Women look at psychiatry.* Vancouver: Press Gang.

Soldatic, K., & Fiske, L. (2009). Bodies "locked up": Intersections of disability and race in Australian immigration. *Disability & Society, 24*(3), 289–301.

Solomon, P. (2004). Peer support/peer provided services. Underlying processes, benefits and critical ingredients. *Psychiatric Rehabilitation Journal, 27*(4), 392–401.

Spandler, H. (1996). *Who's hurting who? Young people, self-harm and suicide.* Manchester: 42nd Street.

Speed, E. (2005). Patients, consumers and survivors: A case study of mental health service user discourses. *Social Science and Medicine, 62*(1), 28–38.

Spivak, G.C. (2005). Scattered speculation on the subaltern and the popular. *Postcolonial Studies, 8*(4), 475–486.

Squire, L., & Slater, P. (1983). Electroconvulsive therapy and complaints of memory dysfunction: A prospective three-year follow-up study. *British Journal of Psychiatry, 142*, 1–8.

Staff Report. (2011, August 9). Police search for missing schizophrenic patients. *Chicago Tribune.* Retrieved January 21, 2012, from http://articles.chicagotribune.com/2011-08-09/news/chi-police-search-for-missing-schizophrenics-20110809_1_police-search-eyes-and-blond-hair-chicago-police.

St-Amand, N. (1988). *The politics of madness.* Halifax: Formac Publishing.

Standing Senate Committee on Social Affairs, Science and Technology. (2006). *Out of the shadows at last. Transforming mental health, mental illness and addiction services in Canada.* Ottawa: Senate of Canada.

Standing Senate Committee on Social Affairs, Science and Technology. (2009). Report of the Subcommittee on Cities. In *From the margins: A call to action on poverty, housing and homelessness.* Ottawa: The Standing Senate Committee on Social Affairs, Science and Technology.

Stanhope, V., Marcus, S., & Solomon, P. (2009). The impact of coercion on services from the perspective of mental health care consumers with co-occurring disorders. *Psychiatric Services, 60*, 183–188.

Starkman, M. (1981). The movement. *Phoenix Rising: The Voice of the Psychiatrized, 2*(3), 2A–9A.

Stastny, P., & Lehmann, P. (Eds.). (2007). *Alternatives beyond psychiatry.* Berlin: Peter Lehmann Books.

Statistics Canada. (2001, December 6). Personal communication from Lori Anderson.

Sterling, A., & Farrow, K. (2011, October 15). The feministing five: Kenyon Farrow. Feministing. Interview. Retrieved November 8, 2011, from feministing.com/2011/10/15/the-feministing-five-kenyon-farrow/#more-39790.

Sterling, P. (2002, October 22). Comments on brain damage and memory loss from electroconvulsive shock. Dublin: The Wellbeing Foundation; paper presented at the New York State Assembly Public Hearing on Forced Electroshock.

Stromwall, L., Holley, L., & Bashor, K. (2011). Stigma in the mental health workplace: Perceptions of peer employees and clinicians. *Community Mental Health Journal, 47*(4), 472–481.

Sunshine, F. (2011, October 31). Lawrence Heights redevelopment plan awarded for excellence. *Inside Toronto.* Retrieved from www.insidetoronto.com/news/local/article/1233655.

Supeene, S.L. (1990). *As for the sky, falling: A critical look at psychiatry and suffering.* Toronto: Second Story Press.

Sweeney, A. (2009). So what is survivor research? In A. Sweeney, P. Beresford, A. Faulkner, M. Nettle & D. Rose (Eds.), *This is survivor research* (pp. 22–37). Ross-on-Wye: PCCS Books.

Sylvestre, J., George, L., Aubry, T., Durbin, J., Nelson, G., & Trainor, J. (2007). Strengthening Ontario's system of housing for people with serious mental illness. *Canadian Journal of Community Mental Health, 26*, 79–95.

Szasz, T.S. (1960). The myth of mental illness. *American Psychologist, 15*, 113–118.

Szasz, T.S. (1961). *The myth of mental illness: Foundations of a theory of personal conduct.* New York: Harper & Row.

Szasz, T.S. (1997). *The manufacture of madness.* Syracuse: Syracuse University Press.

Szasz, T.S. (2001). *Pharmacracy: Medicine and politics in America.* Westport: Praeger.

Takahashi, L., & Dear, M. (1997). The changing dynamics of community opposition to human service facilities. *Journal of the American Planning Association, 63*(1), 79–94.

Tanasan, G. (2011). Building the European network. *European Network of Users and Survivors of Psychiatry Bulletin, 1,* 4–6.

Teelucksingh, C. (2002). Spatiality and environmental justice in Parkdale. *Ethnologies, 24*(1), 119–141.

Teghtsoonian, K. (2008). Managing workplace depression: Contesting the contours of emerging policy in the workplace. In K. Teghtsoonian & P. Moss (Eds.), *Contesting illnesses: Processes and practices* (pp. 69–89). Toronto: University of Toronto Press.

Thobani, S. (2007). *Exalted subjects: Studies in the making of race and nation in Canada.* Toronto: University of Toronto Press.

Thompson, P. (1978). *The voice of the past: Oral history.* Oxford: Oxford University Press.

Titchkosky, T., & Michalko, R. (Eds.). (2009). *Rethinking normalcy: A disability studies reader.* Toronto: Canadian Scholars' Press Inc.

Titchkosky, T., & Aubrecht, K. (2010). The anguish of power: Remapping mental diversity with an anti-colonial compass. In A. Kempf (Ed.), *Breaching the colonial contract: Anti-colonialism in the US and Canada* (pp. 179–199). New York: Springer.

Topp, L. (2007). The modern mental hospital in late nineteenth-century Germany and Austria: Psychiatric space and images of freedom and control. In L. Topp, J. Moran & J. Andrews (Eds.), *Madness, architecture, and the built environment: Psychiatric spaces in historical context* (pp. 241–261). New York: Routledge.

Trainor, J., & Church, K. (1984). *A framework for support for people with severe mental disabilities.* Toronto: Canadian Mental Health Association (National).

Udegbe, O., & Vo, T. (2013). Native informants? Disability justice, the caring mission, and the reproduction of the racial state. Paper to be presented to the Critical Ethnic Studies Association, September 19–21, University of Illinois at Chicago.

United Nations Educational, Scientific and Cultural Organization. (n.d.). Education: Mission. UNESCO. Retrieved September 24, 2011, from www.unesco.org/new/en/education/themes/education-building-blocks/literacy/mission/.

Ussher, J.M. (1992). *Women's madness: Misogyny or mental illness?* Amherst: University of Massachusetts Press.

Ussher, J.M. (2005). Unravelling women's madness: Beyond positivism and constructivism and towards a material-discursive-intrapsychic approach. In W. Chan, D.E. Chunn & R. Menzies (Eds.), *Women, madness, and the law: A feminist reader* (pp. 19–40). London: GlassHouse.

Ussher, J.M. (2011). *The madness of women: Myth and experience.* London: Routledge.

Vanheule, S. (2011). A Lacanian perspective on psychotic hallucinations. *Theory and Psychology, 21*(1), 86–106.

Van Os, J., Kenis, G., & Rutten, B.P. (2010). The environment and schizophrenia. *Nature, 468*(7321), 203–212.

Victorian Government Department of Health. (2011). *Framework for recovery-oriented practice.* Melbourne: Mental Health Drugs and Regions Division, Victorian Government Department of Health.

Vogt, S.C. (2011). Practicing creative maladjustment: The Mental Health Political Action Group. Master's thesis, Simon Fraser University.

von Schulthess, B. (1992). Violence in the streets: Anti-lesbian assault and harassment in San Francisco. In G. Herek & K. Berrill (Eds.), *Hate crimes: Confronting violence against lesbians and gay men* (pp. 65–74). Newbury Park: Sage.

Voronka, J. (2008a). Making bipolar Britney: Proliferating psychiatric diagnoses through tabloid media. *Radical Psychology, 7*(2), 1–19.

Voronka, J. (2008b). Re/moving forward: Spacing mad degeneracy at the Queen Street site. *Resources for Feminist Research, 33*(1,2). Retrieved from http://findarticles.com/p/articles/mi_hb6545/is_1-2_33/ai_n31524744/.

Voronka, J. (2010, June). Consuming consumer narratives: A struggle over how to eat and how to be eaten. Opening plenary presented at the Critical Inquiries Workshop, Centre for the Study of Gender, Social Inequities, and Mental Health, Simon Fraser University, Vancouver, BC.

Wacquant, L. (2006). *Pierre Bourdieu*. Retrieved December 27, 2011, from www.umsl.edu~keelr/3210/resources/PIERREBOURDIEU-KEYTHINK-REV2006.pdf.

Wahl, O. (1995). *Media madness: Public images of mental illness*. New Brunswick: Rutgers University Press.

Walia, H. (2012, January 1). Decolonizing together: Moving beyond a politics of solidarity toward a practice of decolonization. Briarpatch. Retrieved January 7, 2012, from briarpatchmagazine.com/articles/view/decolonizing-together.

Walker, R., & Seasons, M. (2002). Planning supported housing: A new orientation in housing for people with serious mental illness. *Journal of Planning Education and Research, 21*, 313–319.

Warme, G. (2006). *Daggers of the mind: Psychiatry and the myth of mental disease*. Toronto: House of Anansi Press.

Warsh, C.L. (1989). *Moments of unreason: The practice of Canadian psychiatry*. Montreal: McGill-Queen's University Press.

Wastasecoot, B.I. (2000). Culturally appropriate healing and counselling: One woman's path toward healing. In R. Neil (Ed.), *Voice of the drum: Indigenous education and culture* (pp. 121–138). Brandon: Kingfisher Publications.

Watters, E. (2010). *Crazy like us: The globalization of the American psyche*. New York: Free Press.

Weininger, O. (2005 [1903]). *Sex and character: An investigation of fundamental principles*. Bloomington: Indiana University Press.

Weisser, J., Morrow, M., & Jamer, B. (2010). *A critical exploration of social inequities in the mental health literature*. Vancouver: Centre for the Study of Gender Social Inequities and Mental Health. Retrieved from www.socialinequities.ca/wordpress/wp-content/uploads/2011/02/Recovery-Scoping-Review.Final_.STYLE_.pdf.

Weitz, D. (1984). Shock case—A defeat and victory. *Phoenix Rising, 4*(3/4), 28A–30A.

Weitz, D. (1986). Schizophrenia: Exploding the myth. *Phoenix Rising, 6*(3), 8–9.

Weitz, D. (1988). Notes of a "schizophrenic" shitdisturber. In B. Burstow & D. Weitz (Eds.), *Shrink resistant: The struggle against psychiatry in Canada* (pp. 285–302). Vancouver: New Star Books.

Weitz, D. (1994). Call us survivors, not consumers. *Second Opinion, 2*, 16–19.

Weitz, D. (1997). Electroshocking elderly people: Another psychiatric abuse. *Changes: International Journal of Counselling Psychology and Psychotherapy, 15*(2), 118–123.

Weitz, D. (2002). Call me antipsychiatry activist—not "consumer." Retrieved August 11, 2010, from http://radicalpsychology.org/vol3-1/don.html.

Weitz, D. (2003). *Insulin shock*. Retrieved October 31, 2011, from www.psychiatricsurvivorarchives.com/people2.html.

Weitz, D. (2008). Struggling against psychiatry's human rights violations—An antipsychiatry perspective. *Radical Psychology: A Journal of Psychology, Politics, and Radicalism, 7.* Retrieved from www.radicalpsychology.org/vol7-1/weitz2008.html.

Weitz, D. (n.d.). ECT statistics in Ontario: 2000–2004. Unpublished.

Whitaker, R. (2002). *Mad in America: Bad science, bad medicine, and the enduring mistreatment of the mentally ill.* New York: Perseus Books.

Whitaker, R. (2010). *Anatomy of an epidemic: Magic bullets, psychiatric drugs, and the astonishing rise in mental illness in America.* New York: Crown Publishers.

White, H., Whelan, C., Barnes, J.D., & Baskerville, B. (2003). Survey of consumer and non-consumer mental health service providers on Assertive Community Treatment teams in Ontario. *Community Mental Health Journal, 39*(3), 265–276.

White, K. (2007). *Negotiating responsibility: Law, murder, and states of mind.* Vancouver: University of British Columbia Press.

White, K. (2009). Out of the shadows and into the spotlight: The politics of (in)visibility and the implementation of the Mental Health Commission of Canada. In K. White (Ed.), *Configuring madness: Representation, context and meaning* (pp. 225–249). Oxford: Inter-Disciplinary Press.

Whitehead, M., & Dahlgren, G. (2007). *Concepts and principles for tackling social inequities in health: Levelling up part I.* WHO Collaborating Centre for Policy Research on Social Determinants of Health. Copenhagen: WHO.

Whitwell, D. (2005). *Recovery beyond psychiatry.* London: Free Association Books.

Whitzman, C. (2009). *Suburb, slum, urban village: Transformations in Toronto's Parkdale neighbourhood, 1875–2002.* Vancouver: UBC Press.

Whitzman, C., & Slater, T. (2006). Village ghetto land: Myth, social conditions, and housing policy in Parkdale, Toronto, 1879–2000. *Urban Affairs Review, 41*(5), 673–696.

Wikipedia. Elizabeth Packard. Retrieved January 14, 2012, from http://en.wikipedia.org/wiki/Elizabeth_Packard.

Wilkinson, R., & Pickett, K. (2009). *The spirit level: Why greater equality makes societies stronger.* London: Bloomsbury Press.

Williams, A. (Ed.). (2007). *Therapeutic landscapes.* Aldershot: Ashgate.

Wilson, S. (2010). Voices from the asylum: Four french women writers, 1850–1920. Retrieved December 16, 2011, from www.oup.com/us/catalog/general/subject/LiteratureEnglish/WorldLiterature/France/?view=usa&ci=9780199579358.

Wilton, R. (2004). Putting policy into practice? Poverty and people with serious mental illness. *Social Science and Medicine, 58,* 25–39.

Wipond, R. (1999, June 10–16). For your own good. *Monday Magazine.* Retrieved January 25, 2012, from http://robwipond.com/?p=748.

Wipond, R. (2008). A "patient-centered" path toward ignoring patient rights. *Radical Psychology, 7*(2). Retrieved from http://radicalpsychology.org/vol7-2/Wipond.html.

Wipond, R. (2011, June). Crisis behind closed doors. Focus. Retrieved January 21, 2012, from www.focusonline.ca/?q=node/237.

Wiseman, F. (1967). *Titicut follies.* Boston: Zipporah Films.

Wolfelt, A.D. (2003). *Understanding your grief: Ten essential touchstones for finding hope and healing your heart.* Fort Collins: Companion Press.

Wolframe, P. (June, 2011). The invisible straight jacket: Theorizing and teaching sanism and sane privilege. Paper presented at PsychOUT: A Conference for Organizing Resistance Against Psychiatry, New York, NY.

Wong, I.Y. & Solomon, P.L. (2002). Community integration of persons with psychiatric disabilities in supportive independent housing: A conceptual model and methodological considerations. *Mental Health Services Research, 4*(1), 13–28.

Wong, I.Y. & Stanhope, V. (2009). Conceptualizing community: A comparison of neighbourhood characteristics of supportive housing for persons with psychiatric and developmental disabilities. *Social Science and Medicine, 68,* 1376–1387.

Wong, R. (2008). Decolonizasian: Reading Asian and First Nations relations in literature. *Canadian Literature, 199,* 158–180.

Wong, T. (2007, February 23). Parkdale the hottest real estate play in city. *Toronto Star.* Retrieved January 9, 2012, from www.thestar.com/article/184911.

Wood, D., & Pistrang, N. (2004). A safe place? Service users' experiences of an acute mental health ward. *Journal of Community & Applied Social Psychology, 14,* 16–28.

Woodson, M.M. (1994). *Behind the door of delusion.* Denver: University of Colorado Press.

Worden, J.W. (2009). *Grief counselling and grief therapy.* New York: Springer.

Wotherspoon, T., & Schissel, B. (2001). The business of placing Canadian children and youth "at-risk." *Canadian Journal of Education, 26*(3), 321–339.

Yale School of Medicine. (n.d.). *Patient care peer support services.* Retrieved January 6, 2012, from http://psychiatry.yale.edu/care/services/services/peersupport.aspx.

Yanos, P., Stefanic, A., & Tsemberis, S. (2011). Psychological community integration among people with psychiatric disabilities and nondisabled community members. *Journal of Community Psychology, 39*(4), 390–401.

Yellow Bird, P. (2010). Wild Indians: Native perspectives on the Hiawatha Asylum for Insane Indians. N.P.: Center For Mental Health Services (CMHS).

Zembrzycki, S. (2009). Sharing authority with Baba. *Journal of Canadian Studies, 43*(1), 219–238.

Zippay, A. (2007). Psychiatric residences: Notification, NIMBY and neighbourhood relations. *Psychiatric Services, 58*(1), 109–113.

Zisook, S., Shuchter, S.R., Pedrelli, P., Sable, J., & Deaciuc, S.C. (2001). Bupropion sustained release for bereavement: Results of an open trial. *Journal of Clinical Psychiatry, 62*(4), 227–230.

Case Law and Statutes

Advocacy Act, 1992. Ontario Regulation 33/95. Retrieved December 28, 2011, from www.e-laws.gov.on.ca/html/revokedregs/english/elaws_rev_regs_950033_e.htm.

Alberta Mental Health Act, S.A. 1964, c. 54. Retrieved November 1, 2011, from www.our-futureourpast.ca/law/page.aspx?id=2911315.

Alberta Mental Health Act, R.S.A. 2000, c. M-13. Retrieved September 15, 2011, from www.canlii.org/en/ab/laws/stat/rsa-2000-c-m-13/85055/.

Alcoholism Foundation of Manitoba v. Winnipeg (City), [1990] 69 D.L.R. (4th) 697.

Andrews v. Law Society of British Columbia, [1989] 1 S.C.R. 143.

Aurora (Town) v. Anglican Houses, [1990] 72 O.R. (2d) 732.

Battlefords and District Co-operative Ltd. v. Gibbs, [1996] 3 S.C.R. 566.

Children's Aid Society of the Region of Peel v. Brampton (City), [2003] 122 A.C.W.S. (3d) 1149.

Cinderella Allalouf Ad-Hoc Litigation Committee v. Lucas, [1999] CanLII 18723.

Croplife Canada v. Toronto (City), [2005] 75 O.R. (3d) 357.

Dream Team v. Toronto (City), [2011] O.H.R.T.D. No. 1703.

Dream Team v. Toronto (City), [2012] H.R.T.O. No. 25, CanLII.

Fleming v. Reid, [1991] 4 O.R. (3d) 74 (C.A.).

Law v. Canada (Minister of Employment and Immigration), [1999] 1 S.C.R. 497.

Mazzei v. British Columbia (Director of Adult Forensic Psychiatric Services), [2006] 1 S.C.R. 326, 2006 SCC 7.

Mullins v. Levy, 2005 BCSC 1217. Docket C982449. British Columbia Supreme Court. Retrieved November 6, 2011, from www.courts.gov.bc.ca/jdb-txt/sc/05/12/2005bcsc1217err1.htm.

Ontario Human Rights Code, S. 2. (1).

Ontario Mental Health Act, R.S.O. 1990, c. M-7. Retrieved November 1, 2011, from www.e-laws.gov.on.ca/html/statutes/english/elaws_statutes_90m07_e.htm.

Ontario Planning Act, S. 35 (2).

Pinet v. St. Thomas Psychiatric Hospital, [2004] 1 S.C.R. 528, 2004 SCC 21.

R. v. Bell, [1979] 2 S.C.R. 212.

R. v. Conway, [2010] S.C.C. 22, [2010] 1 S.C.R. 765.

R. v. Swain, [1991] 1 S.C.R. 933 at 973, 63 C.C.C. (3d) 481.

R. v. Turpin, [1989] 1 S.C.R. 1296.

Starson v. Swayze, [2003] S.C.J. No. 33, [2003] 1 S.C.R. 722 (S.C.C.).

Vriend v. Alberta, [1998] 1 S.C.R. 493.

Winko v. British Columbia (Forensic Psychiatric Institute), [1999] 2 S.C.R. 625.

About the Editors and Contributors

Lanny Beckman was a founding member of Vancouver's Mental Patients Association (MPA), Canada's first mental health peer support group and a long-time publisher for New Star Press. He lives in Vancouver, BC.

Bonnie Burstow is a long-time antipsychiatry activist, the chair of the first PsychOUT conference, the chair of the Coalition Against Psychiatric Assault, and a faculty member in the Department of Leadership, Higher and Adult Education at the Ontario Institute for Studies in Education at the University of Toronto. She has published extensively in the area of antipsychiatry organizing, feminist critiques of electroshock, and radical trauma theory. Major works for which she is known include: *Radical Feminist Therapy: Working in the Context of Violence* (authored), and *Shrink Resistant: The Struggle against Psychiatry in Canada* (co-edited with Don Weitz).

Kathryn Church is Director and Associate Professor in the School of Disability Studies at Ryerson University, Toronto. In an early book, *Forbidden Narratives: Critical Autobiography as Social Science* (1993), she addressed the dilemmas of professional practice in relation to the unsettling relations of "user involvement" in the mental health field. She is currently taking up the practical possibilities and challenges of "Mad Studies" as they emerge within disability studies.

Lucy Costa has worked as a systemic advocate with the Empowerment Council in Toronto, Ontario. She is pursuing a Master of Laws Degree at Osgoode Hall Law School.

Andrea Daley is an Associate Professor in the School of Social Work, York University, Toronto. Her research interests include access and equity issues in health care policy and program delivery for members of lesbian, gay, bisexual, transgender, and queer communities; women and mental illness; and sexuality and identity. Works in progress include a retrospective review of women's psychiatric in-patient charts for sexuality content and an exploration of service access and equity issues related to in-home health provision for members of Ontario's lesbian, gay, bisexual, transgender, and queer communities.

Megan J. Davies is a BC historian of health with research interests in old age, madness, rural medicine, and social welfare. She teaches in the Health and Society Program at York University. She is a collective member of the History of Madness in Canada website, historyofmadness.ca.

Shaindl Diamond obtained her PhD in counselling psychology at the Ontario Institute for Studies in Education, University of Toronto. She is a member of the Coalition Against

Psychiatric Assault, and an organizer of Toronto's Psychiatric Survivor Pride. In 2010 she served as co-organizer for PsychOUT: A Conference for Organizing Resistance Against Psychiatry.

Erick Fabris is a psychiatric survivor, activist, and ethnographer. His book *Tranquil Prisons: Chemical Incarceration under Community Treatment Orders* was published by the University of Toronto Press in 2011. In 2012, he completed his PhD on experiences labelled psychotic. Erick lectures at the School of Disability Studies, Ryerson University.

Lilith "Chava" Finkler is an independent researcher and former Trudeau Scholar. She has published widely in areas pertaining to mental health, disability, and human rights and, more recently, about land use law and affordable housing.

Rachel Gorman is Assistant Professor in the Graduate Program in Critical Disability Studies at York University. Her recent publications focus on postcolonial representations of disability and racial hybridity. Since receiving her PhD from the University of Toronto in 2005 with a dissertation on disability and class-consciousness, she has held a SSHRC Postdoctoral Fellowship and Lectureship at the Women and Gender Studies Institute of the University of Toronto, and Research Fellowships at Manchester Metropolitan University and the University at Buffalo (SUNY). She has worked on antipsychiatry, Palestine solidarity, and anti-violence campaigns, and has been active in the Disability Arts and Culture movement since 1999.

Eugène LeBlanc is director of a peer-run activity centre in Moncton, New Brunswick, and publisher and editor of the internationally circulated *Our Voice/Notre Voix* since 1987. He is co-author of the 2008 book *Dare to Imagine: From Lunatics to Citizens,* and he received the New Brunswick Human Rights Award in 2003 for his grassroots contribution to mental health issues.

Ji-Eun Lee is a Korean psychiatric survivor who graduated with a unique interdisciplinary undergraduate degree from the University of Winnipeg, where she designed her own program in the field of mental health and psychiatric survivor movement. Also, as of June 2011, she holds an M.Ed. degree in Sociology and Equity Studies in Education from the Ontario Institute of Studies in Education, University of Toronto. So far, her academic studies have been an intellectually useful way of making sense of her experience, even though it is an ongoing struggle on the emotional level.

Brenda A. LeFrançois is an Associate Professor and director of the PhD Program in the School of Social Work, with a cross-appointment to the Faculty of Medicine, at Memorial University of Newfoundland. She has been an activist within the psychiatric survivor movement in the UK and Canada over the past 20 years. With a primary concern for the violence and oppression inherent to psychiatry, her research and writing have focused on the interface between childhood studies and Mad Studies in exploring power relations and children's rights within psychiatry, children's direct involvement in social activism, as well as post-structural feminist theoretical understandings of psychiatrization, sanism, adultism, and abjection. She was one of the founding members of the journal *Radical Psychology*.

Maria Liegghio is a doctoral candidate in the Faculty of Social Work at Wilfrid Laurier University. Based on the principles of youth engagement and participatory action research, her doctoral research involves training a group of youth diagnosed with a mental health issue to collaborate as research assistants in the study of self and family stigma of mental illness.

Robert Menzies teaches Sociology at Simon Fraser University, where he was formerly J.S. Woodsworth Resident Scholar in the Humanities. In addition to his role in organizing the 2008 Vancouver event Madness, Citizenship and Social Justice: A Human Rights Conference, he is currently a member of the collective for the History of Madness in Canada website historyofmadness.ca. Among his book publications are *Survival of the Sanest: Order and Disorder in a Pre-Trial Psychiatric Clinic* (1989), and *Women, Madness and the Law: A Feminist Reader* (co-edited with Wendy Chan and Dorothy E. Chunn, 2005).

Marina Morrow is the Director, Centre for the Study of Gender, Social Inequities and Mental Health and Associate Professor, Faculty of Health Sciences, Simon Fraser University in Vancouver. Marina strongly supports public scholarship and collaborative research partnerships with community-based organizations, health care practitioners, advocates, and policy decision-makers and has been published in a wide range of academic journals and policy reports.

Ryan Pike graduated with a BA in International Development Studies from Trent University and recently completed an MA in Socio-Legal Studies from York University. He currently works as a freelance interdisciplinary researcher and is based in Toronto, Ontario.

Jennifer M. Poole is Mad Associate Professor in the School of Social Work at Ryerson University. Originally from the UK, these days she spends a lot of time thinking about mental health recovery, sanism, and community-based research in Toronto.

Geoffrey Reaume has been involved in the psychiatric survivor, consumer, and Mad community since 1990 and is a co-founder of the Psychiatric Survivor Archives, Toronto. He introduced and has taught Mad People's History at all three universities in Toronto. Currently, he is Graduate Program Director of the Critical Disability Studies MA and PhD program at York University.

David Reville is a long-time Mad activist; he teaches courses related to Mad history at Ryerson University in Toronto.

Irit Shimrat calls herself an escaped lunatic and is a long-time antipsychiatry activist and advocate of alternatives to psychiatric treatment. She served as editor-in-chief of the national magazine *Phoenix Rising: The Voice of the Psychiatrized*; co-founded and coordinated the Ontario Psychiatric Survivors' Alliance; presented two programs ("Analyzing Psychiatry" and "By Reason of Insanity") on the CBC *Ideas* radio show; and wrote *Call Me Crazy: Stories from the Mad Movement* (Vancouver: Press Gang Publishers, 1997).

Nérée St-Amand, Professor, School of Social Work, University of Ottawa, has researched the New Brunswick mental health system for more than 30 years and has proposed alternatives to the institutional and professional models of care. After publishing *The Politics of Madness* (1988), he has authored several books and articles on the subject, with particular attention to the cultural and political dimensions of mental health. He is also a member of the Mental Health Commission of Canada, where he represents the voices of caregivers and victims.

Mel Starkman was the first person in Canada to advocate for the creation of an archive on Mad movement history in the early 1980s. Not long after the chapter that appears in *Mad Matters* was first published as an article in *Phoenix Rising*, he was confined in Queen Street Mental Health Centre, Toronto, where he was an in-patient and outpatient for 13 years from 1982 to 1995. During this time, the Public Guardian and Trustee discarded his personal archive of primary source material, which he had collected on the history of the early Mad movement in Toronto. In 2001, Mel Starkman co-founded the Psychiatric Survivor Archives, Toronto, an organization with which he continues to work a decade later.

Louise Tam completed her MA in Sociology and Equity Studies at the University of Toronto in 2012. She is currently a PhD student in Women's and Gender Studies at Rutgers University. In her master's thesis, she explores how ethnoracial mental health outreach governs communities of colour through tethering anti-racist theory to psychiatric epidemiology.

Jijian Voronka is a PhD candidate in Sociology and Equity Studies at OISE/University of Toronto. She works as a consumer research consultant for the Mental Health Commission of Canada, and as an instructor at Ryerson University's School of Disability Studies. Her current research involves mapping the conditions, limits, and possibilities of peer involvement within a national research demonstration project on homelessness and mental health.

Jennifer Ward is a graduate student of Social Work and also a suicide interventionist and survivor support counsellor. In addition to grief and loss, Jennifer's research interests include suicide, "survivor" discourse, organ donation, and madness/mental health. Jennifer identifies as an ally, suicide survivor, mother, lover, and friend. She lives in Peel Region and believes she has the most wonderful dog in the world.

Gordon Warme MD, University of Toronto, is the author of four books: *Reluctant Treasures*; *The Psychotherapist*; *The Cure of Folly*; and *Daggers of the Mind*.

Don Weitz is an antipsychiatry activist and insulin shock survivor. He has been protesting against electroshock for over 25 years and wants it banned. Don is co-editor (with Dr. Bonnie Burstow) of *Shrink Resistant: The Struggle against Psychiatry in Canada*, co-founder of *Phoenix Rising* magazine, coordinating committee member of the Coalition Against Psychiatric Assault (CAPA), former host/producer of *Antipsychiatry Radio* on CKLN, and author of the e-book *Rise Up/Fight Back: Selected Writings of an Antipsychiatry Activist*.

Kimberley White is a painter and Associate Professor of Law and Society in the interdisciplinary Department of Social Science at York University in Toronto. Recent books include *Negotiating Responsibility: Law, Murder and States of Mind* (UBC Press, 2007); and *Configuring Madness: Representation, Context & Meaning* (Inter-Disciplinary Press, 2009). Scholarly research over the past four years has focused in general on the production and dissemination of top-down knowledge on "mental illness" and "mental health literacy" in Canada, and more specifically on how the use of social marketing and corporate governance frameworks has influenced the structure and mandate of the Mental Health Commission of Canada. Other ongoing research examines the aesthetics and politics of anti-stigma work, and the cultural significance of graffiti/street art.

Rob Wipond has been a professional freelance writer, researcher, journalist, and commentator on community issues and media for over 20 years, specializing in psychiatric civil rights issues within vulnerable populations. His publication credits include *Explore*, *Adbusters*, *Rabble*, *Radical Psychology*, *Monday*, *Georgia Straight*, and *Focus*. He has received several National and Western Magazine Awards nominations for health and science writing, and won a WMA for business writing. He has also worked as an instructor in journalism and creative nonfiction at the University of Victoria and Royal Roads University.

Copyright Acknowledgments

Index

Page numbers in boldface type indicate glossary entries defining the term named. Page numbers in italics refer to illustrations and tables.